SELF-CARE AND HEALTH IN OLD AGE

SELF-CARE AND HEALTH IN OLD AGE

HEALTH BEHAVIOUR IMPLICATIONS FOR POLICY AND PRACTICE

Edited by

KATHRYN DEAN,
TOM HICKEY,
& BJORN E.
HOLSTEIN

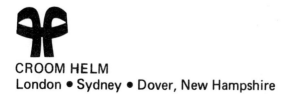

CROOM HELM
London • Sydney • Dover, New Hampshire

© 1986 Kathryn Dean, Tom Hickey and Bjorn E. Holstein,
Croom Helm Ltd, Provident House, Burrell Row,
Beckenham, Kent BR3 1AT
Croom Helm Australia Pty Ltd, Suite 4, 6th Floor,
64-76 Kippax Street, Surry Hills, NSW 2010, Australia

British Library Cataloguing in Publication Data

Self-care and health in old age.
   1. Aged – Care and hygiene   2. Self-care, Health
   I. Dean, Kathryn   II. Hickey, Tom
   III. Holstein, Bjorn, E.
   613'.0438   RA777.6
   ISBN 0-7099-0881-4

Croom Helm, 51 Washington Street, Dover,
New Hampshire 03820, USA

Library of Congress Cataloging in Publication Data
applied for:

Printed and bound in Great Britain
by Billing & Sons Limited, Worcester.

CONTENTS

RA564
.8
.S46
1986

List of Tables
List of Figures
Acknowledgements
Preface, Raymond Illsley

TABLES AND FIGURES

Figures

ACKNOWLEDGEMENTS

This book grew out of an international project on the role of professionals in promoting health behaviour in late life, initiated by the Kellogg International Scholarship Programme on Health and Aging. In 1982, the editors were invited to participate in a project to identify the state of knowledge in self-care and aging in order to translate what is known to a facilitation of the application of knowledge in health planning and the provision of health care.

The editors convened several times to consult with the W.H.O. and other international and national organisations and with a large number of experts in this area of interest. In addition to reviewing the relevant literatures of research, policy, and practice, we visited model programmes in North America and Western Europe and elicited the ideas of many professional colleagues.

The editors are indebted to the W.K. Kellogg Foundation for providing economic support for this project, to the German Marshall Foundation of the United States, to Pfizer, Inc., of New York, and to the Danish Medical Research Council for additional economic support for an international symposium in Oxford, England, in 1983.

It is not possible to acknowledge all the individuals who have aided or facilitated the preparation of this volume. We are, however, especially indebted to the directors of the Kellogg Programm, Erik Holst and Harold Johnson, and to the programme coordinators, Larry C. Coppard and Patricia Sohl, for their support and encouragement.

We would like to acknowledge the many people with whom we met in the preparatory phase of the project for their contribution to the ideas which were developed. During this process experts in areas relevant to the subject were identified to prepare manuscripts for this monograph. The contributors assembled at an international symposium on self-care and aging in Oxford in May 1983 to present the first draft of their manuscripts. Furthermore, we are indebted to Marie R. Haug, Alfred Katz and Roger Ritvo for subsequently agreeing to prepare manuscripts to cover subjects which the symposium participants identified as important for this monograph.

We are indebted to Raymond Illsley, who chaired the symposium, and to Jan Branckaerts, Hans Habils, Uffe Juul Jensen, and Una Maclean who prepared formal presentations which provided invaluable background in cultural, philosophical and sociological aspects of self-care and aging.

We would like to express our special appreciation to J.A. Muir Gray, who not only contributed to the discussion and development of ideas at the symposium, but was our generous host on two occasions and assisted in the planning of the symposium.

We would like to acknowledge all the participants in the symposium, not only those who prepared formal presentations, but also those who organised the discussion and reacted formally to the manuscripts, stimulating our thinking. The participants were: Bent Rold Andersen, J.A.D. Anderson, Robert Anderson, Stig Berg, Tony de Bono, M.A. Bremer Schultze, Ann Cartwright, Kathryn Dean, Patrice Engelberts, Susan B. Eve, Graeme Ford, Stephen Gehlbach, Adrienne Gommers, J.A. Muir Gray, Betty Havens Wim van den Heuvel, Tom Hickey, Erik Holst, Bjørn E. Holstein, John A. Huntington, Raymond Illsley, Uffe Juul Jensen, Malcolm Johnson, Alex Kalache, Robert Kane, Rosalie Kane, Ulrich Laaser, Ronald Liddiard, Una Maclean, Marsha Ory, William Rakowski, Inger Rosenkvist, Cynthia Savo, and Donald L. Spence.

An excellent technical and editorial staff backed up the whole project and made the wheels turn. Our special appreciation is offered to Annelise Nielsen who provided administrative and technical assistance throughout the project, to Thomas Kennedy for his editorial management of the manuscript which has clarified and focused the language of this book, and to Connie Olsen who helped prepare and typed the manuscript.

Kathryn Dean, Tom Hickey, Bjørn E. Holstein

Like many professionals and self-defined radicals, I was at first suspicious of the notion of self-care. I had two main worries. Firstly, the concept was fuzzy. Sometimes self-care, which has an evident and precise meaning, was used interchangeably for self-help, family care, community care, or informal support, and sometimes it was used aggressively as an alternative to a derided professional care. Sometimes it was a descriptive term, sometimes the badge of a social movement. Secondly, the idea was dangerous, likely to be adopted gleefully by a cost-cutting Government unimpressed by welfare arguments. My general feeling was: Please don't put bad thoughts into the minds of anti-welfare politicians; they have enough already.

But the concept persisted and, in its development, outgrew my suspicions. This volume of mature thought and experience illustrates how far the concept has become refined and focused in recent years. I suspect that many deep-rooted social movements start as fuzzy concepts because they represent an early, groping awareness of something that is wrong and something that needs to be done.

If they are innovative and, particularly, if they challenge current values and practice, an accurate terminology may not exist and terms may be overladen with unwanted meanings from the past. The more the idea expresses some widely felt experience or value, the more likely it is to be seized upon by diverse groups and become a broad movement, encapsulating many different but generically related ideas.

In this volume, the meaning of self-care is clear. It is concentrated upon the individual and upon the individual's knowledge, motivation and actions to nurture body and mind by preventive behaviour and by treatment, autonomously, but in cooperation with others. Definitions are attempted in this book but, in their dictionary sense, cannot capture the social connotations which gave rise to and which inform and sustain the concept. Because such connotations are integral to the usage of the term in this volume and elsewhere, I review briefly those few which seem most important to me.

First, self-care emerges not merely as a health device (like jogging for the sedentary affluent city dweller), but as a reaffirmation of the dignity and autonomy of older persons, of a wide age-band which has lost the traditional power, status and respect which it once possessed and which still attaches to the majority of individuals within the age-band in the eyes of people close to them. Too frequently, older persons are mentioned as individual and social problems (what shall we do about the elderly?) and the very act of urging that more, and more appropriate, services be provided may strengthen the popular image of a frail, helpless confused group which needs to be looked after. Many contributions in this volume re-emphasise and document the capacities of older persons and view self-care as a response and a defence against ageist views and behaviour.

Services and professionals emerge as one source of agism, and non-compliance with professional treatment is seen by Haug as a possible indicator of self-respect and of self-care. Failure to use formal services can be conceptualised as rational behaviour based on past experiences of inappropriate and incompetent care. The emphasis in this volume, however, is not anti-professional, not on self-care as an alternative to professional care. On the contrary, it recognises the complementarity of self-care and professional care, but suggests a righting of the current power imbalance in client-professional interaction and a rethinking of profes-sional education and of service provision and organisation. The widespread adoption of self-care is, therefore, not an invitation to cut services, but to change and improve them.

What also emerges clearly is the individuality and the variability of the aging process. Given that young families tend to complete childbearing in their late twenties, that the retirement age is being lowered by a mixture of new technology, economic depression, and agism, and that the length of life and of competence is increasing, the formal duration of old age is now the equivalent of the period from birth to the end of childbearing. This

is a long period of great inter-individual variation, of decline, but also of growth. One theme of
great importance recurring in this book is that the
aging process is continuous and not a dichotomy
between being young and being old. The lives and
cultural values of older persons are, thus, an
amalgam of past historical periods and possibly of
age itself - although specific age-effects, outside
the biological sphere, should be treated with some
suspicion. There are also references to the way in
which age is a socially constructed phenomenon, and
even some speculation about how the numerical
increase in the older population may lead to
increased status and power. For me, the crucial
issue is the regeneration and re-shaping of our
economies and the sensible employment of human
talents at any age. In a depressed economy, the
tendency to reject older persons and make them the
scapegoat of our political and economic incompetence
is too tempting to be avoided. For the foreseeable
future, I doubt that older persons will enjoy status
and power in a society plagued by unemployment.

The maturation of the concept of self-care is
evidenced by the still slight but now growing volume
of innovatory educational, health and social services - some of which appear in this volume. When a
social movement turns into an organised service,
there is cause for rejoicing. There is also cause
for caution. Self-care freely adopted as a philosophy and integrated into a healthy life-style is
characteristic of those educated and relatively
affluent socio-occupational groups which continue,
across Western nations, to have the highest expectation of life and of independence. Its manufacture
and provision by professionals, and its adoption and
administration by the health service managers for
poorer and less educated groups as a substitute for
the comprehensive enhancement of welfare could be a
different matter. What is now needed, as the earlier
positive vision becomes a reality, is evaluation,
not only to discover how best we can extend and
apply the concept but how it fits into and interacts
with formal services. If the authors in this volume
are correct, and I believe they are, one by-product
could be the humanisation of professionally dominated and routinely administered services.

Chapter 1

HEALTH BEHAVIOUR AND SELF-CARE IN LATE LIFE:
AN INTRODUCTION

Tom Hickey

Health care has been viewed traditionally as the
domain of health care professionals and medical care
systems. Health policies have not typically encompassed lay care and personal health behaviour as
key factors in the health care of individuals.
However, lay care has always been the most fundamental form of health care. Recently, consumers of
health care services have become more enlightened,
if not more assertive, by actively participating in
making decisions about their health care and in
following various treatment regimens (Levin, Katz &
Holst 1976).
    Several obvious reasons account for this
gradual shift from what might be called physician-
dominated health care:

1. An increase in the level of education and
   knowledge among the general population;
2. A broader dissemination of basic information about illness and health care via
   popular periodicals and television -- at
   least in developed nations;
3. A greater focus in many countries on the
   rights of consumers in the market-place;
4. An increasing interest in self-help and
   self-improvement techniques and strategies
   for modifying life-style;
5. A greater general awareness of the falli-
   bility and error rate in medical care;
6. A rapid acceleration in the costs of
   medical care; and
7. The continuing predominance of hospital-
   based and institutional care in health care
   systems.

These and related issues provided a starting

point for collaborative study by the three editors of this volume. In addition to reviewing the relevant literature in research, policy, and practice, we visited model programme sites in different countries and elicited the ideas of many professional colleagues. In May, 1983, most of the invited contributors to this monograph convened at Oxford University in England to present draft manuscripts and to discuss significant issues concerning self-care and health behaviour in late life. The contributions by Alfred Katz, Marie Haug, and Roger Ritvo were invited after this symposium to add to the monograph additional important aspects identified at the meeting in Oxford.

HEALTH CARE AND THE ELDERLY

In regard to the health concerns and extended care of the chronically-ill elderly, an additional explanation for the evolving changes in geriatric health-care perspectives can be found in the preoccupation of physicians and traditional medical care with acute illnesses and organic problems of uniform aetiologies. The complexity and duration of illnesses in late life do not typically conform to the traditional medical and acute care models. Thus, self-care and personal health behaviour have gradually assumed a more visible and, with increasing consumer knowledge and skills, perhaps more important role in individual health care -- not as a replacement for traditional medical care, but as its complement and compensation. Informal systems and methods of care and support, including self and lay care, mutual aid and peer support, have long been essential to the overall long-term health care of functionally impaired elderly persons.

The direct involvement of older persons in improving their functional capacity and personal well-being has attracted considerable attention in both Europe and North America. This growing interest has been generated, at least in part, by an increasing awareness of the benefits of personal health behaviour. In addition to numerous descriptive and empirical studies with very specific focus, several articles and books have dealt more generally with health education, self-care, and older patients' health behaviour. As director of the National Institute on Aging in the United States, Dr. Robert Butler reviewed the development of self-care and self-help programmes for the elderly, and found both a wide range of available programmes and increasing interest on the part of older health care consumers (Butler & al. 1979). A similar review conducted at The University of North Carolina's Health Services Research Center focused more specifically on the implications of the self-care movement for the elderly (DeFriese & Woomert 1983). In the Sixth Nordic Congress of Gerontology, held in Copenhagen in 1983, self-care was the focus of several presentations for the first time in this forum. Also, in many northern European countries, health education has grown in importance in national health policies.

Other prominent health professionals and scientists have stressed the importance of preventive health care and lifelong health behaviour in predicting chronic disease risk, and the role and responsibility of individuals in determining the course of their health over the extended period of adulthood (Breslow 1979, Knowles 1977). Another example of the importance of health behaviour in late life can be found in a book by Haug (1981) which deals with the relationships between older persons and their doctors, and the implications for medical treatment and personal health care behaviour. More recently, an international group of scholars developed a report regarding the role and contributions of general practitioners to the medical care of the elderly in the community (Almind & al. 1983).

SELF-CARE BEHAVIOUR

What is self-care behaviour? Specifically, it is the individual's immediate and continuing behavioural reactions to illness, his basic coping strategies, as well as the steps taken to preserve and maintain personal health (Hickey 1980). The initiatives which individuals take on behalf of their own health encompass preventive health care and behavioural and other health interventions. These include:

1. The most basic daily health maintenance behaviour such as good nutrition and dental hygiene;
2. The recognition and interpretation of symptoms;
3. Interaction with social support networks and with the health care system, including taking an assertive role in health care decision making;

3

4. Various forms of self-treatment;
5. Compliance with prescribed or other re-
    medial efforts; and
6. Health education, including the application
    of health skills such as taking one's blood
    pressure or administering injections.

Negative examples might involve harmful behaviour through neglect or avoidance of necessary
health promotion and care such as failure to consult
professionals or modifying an important health
regimen (Dean 1981, Hickey 1980).

Personal habits of health behaviour form the
basis of health care decisions, including self-care,
and determine the points of entry into professional
health care systems as well as compliance with
professional directives.

Health behaviour is an important manifestation
of a person's psychological perspective. It
reflects the individual's perception of his or
her health status and the person's concerns
about health; over time it reveals a pattern of
views about health and some consistency in the
way the person deals with health problems
(Hickey 1980, p. 92).

Older persons' health care decisions, health
behaviour and compliance may be influenced significantly by the accumulated experience of a lifetime
with their own health and illness and with the
health care system as well as by their beliefs and,
perhaps, fears about chronic illness. Individual
self-care initiatives and personal health behaviour
are undoubtedly major determinants of the type and
amount of professional services utilised. Thus, the
known variability among older persons in a number of
domains suggests a comparable diversity in health
behaviour. Curiously, despite the importance of its
role in the use of health services, individual
variability in health behaviour has been largely
neglected in research investigations, public policy,
and programme development.

Stereotypes of older people as generally
incapable and incompetent have resulted in only
minimal recognition of their capacity for self-care.
In fact, the potential for interaction between
self-care and health care systems are not typically
reflected in policy statements about the elderly.
More attention is given to the extensive need for
health care among the most chronically impaired

elderly than to the well-documented evidence that most older people function well in the general community up to a very advanced age -- despite the presence of at least one serious condition (Hickey 1980). For many of these people, personal health behaviour and capacity for self-care, often with informal care and support from others, are of greater day-to-day significance than formal medical services. In fact, many older people quickly learn that their functional health problems are improved only minimally with medical treatment. Thus, behavioural strategies other than seeking professional care and help are often their first and continuing recourse.

LATE-LIFE HEALTH BEHAVIOUR: CULTURAL AND MULTI-DISCIPLINARY PERSPECTIVES

The intent of this monograph is to focus on the broad context of health behaviour in late life from the perspectives of different cultures and professions which affect our interpretations of this area of interest. To accomplish this, scientists and professionals representing various disciplines and cultural viewpoints have been invited to address different aspects of self-care and health behaviour in late life including: philosophical, historical, and economic issues; self-medication, illness and health dependencies; mutual aid, informal care, and support by peers and families; health attitudes and beliefs; and the relation of self-care to professional care and formal health care systems, including enlightened and assertive behaviour when interacting with health care professionals. Several other aspects of this topic could have been selected for special emphasis, including medical and nursing care and the impact of various socio-economic factors and living conditions. Similarly, the health problems most prevalent among older persons have been the focus of many other books and thus are omitted here. We recognise that others may not concur with the incorporation of such issues and priorities within the behavioural focus of most of the papers contributed.

At the outset, we determined that environmental and social conditions represent potentially significant factors in determining individual health behaviour. Therefore, the focus overall and in each of the following written contributions cut across different social groups and cultures. Considerable attention is given to identifying similarities and critical differences in the health behaviour of elderly people in the countries of northern Europe and North America with their varying health care systems. Our hope is to synthesise what little is known generally about this important issue and to suggest applications which might transcend cultures and be adaptable to a wide range of circumstances, situations, and health care systems.

The potential contribution of this cross-cultural perspective lies in its efforts to address an important aspect of a major health crisis facing many nations of the world. Various recent reports and findings from the World Health Organization (W.H.O.) and from the 1982 World Assembly on Aging have stressed the critical health care problems faced by many countries whose population of chronically-ill elderly is burgeoning. One offshoot of past medical and public health efforts to eradicate major infectious and communicable diseases, combined with advances in pharmacology and sanitation, has been increased longevity throughout the world. Gradual declines in morbidity, mortality, and fertility have resulted in higher proportions of older people in the world's population and in much greater numbers of people living and remaining healthier to a very old age. Paradoxically, this burgeoning growth in the numbers of healthy older persons causes concern for health care systems, given that health risks increase sharply in old age.

In the period 1980-2000, the world's population over age 65 will increase by approximately 140 million. Countries to experience the largest growth include China, with an estimated increase of 5.7 million people aged 65 and over; Russia, three million; India, 2.2 million; and Japan, 1.1 million (W.H.O. 1982). In the United States, the population over age 75 is increasing four times faster than those under age 65. Such growth patterns have a parallel in the industrialised nations of Europe. Of greatest significance here is the increase in the numbers of people at maximum health risk -- the population over age 80, whose number is expected to double between 1970 and 2000 throughout the world. These growing populations of very old people are most likely to be health impaired and dependent upon others and in greatest need of health services.

Most countries would seem unprepared to meet the health care needs of their increasingly larger populations of older persons. The world's less developed nations presently spend only about one percent of their gross national products on health care for the elderly. For the most part, this small expenditure is unevenly distributed, leaving large numbers of older people unserved. In the developed nations, three to four percent of national revenues go for health care of the aged, although with uneven patterns of eligibility for care and services. A study by Terris (1980) indicated that 23 countries have health insurance systems which cover only 18 percent of the world's population; 14 countries maintain national health services, bringing the total number of people served to only one out of three. When one includes general programmes of public assistance (108 countries), no more than half of the world's population have access to resources for health care and services beyond themselves and their families.

W.H.O. and various other international bodies, however, have gone beyond merely documenting the demographic concerns. In its Alma-Ata declaration of 1978, W.H.O. emphasised the critical importance of integrating primary medical care with the social context in which people live. This report also noted the importance of many different sources of support for late-life health care.

> Aging people and their families should be more involved in their own care. Health educational information on the promotion of health and prevention of disease is required, as are simple handbooks of personal care (W.H.O. 1982, p. 8).

Other key points in this policy framework include the importance of home care, reducing dependence on the more cost-intensive forms of medical care delivery systems, and providing access-ible health care choices for the at-risk elderly population. W.H.O. seems to have recognised both the error and the inadequacy of attempting to meet the health concerns of older persons with what has been called the "serviced society" model, where health professionals attempt to match a professional service with every health care need (McKnight 1977). Such an approach clearly will not work -- either curatively or fiscally -- given the functional and protracted nature of the health problems of a growing elderly population.

Recent studies and reports from the United States and various European nations have emphasised these same points, noting that seven out of the 10 major causes of death are predominantly behavioural, rather than pathological, in aetiology (Breslow 1979); this suggests again the importance of strategies of prevention, self-care, and environmental supports. Brody (1979) reported that eight out of every 10 persons over age 65 in the U.S. are suffering from chronic and degenerative disease; half this population is severely limited in their activities of daily living and dependent upon others for support and care.

Older people account for a relatively high proportion of the total health care expenditure in the industrialised nations of the world. In the U.S., older people comprise less than 11 percent of the total population, but account for at least 30 percent of health care expenditure and 40 percent of inpatient hospital care. A legitimate concern that public resources and acute medical care strategies are inadequate to meet the elderly's health care requirements makes clear the need for other approaches, including the integration of social support with health care services and additional emphasis on self-care and assistance to family care-givers in the form of education, subsidies, and tax credits. Between 70 and 80 percent of the elderly in the U.S. and Western Europe have been estimated to receive care and support from related household members.

Family care, however, cannot be regarded as a replacement or compensation for lack of service. The degree to which family care is denied by the elderly or is a burden to the care-giver is not known. Therefore, family care is not discussed here as a substitute for health care or self-care. Rather, the focus is on the interactions between the various forms of care and how families and health care professionals can stimulate the development of health behaviour and self-care in older people. Thus, the issue of social networks is integrated with the discussion of other issues rather than being treated as a separate topic.

CONCLUSION

The potential value of this monograph is anticipated to be in its implications for research, policy, education, and practice, and cross-cultural exchange. Collective efforts must be found to stimulate developments in at least five major areas:

1. To determine predictors of self-care and positive health behaviour;
2. To determine and develop methods for teaching and/or influencing people to better help themselves as a means of maintaining control over their personal health;
3. To find ways to effect changes in utilisation rates and in supplementing limited formal health care services;
4. To study various strategies and approaches for their efficacy in teaching clinicians to facilitate self-care behaviour among the elderly; and
5. To disseminate and adapt what we presently know about self-care and preventive health behaviour for countries with even fewer resources and formal systems for the health care of the elderly.

In summary, the health status of most older people in industrialised nations is better than it has ever been, with greater numbers of people living longer and the onset of chronic impairment delayed until the later years. This optimistic picture however, is incomplete, given the dramatic worldwide increases occurring in the numbers of "very old" (i.e., over age 75) persons and the corresponding inadequacies in health care policies and mechanisms to deal with the long-term care needs of that age group. Thus, the importance of self-care behaviour and family care for a cohesive and effective health care system increases.

The opening chapters of this monograph lead the reader through the more salient theoretical and conceptual issues which provide a context for self-care and health behaviour in late life. Holstein broadly explores conceptual issues related to behavioural variability in health perceptions and practices. Johnson questions the validity of commonly accepted age norms and their inherent relationship to a pathology model. In their individual contributions, Dean, Rakowski, and Ford have carefully analysed and integrated the rich, extensive research literature surrounding the investigation of self-care, health maintenance priorities, and illness behaviour. The chapter by Katz attempts to define more precisely the practice aspect of this literature as it translates to self-care and self-help programmes for the elderly. Cartright, Anderson and Eve present interesting contrasting data on the use of medications and related self-care practices by the elderly in different countries. The closing chapters of this volume examine self-care and health behaviour in the context of the health care system. Haug looks at the emerging literature on doctor-patient relationships and their impact on self-care and health behaviour among the elderly. Kane and Kane view self-care as one of many types of health care which should be integrated with formal care. Ritvo and Liddiard view it from the policy perspective of different types of health care systems. In the final chapter, the three principal contributors have integrated the major themes of this volume with a focus on policy, practice, education, and research.

As in the discussion at Oxford, this book deals with the international scope of the issue of late-life health behaviour, which suggests that in both social welfare and market health economies, policy-makers are faced with the same demographic and economic challenges in planning care and services for the elderly. Research scientists in the different countries represented at the Oxford meeting and in this volume have raised similar questions about the behavioural predictors of health status; the social epidemiology of illness in late life; physical impairment and pathology in the context of functional capacity; and many others, including questions of method and application, decision-making, and informal support and public service configurations. Educators and practitioners are similarly challenged in different countries by the interface between the narrowly conceived technological models of medical care and the much broader social context of extended chronic illness and personal health dependency in late life.

REFERENCES

Almind, G., Freer, C.B., Gray, J.A.M., and Warshaw, G. (1983) 'The Contribution of the Primary Care Doctor to the Medical Care of the Elderly in the Community,' University of Michigan Institute of Gerontology, Ann Arbor

Breslow, L. (1979) 'A Positive Strategy for the Nation's Health.' Proceedings of the National Health Forum. National Health Council, New York

Brody, S.J. (1979) 'The Thirth-to-One Paradox: Health Needs of the Elderly and Medical Solutions,' National Journal, pp. 1869-73

Butler, R.N., Gertman, J.S., Oberlander, D.L., and

Shindler, L. (1979) 'Self-Care, Self-Help, and the Elderly,' International Journal of Aging and Human Development, Sept. pp. 95-119

Dean, K. (1981) 'Self-Care Responses to Illness: A Selected Review,' Social Science and Medicine, 15A, pp. 673-687

DeFriese, G.H. and Woomert, A. (1983) 'Self-Care Among U.S. Elderly: Recent Developments,' Research on Aging, 5, (1) pp. 3-23

Haug, M.R. (ed.) (1982) 'Elderly Patients and Their Doctors,' Springer, New York

Hickey, T. Health and Aging, (1981) Brooks/Cole, Monterey, California

Levin, L.S., Katz, A.H., and Holst, E. (1976) Self-Care. Lay Initiatives in Health. Prodist, New York

McKnight, J. (1977) Social Policy, 8 (3), p. 110

Terris, M. (1980) 'The Three World Systems of Medical Care: Trends and Prospects,' World Health Forum, 1 (2), pp. 72-86

World Health Organization Report, (March 26, 1982) 'Health Policy Aspects of Aging,' v. 82-23752, United Nations, New York

Chapter 2

AGE AS A LABELLING PHENOMENON

Malcolm L. Johnson

"TWENTY THREE"

I shall hate growing old
I dread the sagging flesh, the stiffened joints,
The laborious puffing up the shadeless hill
Where once I leaped and listened to the wind,
Blew kisses to the stars, and wept
Because the world was old and wise, and I
So young.

I shall hate growing old.
I dread the enfeebled bones, the tired mind,
The quiet colours of maturer gowns;
The knowledge that no more the tolerant smile
Will greet the foolish act, the spoken word,
The rapid birth and death of live -- and love.

But when I have grown old, and numbered years
Bid me heed youth's swan song, and be sad,
I shall not mourn its passing and despair,
Not bitterly reflect on past delight;
I shall not wish the gay years back, nor sigh
Regretfully and murmur "limbs you once were strong"
and "hair you saw more sun when gold than grey".

For all that I have now and all I am
I shall be proud to pay the price of age.
The knowledge that I seek -- the kiss of fame -
The elusive human mind, its hopes and cares,
Its boundless depths which fill me with such fire
That I must laugh and cry and dance -- or die .....
All these will be the fault of withered skin.

The world may smile and pass its pitying way
And see me for a waste and useless tool
In nature's cruel hand. A thing
That lived its little life, then welcomed death.

Yet shall I have my riches and my dreams,
The summer nights, the rainsong, and content.
Yet shall I wrap my aged body round
With all the life I've lived, and so be young -
And so remain unjealous, unafraid.

Mary Crowe

That generational factors exist and life experience
makes some difference has always been somewhat
recognised, but the assumption now has become
widespread that the characteristics of the elderly
population are indeed characteristics of old age.
Old is as old does. To the morbid picture of later
life drawn for us by poets (and Mary Crowe's poem is
a good example of its genre), novelists and
historians, researchers across the whole spectrum of
social and medical sciences have contributed yet
more evidence of pathology and incompetence. Against
this apparent conspiracy of data, attempts have been
made to call its bluff and assert (equally er-
roneously) that all is beauty and light at the
further end of life.

This paper is not part of the growing movement
against ageism, nor does it take an ideological
position which declares the rights of older people
to equality of treatment and esteem with those who
are younger. It is not out of sympathy with these
concerns, but its purpose is analytic rather than
emotive. The central question to be addressed here
is: If it is not axiomatic that the characteristics
of those who are at present old are the inherent
features of old age, which elements appear to have
universal significance and which might be seen as
artefacts of personal and group history? To put it
in terms of the title, how far is age -- and old age
in particular -- merely a label which denotes
socially constructed attitudes within a given
cultural context at a specified point in time?

The lexicon of words commonly available to
describe old age is growing. Some of the growth
derives from a desire to leave behind contaminated
language with all its negative stereotypes in favour
of finding words of more positive effect. Thus,

terms like "elder" have been polished up and put back into use to denote seniority, respect and life-hardened wisdom. Some writers now adopt the form "older people" rather than the aggregate term "the elderly." Yet they do so against an infiltration into common speech of words like geriatric, senile and demented, drawn directly from medical vocabulary to mark out broad fields of pathology. The fact that the incorporation of these words takes little account of their true meaning is immaterial. What is of importance is the way they are employed as powerful labels indicating serious physical and mental incapacity which renders people (or things) worthless.

It is in the conjunction of these linguistic patterns and their lack of congruence with the realities of old age that our interest lies. For if labels are being applied in a socially powerful way without regard to their veracity, we are observing a further feature of the social construction of age stereotypes. The consequences of stereotyping are considerable, not only in the everyday world but also in the way policy is conceived and research is formulated and executed. Thus, there is a danger that current preoccupations will create a socially manufactured and distorted view of old age which will be mistakenly seen as a permanent feature of life in so-called developed societies.

To pursue the twin themes of conceptual clarity and historiography, we must first offer an account of the emergence of a research-based pathology model of old age and make some observations about cohorts, generations and the links between personal and group history. On these bases it will be possible to build an argument about the changes already evident in retired populations which have implications for policy, service provision and research.

RESEARCH ON OLD AGE

Studies of ageing and old age are no longer rare, as might have been claimed confidently as little as 20 years ago. But in the intervening period the growth of geriatric medicine, the expansion of academic and policy related research, along with changes in the demographic structure, have made later life more important and better understood. However, a recognition that gerontology is still very youthful as a field of study is important. Much material has been gained through recent research which has aided our social and medical understanding of old age, but it remains very partial and skewed in favour of the maladies which come with age.

CONTRIBUTIONS TO THE PATHOLOGY MODEL

The history of research into old age over the past hundred years tends -- as do contemporary studies -- to be linked to the resolution of problems connected with the rising proportion of elderly people in the population and their absolute numbers. In 1881, people over the current retirement ages in England and Wales formed little more than five percent of the population. By the turn of the century this proportion had risen to more than six percent. At the last published census in 1981 it had advanced strikingly to over 17 percent with the greatest expansion taking place in the 75 plus age groups. A century ago, the great concerns brought to public attention by the growing school of social surveying reformers involved poverty, illnesses and institutional care of the aged. These culminated in the report of the Royal Commission on the Poor Law of 1905-9, which laid down a blueprint for the welfare state, and more immediately led to the introduction of old age pensions (1).

During the next half century, the interests put so firmly on the British political agenda by Booth (2), Rowntree (3), Webb (4), Bowley, and Burnett-Hurst (5) remained fixed. Between them, these pioneers had uncovered areas of ignorance so vast and forms of need so fundamental that few of their successors reached out beyond the territory they had defined. As a result it became a commonplace that old age for those from all but the most privileged classes was characterised by physical illness, poor nutrition, inadequate housing, and fear of the pauper's death. Thus, whilst important basic scientific research proceeded slowly on the biological bases of ageing, the greatest efforts of medical research were to do with ill health, both physical and mental (6).

This small, but consistently growing body of knowledge provided a basis for Sheldon (7) to complete his important study of old people in Wolverhampton early after the Second World War. In the resulting book he was able to provide a taxonomy of the sicknesses which were attributed to old age and to suggest ways in which these could be medically managed. Significantly, the studies which followed have been developments of specialist areas of his broad-ranging studies. Incontinence, falls, strokes, dementia, confusion, and depression remain high in the profile of medical research.

Social scientists in Britain have always been fewer in number in the gerontological field, despite that their work has had enormous impact both on the public consciousness and politically. They, too, have been preoccupied with the causes and consequences of poorer physical health and the social deprivations which appear to follow retirement from work. After the major policy reforming studies at the turn of the century there, was a lull in activity. The inter-war years produced a very modest literature about the effects of retirement, but it failed to leave any permanent mark.

The resurgence of interest in social welfare provision occasioned by the Second World War and the war-time planning for a welfare state served to re-focus attention of old age. Beveridge's pension plan revived the debates of the first decade of the century about the quality of life after retirement (8). Income, health, and housing resumed their position at the head of the agenda -- an agenda which has survived almost intact to the present day. But as empirical studies of the life circumstances of old people began, they soon developed specialist orientations (9). Apart from Peter Townsend's The Family Life of Old People (10), few notable studies have looked at the subject in the round. In particular, research of a social and medical kind alike gave price of place to studies of "need." As a result, the enormous output of research which has been produced since the early fifties has provided a highly detailed account of the structural characteristics of the retired population, the illnesses which are likely to afflict them, the sources of their income, the quality of their housing, their occupancy of hospital beds and consumption of general practitioner services, their need for social support services at home, the changes in family support which have necessitated increased public provision and the quality of institutional care. More recent work has turned to the effectiveness of social policy provision to meet the needs of elderly people, particularly as the rising and ageing of this sector of the population became apparent. Studies of geriatric care, old peoples' homes and the whole range of domiciliary services, both statutory and voluntary, became increasingly common (11).

The pathology model of ageing argument can, of course, be extended too far, for studies within what is here called normal ageing do exist. Psychologists, although equally afflicted by the desire to depict old age as a deviance from the arbitrary norms of early adulthood, have nonetheless done much to identify the general characteristics of retired populations. Yet until very recently their explanations of normal cognitive functioning, personality integration, memory retention and learning skills have served to reinforce the image of old age as a period of chronic decline. These studies have formed the main stream of "human growth and development" studies which map the whole life as a series of age related stages. Until the upsurge of "lifespan" studies in the US, influenced by the work of Goulet and Baltes (12), Nesselroade and Reese (13), and Baltes and Schaie (14), the last stages of any volume or taught course on human development present a picture of expected (and therefore normal) decline on all major parameters. Only in the past five years has this orthodoxy been firmly challenged, drawing its strength from a close scrutiny of prior assumptions and inappropriate methodologies (15). Thus, for example, it is now claimed that the agreed view of decrements in memory function with age are in some measure due to the inappropriate nature of the tests (older people find them meaningless) and the failure to recognise that as people grow into middle age and beyond, they sift information more carefully and story only the essence of what they need, rather than whole chunks of undigested material (16).

LIFE HISTORY APPROACHES

Equally there are shifts of interest to be observed across the social sciences. As the Editor of an international and multi-disciplinary journal, Ageing and Society, I receive and read over a hundred articles a year, submitted for publication. The bulk remain in the mould outlined, but increasingly there is an awareness of the need to theorise, to examine the political economy of old age, and to view old age as a product of a life lived (17).

It would be possible to further document and classify the output of age related research as part of this document, but this would be lengthy and unnecessary. Convincing evidence of the pathology orientation of studies in old age can be readily found in the series of annual publications produced by the Centre for Policy on Ageing (formerly NCCOP), Old Age: A Register of Social Research. This annual compendium contains details of all the serious work being undertaken in the field. Each year, an analysis is produced by Hedley Taylor of the main subject areas and the percentage of projects under each heading. The volume for 1979-80 identified 165 studies under 40 headings. Of the headings themselves, only three could be classed as a non-problem centred kind -- eight percent of the total. Typical headings are labelled: rehabilitation, sheltered housing, information needs, mental disorder, residential care, etc.

Too much emphasis on these features of the body of research on ageing could lead to a misunderstanding of the purpose of drawing attention to them. There is no implication that this work is in any important sense bad, only that it is providing us with a distorted picture of later life which lacks congruence with my own studies and experience of work with older people. It has led both policy makers and the world at large to see old age as synonymous with sickness, poverty and mental decrepitude. The fact that these conditions do occur amongst the older members of our society is neither to be denied nor ignored. What is important, however, and a central proposition of this, is to recognise that much of what professional observers and helpers see as pathological and problematic is not seen in that way by older people themselves.

For some years, now I have been involved in both theoretical writing and empirical studies of social ageing, as well as in social policy issues in old age. Throughout this period, I have been anxious to encourage researchers and analysts to take more account of how elderly people see and value their own lives, particularly in the context of their life histories. In other places, I have written at length about the relationship between life experience and the experience of old age (18). Inevitably, former life-style and practices are powerful and formative factors, not only in the material conditions of life in retirement, but also in the way it is perceived and interpreted. All too little account is taken of these factors in determining what society will do for its older members. Indeed, I frequently use a metaphor which compares the social and medical pathologist with spectators in the arena at the end of a marathon race who see the runners enter, tired and bruised, for the last lap. They see their task

18

as attending to relieving the weariness and the pain without ever asking how the race was run or what plans they may have for further racing.

It is no longer necessary to defend the biographical approach as a technique. Its roots can be found, as Rosenmayer (19) has reminded us, in the European tradition of sociology and exemplified in such classic studies as The Polish Peasant (20). The literature of psychology and the processes of life development go back to Freud and Jung, taking a specific biographical form in the work of Erikson (21). More recently there is evidence of its impressive application in studies of middle age by Neugarten (22) and Valliant (23) amongst others. At the same time, increasing sociological attention has been given to life stories, particularly in relation to ageing and old age. In America, Glen Elder's retrospective accounts in Children of the Great Depression (23) and Tamara Hareven's recent volume (24) are testimony to the confident and increasingly sophisticated analysis of whole or partial biographies. In France Anne-Marie Guillemard's study of retirement (25) has been followed by others in this form, the latest to be reported being Gaullier's researches on redundancy experience of men in their fifties (26). The most widely read life history studies of recent years have been Dan Levinson's The Seasons of a Man's Life (27) and the linked volume of more dramatically depicted accounts in Gail Sheehy's best selling book Passages (28). Their success has served to legitimise an approach which has had to struggle for respectability, despite its long and honourable history. This may explain the dearth of such studies in Britain where the prevailing views about suitable methodologies for the study of ageing processes have favoured more structured approaches.

Cohorts, Generations, and History

The essential argument for viewing ageing throughout the life span as a continuous and ever changing process, which takes different forms in each successive cohort, has already been briefly made. But before going on to look at the practical issues which arise out of these shifting patterns, we must give some attention to conceptual tools and the ways they are to be applied.

The notion of generation as a description of biological and lineage relationships goes back into ancient history. It provides much of the organising work of Jewish history as recorded in the Old ment and was an equally well developed set of ᵣₑ_ ːionships in classical Greece. It served then as a system of age-grading which made possible the allocation of roles, relationships, economic tasks and patterns of authority. In modern societies, the temporal aspects of generational differences have come to the fore. Social organisation no longer rests on lineage, nor does it indicate any universal attribute of authority or status. Indeed, as we have already observed, the longer lived generations are more likely to find themselves suffering from status deprivation than from glory in their seniority. Within studies of ageing, it has been common to avoid the wider applications of the term generation and to confine attention to the social membership category which is formed by the different layers of family formation.

In its looser usage, generation can mean a group of individuals who share a common experience such as "the Second World War generation" or Glen Elder's (29) collective term "Children of the Great Depression." Within the setting of this paper, the pioneering work of Leonard Cain (30) used the term in this way. In writing of "the new generation of elderly people," he was referring to a demographic cohort rather than a socio-biological category. To avoid confusion and because it appears to be a heuristically more valuable device, attention here will be confined to age cohorts. In making this choice of words and associated ideas, I am conscious of a highly developed tradition of discourse which deals with generations as sociological entities defined by common experience. This includes Mannheim (31), Elkins (32), and the formative work of Erikson (33). Therefore my choice is based on convenience and the wish to avoid ambiguity as far as possible.

A cohort is constituted by the coincidence of the birth of its members within a specified time period. This is not to say that a cohort is merely an age-group in the manner commonly adopted when presenting population based data in tabular form. The routine analysis of data by dividing subjects into five or ten year age groups is one of the principal practical reasons why we have neglected the historical dimension in social science and medical empirical research. This leads to the comparison of arbitrary age segments in a way which assumes that any differences are attributable to age. The unconsidered use of that practice leads to the age labelling this paper is attempting to challenge.

What constitutes the organising experience of a cohort which will allow its proper segregation (for analytical purposes) from the rest of a given population is a matter of historical judgement -- a judgement which acknowledges the unifying influence of social structure on the experience of individuals. An elaboration of the long-standing debate about the duality of ego and community in the lives of individuals which has absorbed social scientists for many decades cannot be undertaken here; readers are referred to the excellent summary of it by Philip Abrams, who in his volume Historical Sociology also provides a most coherent argument for the combining of historical and sociological analysis.

Abrams's concern is with the refinement of sociological generations; his argument employs that term, but can equally serve the more specific sub-set -- the cohort. In identifying the peculiar configuration of biographical experiences which arise from common history, he writes:

> But sociological generations are not made ad lib. New styles of identity can only be made within the specific historically constructed possibilities of the world entered by any given biological generation. If a new sociological generation is to emerge a new configuration of social action, the attempts of individuals to construct identity must coincide with major and palpable historical experiences in relation to which new meanings can be assembled. Creativity feeds on experience not will. Biological age gives individuals distinctive problems and distinctive resources for solving these problems ... But it is historical events that seem to provide the crucial opportunities for constructing new versions of such meanings. (35)

Using this approach, a sociological generation could include people drawn from a variety of age groups, and for this reason I choose to confine attention to age-based cohorts for use in relation to old age.

In considering the parameters of a cohort, we must consider the pervading influences in the lives of those encompassed. In her study of Canadian family patterns of people born in the last decade of the nineteenth century and in the early twentieth, Jane Synge (36) lays particular stress on the need

to integrate personal and historical factors in
family life for a group which were born in a
specific and transitional historical phase. She
continues: In addition, data from these sources may
also indicate whether characteristics that we
currently associate with ageing may stem in part
from the specific features of the early life
experience of people now in their seventies and
eighties."

Similarly, Martin Kohl (37), in reporting a
study of flexible retirement in Germany, observes:
"Historically, not only the chronological age at
which the socially structured transitions in the
life-course occur, has changed, but the character of
the temporal organisation itself." He goes on to
identify factors relevant to his sample of early
retirees, which include "... the development of an
age-graded school system, of other age-graded
systems of public rights and duties, the transformation from a demographic pattern of random
experience to a pattern of predictable life-span and
the narrowing of the age for the "normative" events
of the family cycle and work career."

Thus, in examining those who now fall into the
groups called old, it is increasingly necessary to
find demarcations of historical identity. My own
markers in this process include the commencement of
the First World War, the points at which universal
education was extended, and -- in relation to health
and social welfare -- the extent of adult working
life completed before the full introduction of the
Welfare State in Britain. (38)

Indeed, it is to such an examination that we
now proceed and where the practical consequences of
cohort changes are to be observed. The world of
"health" in later life is here interpreted broadly,
for one contemporary historical element which needs
to be registered is the wider conception of how
health can be maintained by comparison with the
services available to prior cohorts of old people.
The forms and patterns of service delivery which
change as a result of professional influence might
in the future also have to be more responsive to
changes within cohorts of consumers (39, 40).

CHANGING PATTERNS AMONG THE RETIRED POPULATION

In a book about her views on ageing, Maggie Kuhn
(41), the leader of the Grey Panthers, quotes a
section from Alex Comfort's volume, A Good Age,

which summarises the position well:

> Unless we are old already, the next "old people" will be US. Whether we go along with the treatment meted out to those who are now old depends on how far society can sell the bills of goods it sold them -- and it depends more upon that than upon any research. No pill or regime known, or likely, could transform the latter years as fully as could a change in our vision of age and a militancy in attaining that change (42).

Attention on "the active elderly" usually focuses on the retention of physical and psychological fitness to lead a life much the same as younger people's. It implies being ambulant, capable of walking distances, carrying purchases, negotiating busy roads, and coping with public transport. The notion essentially concerns the retention of functional capacities in dealing with what are known as activities of daily living. Clearly, this is one of the interpretations which must be taken into account for the decline in physical health and strength is a seriously limiting factor for older people. But the severe onset of these conditions is being kept at bay until later in the life span, and this, combined with a less hostile environment, could release a more creative phase during retirement.

So, in addition to functional health, we will need to examine two other forms of increased activity which coincide with and are stimulated by a greater healthiness. The first might be termed corporate consciousness and action; the second, the recolonisation of eldership.

Functional Health

Functional health in old age is well established to be highly correlated with previous life-style and status. Shanas and Maddox sum it up neatly: "In general the lower the socioeconomic position of an individual, the higher the prevalence of disease and the higher the age-specific mortality rate. These commonly observed associations between socioeconomic position, illness and life expectancy have a complex explanation. Indices of socioeconomic position usually include measurements of income, occupation and education. Such factors, singly or in combination, are reflected in different styles of life and differential access to, and use of health resources. For instance, low income, a manual occupation and minimal education generally predict a high incidence of disease and elevated death rates in all industrialised countries (43).

The implication of these relationships is that middle class people are more likely to survive into old age, with artisans whose work has been particularly arduous or dangerous to health dying at earlier ages. In general, this picture is supported by official data on mortality, resulting in a situation whereby those who do survive into retirement can expect to live to 80 and beyond. Population projections indicate that from 1986 until the end of the century, those aged 85 and over will increase constantly and dramatically to a number 60 percent above the current figure (44). The consequences of more people living a full life span are mixed. They are expected to remain independent and living in the community for longer, but in doing so will suffer the accumulated effect of chronic disease.

The detail of age related health status is not an essential part of this paper, but it has been necessary to lay the ground for our understanding of the extended period of physical and psychological well being sufficient to allow adequate social functioning. This can be simply but graphically illustrated, by pointing to the rising average age of admission to Old People's Homes. Ten years ago, average admission age was in the lower 70s with places being given on occasions to people still in their 60s. Now elderly people have difficulty gaining admission to a residential home before their 80th birthday.

As this group of "old old" consolidates its position, changes in the social structure of the retired population as a whole will be taking place. There will be more people within it, at all ages, whose socioeconomic position is higher than previous cohorts -- reflecting improvements in working conditions, the embourgeoisement of mid-twentieth century Britain, with its better nutrition, housing and education. In sum there will be more older people throughout the age ranges which have health sufficient to allow for future and active participation in society. These new cohorts will have experienced relative prosperity, support of the welfare state and the rise of consumerism. A new and more aggressive climate of expectation can be expected to replace the polite acquiescence and minimal expectations to which researchers and practitioners are currently accustomed.

Cohort changes provide the key to many of the likely developments in the future. Life experience for groups of people of the same age group inevitably conditions their expectations and their responses to social and economic circumstances. Those currently over 70 in Britain were born into an Edwardian era which marked the end of Britain's dominance of world trade and led directly into the First World War. The inter-war depression followed, being terminated by the 1939-45 war, which in turn brought several years of continuing hardship. Only in the 1950s, when this group was already moving towards the end of its working (employment) life, did prosperity of a pervasive kind emerge. This historical phase has therefore been one of deprivation followed by relative plenty, creating amongst those who are now old an understandable sense of comparative well-being.

Again, drawing on my own recent life history studies (45), it is clear that relative deprivation is the lynch pin of satisfaction or dissatisfaction in later life. For this generation, their reference groups are principally themselves in the past and their own parents in retirement. Any objective assessment of living standards would give support to the view that Abrams discovered, that the current cohort is comparatively well off and perceives itself as such. Yet for those who saw the welfare state constructed during their mid-life or earlier and particularly those who were young in the immediate post-war period, the comparison will have an increasingly negative effect. Current expectations of income in retirement are having to be radically revised, whilst projections about the costs of future financial support for the retired give little cause of optimism.

In the interstices of frustration and unmet expectations, political reaction grows. For Britain, there is a long way to go, but during the period under consideration in this paper, the strong likelihood is that successive cohorts will not only be more highly motivated to take action, but their higher skills will facilitate an organised lobby of a kind as yet unknown in Britain.

Corporate Consciousness and Action

Corporate consciousness and action can reasonably be predicted than as the response of the increasingly articulate and socially skilful retired population. This group will be less poor, overall, than its predecessors as occupational pensions and home ownership supplement state support. Like its American counterpart, it is likely to seek a better deal for retired people in everyday transactions where prejudice and commercial practice limit their opportunities. There are no immediate signs of a common consciousness emerging amongst older people in Britain. Certainly, no political allegiance is observable yet. But there are signs of an increasing commercial recognition of retired people as a worthwhile market, especially in transport, holidays, domestic equipment, and personal services. Banks, building societies, insurance companies, employers, and the trade unions continue to exercise unremittingly ageist discrimination against retired people in a manner which may not be tolerated for much longer.

The American experience of increasing consciousness by elderly people of their position arose out of their desire to challenge commercial interests and later to act as lobbyists in influencing government policy at state and federal level. Perhaps inevitably those who became involved in organised activity to secure better treatment from those offering goods and services in the marketplace were what Pratt, in his book The Gray Lobby (46) calls the "slightly privileged." In first pursuing preferential treatment amongst traders of all kinds and, then, in the 1960s, focusing more clearly on political influence, a number of influential national groups emerged. The largest and most durable of them are: The American Association of Retired Persons (AARP) and the National Retired Teachers Association (NRTA), which function in national affairs as one body. The National Council of Senior Citizens (NCSC), which was set up in the 1960s to campaign for Medicare and then extended its interests has a less middle class membership than AARP. More cross-sectional in its membership and more campaigning in its approach than either of these are the Gray Panthers.

Together these mass membership organisations (their combined membership is counted in millions) are able to act as foci for political reform within the United States and to directly influence state and federal policy. The U.S. Senate has in recent years passed legislation raising the compulsory retirement age for public employees to 70. Such a development is currently inconceivable in Britain because elderly people are not organised, nor do they appear to wish to be organised on their own behalves. But relative deprivation has proved to be the most powerful force for dissatisfaction in later life. Such dissatisfaction is likely to increase dramatically as those who anticipated a long and comfortable retirement find themselves straitened by inflation and governments which may want to execute a backlash against retired people in favour of employed and unemployed younger people. Should these speculations come to pass, they could be the triggers for mass membership organisations on the American model. If they do arise, these groups will undoubtedly seek re-entry into all the corners of social and economic life to establish a respected place for old age.

Colonisation of Eldership

Colonisation of eldership is an expression of this desire to re-enter the social world on equal or even positively discriminated terms. The phrase adopted here is not meant to denote the return to another golden age, but takes eldership to mean recognition of and due respect for experience. At its core, this "recolonisation" is about self respect and mutual respect across generations. It requires society to make a more generous place for old age, but one which also allows greater opportunity for inter-generational support and cross-generational exchange.

In a newly reported study of early retirement in France, Xavier Gaullier (47) depicts the post war period of policy on old age as having gone through three phases. The first period he saw as the transformation of old age into retirement. The second, in the 1960s, was characterised by the transformation of old age into the Third Age (a period of leisure, autonomy and self-realisation). In the latest stage, dating from about 1976, he sees the policy for old age having become a policy of Employment. Rising unemployment has brought about earlier and earlier enforced retirement (down to 50 years in some parts of the country). Gaullier writes: "An individual is declared "old" by authorities responsible for employment and rejected definitively from the job market uniquely on account of his old age, regardless of his state of health, his biological or psychological ageing ... There is no longer a promotion of a way of life but rather the payment of allowances to the unemployed ... For a long time old age policy favoured the social insertion of the elderly, the new policy brutally excludes them from social life."

These observations have a familiar ring not only in the British context, but in almost all the countries of Europe and North America, where economic recession has led uniformly to early retirement and redundancy, coupled with a reduction of services and monetary benefits. In this account, the author attributes the crisis in old age policy to weaknesses in the capitalist structure as well as to the political allegiance of governments to the "working population." Certainly structural factors are pre-eminent in the situation. The restitution of France's Third Age concept is not likely to be achieved by individual effort. Yet a return to a concept of a society which provides open access to all its major arenas for older people is simply to re-state a tenet of human rights.

Within the reconstructed forms of eldership, there will need to be provision for a great diversity of life-style. Thus, the most important reforming function to be performed would be the systematic removal of constraints on personal decision-making. So the agenda might well include the removal of paternalistic practices amongst health and social welfare practitioners, housing managers, etc., who presently take significant decisions for older people with little or no real consultation. It is, then, a restoration of the civil rights which have become so eroded, as Alison Norman has reminded us (48).

POLICY IMPACT

The foregoing discussion has combined current observation with speculation about the future. It has adopted a more positive and optimistic posture than most commentators would choose. This is not due to excessive hopefulness or misplaced idealism, but because it represents one of the real and likely options for the future. The present pattern of heavy dependency on public provision associated with exclusion from economic work is not one which can be sustained for much longer.

As a beginning (and very selective) agenda for discussion of possible changes of policy which would reduce dependency and capitalise on the capacity for greater activity, the following four topics illustrate the practical possibilities and potentials of greater activity amongst older people:

Education
British education is directed towards the young. But

28

increasingly there is pressure for lifetime education and in particular opportunities for learning after retirement. Both Norman Evans (49) and Eric Midwinter (50) have outlined the rationale for this necessary expansion which both recognises and nurtures the life experience of people in later life. Britain is already under pressure to adjust its models of further and higher education to accept the retired on their own terms. In France, the University of the Third Age is one model. In the USA there are many others. Within this context oral history and the valuation of life histories will have an important place.

Housing Stock/Personal Capital

With increasing numbers of retired people being owner occupiers living on the product of diminishing savings, due to inflation, there will exist opportunities for releasing family housing whilst liberating otherwise unconsumable capital. At present a few insurance companies run Home and Income schemes whilst an even smaller number of property companies offer investment opportunities tied to guaranteed residential accommodation and personal support packages. The extent of the "unavailable" wealth of otherwise poor elderly people in Britain has not, to my knowledge, been computed. It has not yet been recognised either by governments or by commerce as having potential.

In assisting elderly people to remain independent, such developments would unlock funds which could transform their life-styles. The principal drawback, apart from the heavy cost of initial funding, is the deep reluctance currently elderly people have to spending "my child's inheritance." The new generations of old people may find these social obligations less onerous, whilst the housing market itself is likely to become more social in character (51), (52). On a broader canvas, the whole area of inherited wealth and the social taboos which surround it will need to be explored.

Vigour, Leisure, and Work

Active retirement can now be expected to be around twenty years. Traditional leisure pursuits and domestic occupation are proving inadequate for many pensionable people, just as they are inadequate for early retirees and unemployed people. Indeed, this common situation of large groups of people of different ages, aptitudes and experience may be the way of breaking the mould (comfortable for some, but desolate for many) of retirement as a period of economically non-productive leisure activity.

Inter-generational Relations

As indicated earlier, inter-generational relations are not always harmonious or productive. Nonetheless, kinship is still the strongest inducement to provide help and support to others. At present, women, frequently retired themselves, are far and away the largest providers and old people the heaviest consumers. This subject has only just emerged on the policy agenda. Muriel Nissel and Lucy Bonnerjea's report (53) represents one of the first serious British attempts at a time-budget analysis of what family care actually means. Yet, much exploration remains to be done about sex stereotypes, work patterns and family structure which inhibit a larger contribution from men.

CONCLUSIONS

Three broad arguments have been advanced in this paper. The first is that normative notions of old age which are used as labels for powerful negative stereotypes are to a large degree unjustified. They depend upon a pathology model of later life which is partial and skewed. The second is that, as a result of traditional beliefs about the nature of old age, we have confused age and cohort factors. Once a distinction can be drawn between the persistent features of a given age status and the historical influences which shape its form in any given age, it will be possible to speak of old age with more assurance. The third argument concerns areas of the lives of presently older people which show signs of being changed as they are succeeded by the incoming cohort.

To have attempted to bring three such broad themes together in one short paper necessarily means that none of the arguments has been fully fashioned and executed. Nonetheless, it is hoped that the general thesis concerning age labelling has been somewhat clarified. If so, more attention to the historical dimensions of ageing may well be the result.

NOTES

(1) Report of the Royal Commission on the Poor Law (1905-9), HMSO London, 1909.

(2) Booth, Charles, Life and Labour of the People of London, Macmillan, London 1902

(3) Rowntree, B. Seebohm, Poverty: A Study of Town Life, Macmillan, London 1901.

(4) Webb, Beatrice, My Apprenticeship, Longman Green, London, 1926.

(5) Bowley, A.L. and Burnett-Hurst, A.R. Livelihood and Poverty, London 1912.

(6) Handbooks which attempt to provide synthesis of existing work tend to be a sound guide to the pattern and distribution of existing research. In gerontology such a series of handbooks, under the general editorship of James Birren, has been published over the past fifteen years by Van Nostrand Reinhold (New York). In 1981 a new series of Annual Reviews of Gerontology and Geriatrics, edited by Carl Eisdorfer and published by Springer, appeared. The foci of attention noted in the text are clearly identifiable in these volumes, as they are in the leading journal, Journal of Gerontology.

(7) Sheldon, J.H. Social Medicine of Old Age, Oxford, University Press, 1948.

(8) Macintyre, Sally, "Old Age as a Social Problem, some notes on the British experience." In Dingwall, R. & al. (eds.) Health Care and Health Knowledge, Croom Helm, London 1977.

(9) These specialist studies included: Cole, Dorothy, The Economic Circumstance of Old People, Occasional Papers on Social Administration, Bell and Son, London 1962; Brockington, F. and Lempert, S.M. The Social Needs of the Over Eighties, Manchester University Press, 1966; Tunstall, J. Old and Alone, Routledge and Kegan Paul, London, 1966; Townsend, Peter, Last Refuge, Routledge and Kegan Paul, London 1962.

(10) Townsend, Peter, The Family Life of Old People, Routledge and Kegan Paul, London, 1957.

(11) See the series of literature and policy reviews which map this growth of studies, Profiles of the Elderly, Vols. 1-8, Age Concern, Mitcham 1976-.

(12) Goulet, L.R. and Baltes, P.B. (eds.) Life-Span Developmental Psychology: Research and Theory, Academic Press, New York, 1970.

(13) Nesselroade, J.R. and Reese, H.W. (eds.) Life-Span Developmental Psychology: Methodological Issues, Academic Press, New York, 1973.

(14) Baltes, P.B. and Shaie, W. (eds.) Life-Span Developmental Psychology: Personality and Socialization, Academic Press, New York, 1973.

(15) Taub, H.A. "Life-Span Education: A Need for Research with Meaningful Prose," Educational Gerontology, 5, 1980.

(16) Labouvie-Vief, Gisela, and Blanchard-Fields, Fredda "Cognitive Ageing and Psychological Growth," Ageing and Society, 2,2, July, 1982.

(17) See Walker, Alan, "Towards a Political Economy of Old Age," 1,1, March 1981; Townsend, Peter "The Structured Dependency of the Elderly," Ageing and Society, 1, 1, March 1981; Estes, Caroll, "Dominant and Competing Paradigms in Gerontology, Ageing and Society, 2,2, July 1982; Taylor, Rex and Ford, Graeme, "Lifestyle and Ageing," Ageing and Society, 1,3, November 1981.

(18) See for example, Johnson, Malcolm L., "That Was Your Life: A Biographical Approach to Later Life." In JMA Munnichs and W.J.A. van den Heuval (eds.) Dependency and Interdependency in Old Age, Martinus Nijhoff, The Hague, 1976 and An Ageing Population: Relations and Relationships, Open University Press, Milton Keynes, 1979.

(19) Rosenmayer, Leopold, "Age, Lifespan and Biography," Ageing and Society, 1,1, March 1981.

(20) Thomas, W.I. and Znaniecki, F. The Polish Peasant in Europe and America (2 vols) over Publications, New York, 1927.

(21) Erikson, Erik, Childhood and Society, Norton, New York, 1950.

(22) Neugarten, Bernice (ed.) Middle Age and Ageing: A Reader, University of Chicago Press, 1968.

(23) Elder, Glen, Children of the Great Depression, University of Chicago Press, 1974.

(24) Hareven, Tamara, K. (ed.) Aging and the Life Course, Guildford Press, New York, 1981.

(25) Guillemard, A.M. La Retraite-une Mort Sociale, Mouton la Haye, Paris, 1972.

(26) Gaullier, Xavier, "Economic Crisis and Old Age - Old Age Policies in France," Ageing and Society, 2,2, July 1982.

(27) Levinson, Daniel, J. The Seasons of a Man's Life, Alfred Knopf, New York, 1978.

(28) Sheehy, Gail, Passages: Predictable Crises of Adult Life, Dutton and Company, New York, 1974.

(29) Elder, Glen, op. cit.

(30) Cain, Leonard D. Jr. "Life Course and Social Structure." In Faris, R.E.L. (ed.) Handbook of Modern Sociology, Rand McNally, Chicago, 1964 and "Age Status and Generational Phenomena: the New Old People in Contemporary America" The Gerontologist, 7, 1967.

(31) Mannheim, K., "The Problem of Generations." In Essays on the Sociology of Knowledge, Routledge and Kegan Paul, London, 1952.

(32) Elkins, S.M., Slavery, University of Chicago press, 1959 (cited by Abrams - see below).

(33) Erikson, Erik, Childhood and Society, Norton, New York, 1963.

(34) Abrams Philip, Historical Sociology, Open Books, Shepton Mallet, Somerset, 1982.

(35) Ibid. pp. 255-256.

(36) Synge, Jane, "Cohort Analysis in the Planning and Interpretation of Research Using Life Histories." In Bertaux, D. (ed.) Biography and Society, Sage, Beverly Hills, 1981.

(37) Kohli, Martin & al., "The Social Construction of Ageing through Work," Ageing and Society, 3,1, March 1983.

(38) For further elaboration of these claims see Phillipson, C., Capitalism and the Construction of Old Age, Macmillan, London, 1982.

(39) Brown Eve, Susan, "Older Americans' Use of Health Maintenance Organisations," Research on Aging, 4,2, June 1982.

(40) Haug, Marie, "Doctors and Older Patients," Journal of Gerontology, 34, 6, November, 1979.

(41) Hessel, Dieter (ed.) Maggie Kuhn on Ageing, Westminster Press, Philadelphia, 1977.

(42) Comfort, Alex. A Good Age, Mitchell Beazley, London, 1977.

(43) Shanas, Ethel and Maddox, George. Ageing Health and the Organisation of Health Resources. In Binstock, R.H. and Shanas, E. (eds.) Handbook of Ageing and the Social Sciences, Van Nostrand Reinhold, New York, 1976.

(44) OPCS Population Projections 1977-2017, Series PP2 No.9, HMSO, London, 1979.

(45) Johnson, Malcolm L. with di Gregorio, Silvana and Harrison, Beverly. Ageing, Needs and Nutrition: A Study in Community Care, Policy Studies Institute, London, 1981.

(46) Pratt, Henry J. The Gray Lobby, University of Chicago Press, 1976.

(47) Gaullier, Xavier. "Economic Crisis and Old Age: Old Age Policies in France," Ageing and Society 2,2, July 1982.

(48)   Norman, Alison, Rights and Risk, Centre for Policy on Ageing, London 1980.

(49)   Evans, Norman. The Knowledge Revolution, Grant McIntyre, London 1981.

(50)   Midwinter, Eric, Age Is Opportunity: Education and Older People, Centre for Policy on Ageing, London, 1983.

(51)   Webster, David, "A Social Market Answer on Housing," New Society, 12, November 1981.

(52)   Kemeny, Jim, The Myth of Home Ownership, Routledge and Kegan Paul, London 1981.

(53)   Nissel, Muriel and Bonnerjea, Lucy, Family Care of Handicapped Elderly, Policy Studies Institute, London 1982.

Sections of this paper are drawn from Johnson, Malcolm L., "Greater Activity in Later Life." In Fogarty, M. (ed.) Retirement Policy, the Next Fifty Years, Heinemann, London, 1982.

Mary Crowe's poem is quoted from Gray, Barbara, and Johnson, Malcolm, Up the Long Track - Poems of Ageing - An Anthology, submitted for publication.

Chapter 3

HEALTH RELATED BEHAVIOUR AND AGING: CONCEPTUAL
ISSUES

Bjørn E. Holstein

INTRODUCTION

Ideally, this book should answer three questions:
1. How does health related behaviour affect the
aging process? 2. How does the aging process affect
health related behaviour? and 3. What other factors
shape health related behaviour and the aging
process? However, none of these three questions can
be answered satisfactorily today because of lack of
knowledge.

The focal interest of this chapter is to
discuss concepts of health related behaviour in
relation to conceptual frameworks of aging. Two
basic assumptions are inherent in the discussion
throughout this paper and the others which follow.
Firstly, health related behaviour is viewed inter-
actionally, as having been shaped throughout a
lifelong interaction with material living conditions, social support networks, the formal health
and social care delivery systems and its professionals. The behavioural manifestations, in turn,
shape the individual's interaction with the environment. Secondly, responsibility for personal health
cannot be placed exclusively with the individual or
with formal and informal support systems; it is
shared and mutually interdependent. The individual's
health related behaviours determine the use of
services, and the structural and content characteristics of the service provision systems affect the
individual's behavioural response to illness and
health.

Thus, concepts such as self-care and health
behaviour also imply interactions between the health
care system and the elderly. The complexity of the
aging process and of the relation between health and
aging necessitates conceptual clarification to

35

analyse the relationships. This chapter will discuss, firstly, conceptual perspectives of aging and, secondly, conceptual perspectives on health related behaviour. Finally, a few components for future discussion of these issues will be suggested.

CONCEPTUAL FRAMEWORKS OF AGING

Methodological and Theoretical Problems

Understanding the relation between aging and health related behaviour is prerequisite to understanding the normal aging process. The development of a comprehensive model of normal aging has been impeded by several methodological and theoretical problems, which consequently affect our thinking in the area of health behaviour and self-care.

Five problems of special significance should be mentioned:

1. Difficulties in Discriminating Age from Cohort.

Recognition of age-related attributes is often dramatically improved when studies of cohorts supplement knowledge based on cross-sectional studies. Age-related behaviour, health, and living conditions are, thus, related not only to age, but also to the experience of historical events at specific age intervals. This is illustrated by studies of intellectual performance and age (Schaie 1977, Botwinick 1977). Cross-sectional studies show a considerable decrease in intellectual performance with increasing age, suggesting a "natural" decline in these capacities as one grows older. Longitudinal studies, on the contrary, show stable or even increasing intellectual performance from early adulthood to old age. These results from cross-sectional studies were due to differences in educational background of the various age groups, showing the importance of the impact of early life experience on performance and function in late life.

Historical and societal conditions may well have varying impact on the health-and illness-behaviour of different generations of elderly. Longitudinal studies might, therefore, add considerably to our knowledge of normal aging and the interaction between the biological aging process, living conditions, and behaviour. But despite their importance, results based on longitudinal studies regarding normal aging can become obsolete since studies

of subsequent cohorts often show substantial d.
ences from one cohort to another (Svanborg
Svanborg, Bergstrom & Mellstrom 1982).

For both the study and the improvement
health behaviour in late life, this necessitates
caution in the description of age-related habits.
These may be less related to age as to a specific
generation's exposure to specific historical antecedents. Thus, historical preconditions need to be
differentiated from the characteristics of normal
aging.

2. Major Variations in Age-related Functional Loss.

Age-related activities and reserve-capacities vary
according to the specific organ or function (Heikkinen 1982, From-Hansen 1982, Aeldrekommissionen
1980). This statement may be illustrated from
examining physiological changes over time (Figure
3.1).

Evidence exists that some functions such as
glucose-tolerance remain unchanged with age under
optimal life conditions (Figure 3.1 A). Figure 3.1 B
illustrates that other functions such as maximum
heart frequency and capacity of the kidneys and
lungs are reduced in an age-determined way regardless of health, physical exercise, and other habits.

However, this is true for maximum capacity. The
actual level of functioning may still be heavily
influenced by habits and living-circumstances. The
actual lung and heart functions improve with
training even in very advanced age. A physically fit
and well-exercised 65-year-old has the same oxygen-
uptake as an out-of-shape 30-year-old person. The
winning time in Marathon races for pensioners these
days would have won Olympic gold medals at the
beginning of the century.

Curve C illustrates age-conditioned loss in
capacity caused by illness, curve D the combined
effect of age-determined and age-conditioned reduction in maximum function. For both these curves,
the actual decline due to disease is to a large
extent affected by physical fitness, nutritional
conditions, self-care responses to illness, and
other behavioural elements.

The curves indicated in Figure 3.1 are restricted to physiological functions. Psychological
and social functions such as intellectual and
artistic performance, and certain learned skills
(Botwinick 1977) and even mental health (Haug,
Belgrave & Gratton 1984) may not remain stable or

Figure 3.1

Functional capacities and age. Functional level at rest changes only slightly with increasing age. Maximum function changes differently according to age-determined and/or age-conditioned functional loss.

Source: From-Hansen 1982.

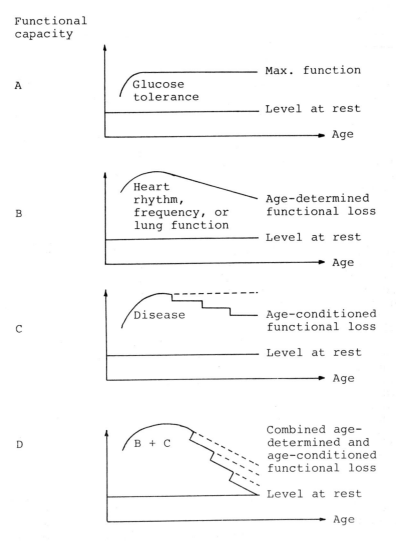

decrease with age, but may even increase. Again, the actual development varies according to individual behaviour and exposure to stimulating environment and experience.

Strategies for improving health behaviour and self-care should adjust to such conditions. The overall effect of biological change is a generally reduced biological reserve capacity (WHO 1984, Almind, Freer, Muir Gray & Warshaw 1983, Heikkinen 1982).

The cumulative result of the normal aging process in biological terms is a decrease in the speed by which the organism will return to homeostasis after stressful episodes such as illness and loss. The effect is also a decreased autoimmunity and thus a decrease in the capacity to fight disease. These biological facts underscore the increasing importance of maintaining health and functional capacity with advancing age by keeping the biological reserve capacity as close to maximum as possible. In very advanced age, however, the biologically determined loss of reserve capacity will also make adequate health behaviour and self-care increasingly insufficient in coping with health problems.

3. Individual Differences Increase with Age. Inter-individual variations in health as well as in habits are evident with increasing age. Many older people maintain optimal health and function until late adulthood, although an increasing proportion will have chronic disease, illness or impairment over time. Thus, the differentiation in health increases with age.

The differentiation in the health profile which increases with age seems also to increase over time. Theories explaining health related behaviours in late life must take into consideration such inter-individual differences to a much larger extent and in a much more dynamic way than in the past. This, again, means that the promotion of adequate health related behaviours in late life requires a variety of means and techniques to be efficient with a heterogeneous population.

4. Age-related Changes in Functional Capacity Vary in both Direction and Origin. Age-related changes in health and habits are not always irreversible and/or continuous in performance decline (Heikkinen 1982).

On the contrary, physical exercise, nutritional improvements, and optimal care might often result in significant gains in health and capacity. Moreover, old people are receptive to health advice to a very advanced age. For example, in a Danish longitudinal study, From-Hansen (1982) described older people's performance in sports and physical exercise as gaining from three percent in 1967 when they were 70 years old, to 20 percent in 1977, when they were 80.

The recognition of the potentials for increased performance in old age is a cornerstone in the argument for the promotion of preventive and rehabilitative actions by lay persons. Unfortunately, environmental factors and sudden life events (e.g., loss of spouse or friends, retirement, illness, relocation) often create discontinuous negative changes in health and/or behaviour. Such events happen more frequently with advancing age, and their negative effects may incorrectly be regarded as attributes of the aging process itself.

In view of the described gains and losses in functional capacity, the process of aging should not be seen as a continuous decline in function, nor as a fixed sequential pattern; rather, it should be viewed as a series of mixed predictable and unpredictable, continuous and discontinuous, desirable and undesirable changes. This may both impede and enable the promotion of adequate health related behaviours, thus entailing a challenge to health professionals working with the elderly in clinical settings as well as to administrators and policymakers in the field of health and social services.

5. Difficulties in Assessing Health with Increasing Age. The pattern of disease among old people is dominated by multiple problems and chronic conditions. Moreover, clinical manifestations of old persons' diseases are often vague and uncharacteristic, making misdiagnoses and mistreatment more likely in the health care system. Medical treatment and cure might then benefit from a consciously planned cooperation with activities performed by the old person and/or his family and social network (WHO 1984, Almind, Freer, Muir Gray & Warshaw 1983).

Optimal functional ability is often considered to be much more important to the old person than good physical health. Whereas the chronic conditions from which many old persons are suffering are not preventable, functional capacities can often be preserved by appropriate health habits. Of major importance are beliefs and perceptions of health (Hickey 1980, WHO 1984). Self-assessment of health status correlates only to a moderate degree with objective or physician rated health status, leaving large groups of elderly feeling quite comfortable with their health, despite obvious chronic illness; similarly, other groups feel negative about their health even where no major illness is detected. Practitioners are generally more pessimistic about the health condition and outcome of treatment than the elderly are themselves (Haug 1981). To some degree, self-assessed health predicts utilisation of health services and the functional ability of the old person (Wan & Odell 1981) as well as mortality (Mossey & Shapiro 1982).

By a careful, systematic assessment of functional status, one can provide the information needed to design optimal health related behaviour. Health-assessment in itself is not necessarily a stimulation of health promotion. In fact, the typical physical health-assessment is often too narrow and might even reinforce the negative expectations and stereotypes of older people. A more holistic approach, however, including assessment of qualities and resources needed to determine adequate health action, may well contribute to health promotion and functional improvement of old persons. Maddox (1981) recommends simultaneous assessment of several functional dimensions: 1. social; 2. economic; 3. mental health; 4. physical health; and 5. activities of daily living.

Old persons' interactions with the health care system are often inefficient, due to barriers in the professional, in the patient, and in the environment. Barriers connected with the physician might be lack of knowledge, skill and proper attitude (Williams 1981; Shanas 1981). According to Maddox (1981), physicians often seem to avoid learning how to communicate with older patients and tend to maintain stereotypic attitudes of the elderly.

Patients often misinterpret illness symptoms as signs of old age (WHO 1984); thus, their attitudes to the physician are not always appropriate for a constructive dialogue (Almind, Freer, Muir Gray & Warshaw 1983). Additionally, families and other social support networks and the health professionals with whom they interact can reinforce the stereotypes of old age (Kuypers & Bengtson 1983). Moreover, environmental factors such as available care facilities and transportation may affect the communication. Therefore, proper use of the health

41

care system is an important issue in promotion of health related behaviours, and an integral part of proper clinical practice to contribute to the situation.

Perspectives on Aging
Behavioural scientists have used different ways to describe old people's interaction with society often with reference to the terms disengagement, activity and continuity. There are implications here for the understanding of health related behaviours.

The Disengagement Perspective. (Cummings & Henry 1961) claims that activities inevitably decline in late life due to personal factors and withdrawal from normal social and community life. Disengagement has been seen as a part of optimal aging. This interpretation of mainly cross-sectional data is today considered disastrous in its consequences. Described in a more interactionistic way, both the individual and the society might or might not disengage in the interaction process. The unhappy situation in modern societies is that society disengages the individual rather than the opposite. The result will often be disengagement, indicating that society is in control. By reinforcing negative stereotypes of the elderly, the health care system and social support networks contribute to this enforced disengagement. From this perspective, the objectives of health behaviour must be to delay this process and to compensate for loss of functional capacity. Relatively little trust can be placed in health promotion and disease prevention. Self-care will be considered to be behavioural responses to illness rather than health maintenance and health promotion.

The Activity Perspective views aging in a more optimistic light, as a period where new skills and activities can be learned and initiated (Neugarten 1977, Neugarten, Havighurst & Tobin 1968).

Aging is not seen as a process of engagement or disengagement, but as a process of adaptation in which personality is the key element. The individual plays an active role in adapting to the biological and social changes that occur with increasing age but also in creating patterns of life that will afford the greatest ego involvement and life satisfaction. This perspective is supported by the recognition of the stable or even improving intellectual performance with increasing age and by the fact that most old citizens have the available time network resources and relatively good health. Activity is seen as a part of optimal aging.

In this perspective, preventive action and health promotion will be seen as a more relevant part of self-care simply because the general belief is that old people have sufficient resources to improve their functions and to gain from continued learning and new experiences. Among the most striking examples are the numerous sports competitions for retired persons, including marathon races and the egalitarian education for old people in the University of the Third Age in France.

The Continuity Perspective refers to the fact that throughout their lives most older people show considerable continuity in their personality, behaviour, and often even living conditions (Aeldrekommissionen 1981, Neugarten 1977). Major discontinuities, of course, also take place: children moving from home; retirement from work; loss of spouse, relatives and friends; illness and impairment, etc. Despite these discontinuities, continuity in beliefs and habits seems to persist.

Policy-makers and practitioners thinking in these terms will see as the task of the elderly-policy and social and medical practice to maintain pre-existing lifestyles and living conditions intact for as long as possible. When change becomes necessary, it should be managed in a way that the best possible relations to earlier stages of life are maintained. One should try to hold the balance between desires and abilities in a situation with an increasing potential for imbalance. Considerable effort should be made to prevent dramatic, undesirable changes in the life situation of old citizens (Aeldrekommissionen, 1982).

This perspective underlines the importance of the environment and policy aspects. It does not, however, deal with the problems created by seeking continuity in an undesirable life situation. Continuity in a life full of perceived and/or objective restraints and unpleasant living conditions would not seem a proper policy objective or goal for providing health care and social support.

The health behaviour and self-care implications of this perspective stress the importance of an early initiation of healthy habits, and early compensation to predicted functional losses. Every health or illness behaviour introduced in advanced age should be in reasonable accord with previous habits as well as with anticipated future situations. This is close to being a description of the actual situation (Ford, this volume). Health and illness-behaviour of old age seem to be basically of the same kind as these behaviours in younger age groups, suggesting a real continuity in behavioural response to health risks and health problems.

By stressing the interaction between environment and coping with aging and the importance of time perspective, the continuity perspective invites thinking in terms of a more dynamic health behaviour model. The planning of health behaviour and self-care in late life should then be affected by what we know about continuities and discontinuities in the living situation in the second half of the life span.

HEALTH RELATED BEHAVIOUR: CONCEPTUAL ISSUES

One of the challenges in the conceptualisation of health related behaviours is the variety of conceptual models of behaviour generally speaking. The behavioural sciences are characterised by at least three different views of behaviour, each having specific implications for our understanding of health related behaviour: The behaviouristic model, the action model, and the socialisation model. The behaviouristic model has some elements in common with the disengagement perspective on aging; the action model reflects some of the components in the activity perspective, and the socialisation model reflects important aspects from the continuity perspective.

The Behaviouristic Model in its basic form implies the recognition of behaviour as a response to environmental stimuli without intervening motives and normative regulations. This perspective suggests that we try to understand health related behaviours as shaped only by obvious stimuli such as health education, symptoms/signs of illness, socioeconomic conditions of life, and available options for preventive action and service provision. Beliefs and motives, future orientation, evaluation of choice-points and other mediating factors are not included

in this behaviouristic model. The operational
variables will then be instruction in health habits
and ways of organising services.

Elderly people's health-related behaviours do
vary according to stimuli such as health education
(Gatherer & al. 1979); type of symptom (Dean &
Holstein 1983); need for services (Wan & Odell
1981); and according to available services and
programmes (Chapman & al. 1979). However, these
stimuli far from explain the whole range of
behavioural responses. The illness itself does not
always act as an effective stimulus. For example,
Byrne & White (1979) describe elderly persons'
illness behaviour as affected more by available
types of treatment, whatever their efficiency, than
by the seriousness of the disease. Barney & Neukom
(1979) describe elderly people suffering from
chronic and complex health problems as not eagerly
waiting to use new health services.

An almost opposite conceptual model of behaviour is the Weber/Parsons/Shils action frame of
reference. This perspective regards action as
including all human behaviour, overt or inward. The
crucial factors are: 1. the motivation to conscious
direction of the action, and 2. the influence of
normative regulations and other interactions with
situational and contextual factors. This model
emphasises the importance of intellectual fuel for
development such as motives. Promotors of adequate
health-related behaviours who understand behaviour
in this way will probably work consciously with
motives, values, attitudes, and beliefs, trying to
alter these psychological factors and behaviour
simultaneously.

The association between health-related beliefs
and health-related behaviours has been studies
intensely at least since the 1960s (e.g., Kasl &
Cobb 1966, Rosenstock 1967), but no strong and
consistent documentation of the importance of health
beliefs on health or illness behaviour has yet been
presented (Dean 1983). A lack of consistency between
health habits and health beliefs is often reported,
especially in the health education literature
(Gatherer & al. 1979, Baric 1980) indicating that
the action-model is insufficient to explain behaviour.

The Concept of Socialisation, denoting the process
by which individuals learn or develop socially and
culturally accepted social behaviours as a means of

45

adjustment, may be a more appropriate model for discussing health-related behaviour. This approach stresses the important influence of the social context in which behaviour takes place and the aspect of continuous adjustment to changing situations (e.g., as in advanced age).

People continue to socialise all their lives: to retirement; to loss of spouse and friends; to decreasing economic power and influence on society; and to chronic illness. Because of the emphasis on continuous adjustment, this model is suitable for explaining health behaviour in age groups facing changing social and health conditions.

The interactionistic basis of this theoretical perspective has been formulated in various ways in medical psychology and sociology in recent decades. A classical contribution is Szasz & Hollender's (1956) description of three models of relationships between doctors and patients, suggesting the role of the doctor as an important determinant of patient-involvement in decisions regarding their health and, thus, a major determinant of patient-socialisation. Another classical contribution is Bloom's (1963) concept on patients' negotiations with their doctors, their social network and their work colleagues. Bloom and Speedling (1981) develop the socialisation model view further. One of their main points is that the role of advanced adulthood is sharply discontinuous. Thus, continued socialisation in old age - including the health aspect - might be necessary.

Documentation is available regarding benefits for elderly persons from programmes building on this socialisation viewpoint, although only to a limited extent (e.g., Lieberman & al. 1979).

Definitions of Self-care and Health Behaviour.
The concepts with relation to this area are numerous: Health behaviour, illness behaviour, sick role behaviour, lay-care, self-care, self-help, defensive health behaviour, self-treatment, self-medication, health-maintenance, etc. Moreover, there is no concensus regarding definitions of these concepts.

Parsons' (1951) classical description of the sick-role is one of the basic inspirations to the study of behavioural responses to illness. The concept of sick-role and sick-role behaviour has been modified, for example by Coe (1981) and by Kasl & Cobb (1966) and new concepts developed.

Mechanic (1962) was one of the first scholars to define illness behaviour as referring to the ways in which given symptoms may be differentially perceived, evaluated, and acted or not acted upon by individuals. Suchman (1965) later separated five stages of illness experience closely related to behavioural responses but, in contrast to Mechanic, extended the process further than the seeking of professional help: 1. symptom experience; 2. assumption of the sick-role; 3. medical care contract; 4. dependent-patient role; and 5. recovery or rehabilitation.

Kasl & Cobb in 1966 gave the widely known definitions of three separate concepts:

Health behavior is any activity undertaken by a person believing himself to be healthy, for the purpose of preventing disease or detecting it in an asymptomatic state. Illness behavior is any activity undertaken by a person who feels ill, to define the state of his health and to discover a suitable remedy ... Sick-role behavior is the activity undertaken by those who consider themselves ill, for the purpose of getting well (Kasl & Cobb 1966 p. 246).

Common to the definitions was the relatively individualistic and static approach to a phenomenon which basically should be considered dynamic and holistic. There was no explicit statement whether these behavioural responses should be regarded as continuous or episodic/discrete. The definitions of illness behaviour and sick-role behaviour seem better suited to acute or episodic than to chronic illness, because of the lack of a temporal perspective.

The lack of a proper definition of the role of the chronically-ill is not just a problem in the literature of the behavioural sciences; it probably reflects the lack of such a well-defined and proper role in the society.

The role of the chronically-ill has been described in terms of the five characteristics of the at-risk role (Kasl 1974, Hickey 1980). According to this description, the chronically ill older person: 1. has no institutionalised position; 2. has only duties attached to his role, but no privileges; 3. has an indefinite time span; 4. lacks continuous reinforcement from health professionals and the social environment; and 5. lacks the feedback provided by changes in symptomatology and in

treatment procedures. The effect of these characteristics, indicating a total lack of social and
psychological acceptance, will most likely be that
"... the expected standard of behavior seems to be
that of health, in contrast to the acceptability of
an illness norm in a sick role context" (Hickey 1980
p. 95). When chronically-ill, one is not "allowed"
to complain over pain and discomfort in the social
context; health providers will probably not seriously try to help avoid discomfort, and even the
performance of self-care is not really "allowed."
This situation, of course, is not promotive of
self-care and health behaviour.

The recognition of the important role of the
social situation and the family in the rehabilitation and care of chronically-ill patients (Litman
1974) and the important role of the doctor (Haug,
this volume) suggest a need for a special initiative
from health providers and social networks to cope
with the situation of chronic illness in a constructive way.

In his textbook of medical sociology, Mechanic
(1968) introduced the holistic and dynamic aspects
of the concept of illness behaviour, but without
touching upon chronic illness. At the same time he
pointed out two different basic viewpoints regarding
illness behaviour which are of practical applica-
bility to health education:

> Such patterns of behavior may be seen as a
> product of social and cultural conditioning
> since they may be experienced and enacted
> naturally in the social contexts within which
> they appear relevant - one in which illness
> behavior may be seen as part of a coping
> repertory, as an attempt to make an unstable,
> challenging situation more manageable for the
> person who is encountering difficulty (p. 117).

This cultural context view suggests that health
behaviour and self-care should be understood as an
integral part of the elderly and older person's
natural environment by their providers of social and
medical services, and by groups of people with whom
they are familiar, focusing on perceived relevant
action. The coping-strategy view suggests that
health behaviour and self-care should be promoted in
these particular situations where coping is needed -
probably by individual counselling and support. Both
of these general strategies may well solve some of
the problems in establishing a proper role for the

chronically-ill.

A few scholars have subsequently developed the definitions of this area in harmony with the socialisation model of behaviour and integrated them into psychological and sociological frames of reference. For example, Hickey (1980) in his definition of health behaviour comes close to the concept of a dynamic coping-strategy:

> Health behaviour is an important manifestation of a person's psychological perspective. It reflects the individual's perception of his or her health status and the person's concerns about health; over time it reveals a pattern of views about health and some consistency in the ways the person deals with health problems (p. 92).

The concept of self-care first appeared in the professional literature in the early 1970s, and was presented by Levin, Katz & Holst (1976) as:

> ... a process whereby a lay person functions on his/her own behalf in health promotion and prevention and in disease detection and treatment at the level of the primary health resource in the health care system.

Several scholars developed definitions of self-care for research purposes in these years. Dean (1980) expanded the understanding of self-care by specifying several behavioural elements, including the aspects of professional consultation and the possible interaction between self-care and professional care. She included the following elements: preventive/health-maintaining activities, recognition of symptoms and signs of illness, the decision whether to do anything about it or not, seeking advice from friends and relatives, seeking medical or other professional advice, self-medication, and non-medical self-treatment.

Another example is Kane & Kane's concept of defensive health behaviour (Kane & Kane, this volume), introducing aspects of the decision process.

Other aspects of health related behaviours have been stressed by other scholars. For example, Fabrega (1973) proposed a definition pointing to a problem-solving/decision-making process. A different, but equally relevant research tradition is the research on coping with crisis or stress, including disease and disability. Coping refer to activities that an individual engages in that are intended to control the outcomes of events perceived as physically or psychologically threatening. Some coping behaviours are active and concentrate on changing the situation itself. Others are cognitive and focus on changing the meaning of the situation. And still others are designed to permit avoidance of the situation (Pearlin & Schooler 1977).

Coping, parallel to health-related behaviours, is often described in terms of a number of behavioural elements or in terms of differentiated behavioural patterns or strategies (Viney & Westbrook 1982, Menaghan 1982).

In accordance with our perception of health behaviour and self-care also the coping literature reflect the interactionistic and the context-related approach.

It has been suggested that adequate coping techniques can be promoted by training (Abrahams & al. 1979, Thompson & al. 1983) and several techniques are suggested: Self-regulation (Fisseni 1982), and active problem-orientation (Schmitz-Schertzer & al. 1983). Training of therapists and other supporters of the elderly may increase the coping-ability of the elderly (Thompson 1983, Wang & al. 1977).

Basic sociological variables such as social class, sex, and marital status are associated with coping ability although the nature of the association is less clear (Menaghan 1982). The docility-hypothesis, suggesting that less competent persons have less variety of coping abilities and lower threshold for stress, has been presented with some documentation (Morgan & al. 1984). Also, subjective assessment of having supportive social network, being in excellent or good health, not being lonely, and experiencing few signs of aging are associated with active or positive coping (Ward & al. 1984, McDonald & Suchy 1980, Dooghe, Vanderleyden & VanLoon 1980, Fisseni 1982).

A number of psychological factors have been suggested as powerful in the mechanism of coping. The concept "locus of control," developed from psychological theory, is one of the variables which shows the most consistent association with health related behaviours (Dean 1984). The usual behavioural science understanding of this term is the individual person's perception of whether or not she or he has control over reinforcement of activities. External control, then, refers to the perception of activities being the result of other more powerful people, pure luck, or destiny. Internal locus of control refers to the perception of being in control over activities oneself (Cicirelli 1980, Rotter 1966).

COMPONENTS OF A NEW PERSPECTIVE OF AGING AND HEALTH RELATED BEHAVIOUR

As we have discussed in this chapter the development of models and theories of aging and health-related behaviours is a difficult but important task for the future elderly policy. The components of such models must be in harmony with knowledge on both aging and self-care perspectives. The aging perspective should include the recognition of the aging process as a series of mixed predictable and unpredictable, continuous and discontinuous, desirable and un-desirable changes. At every point in the aging process behavioural procedures should be identified: 1. to stimulate and promote health and function, and 2. to react adequately, behaviourally as well as psychologically, to symptoms and incapacities.

The self-care perspective should include con-siderations on at least four dimensions regarding the content and context:

1. Who's involved? This can be described as a continuum from lay initiatives to professional determinations (DeFriese & Woomert 1983). An alternative description is a continuum from indi-vidualistic to collectivistic, including the phenom-enon of self-help groups and collective actions for health (Robinson 1980, Lieberman & al. 1976, Katz - this volume). Even the relation to social networks should be included.

This dimension should ideally specify the health responsibility of the old person, of her/his social network, and of the professional providers of health and social services. The interaction between the health system and the individual behaviour should likewise be specified, because this inter-action between self-care and health care is the main gateway for the health care professionals when improving old peoples' abilities to cope with health problems.

2. What's involved? Butler & al. (1979-80) describe three levels of self-care education and practice: acts performed as part of daily living; consciously

augmented health knowledge and awareness; assumption of tasks formerly the domain of the professional care giver. Each of these levels could be performed at different stages from healthy to ill or vice versa. They could be performed by the lay individual alone or in cooperation with the providers of care.

3. For what purpose? Several purposes could be defined, one by one or in combination. DeFriese & Woomert describe the possible purposes as a continuum from health promotion to management of chronic or post-surgical conditions. Any specific purpose, of course, requires its own specific action. Amann (1980) discusses the purpose from the need point of view, as whether the actions should serve as a substitution, a compensation, or a supplement to professional care.

4. In what context? There are considerable variations within and between communities regarding health beliefs, health policies, and availability of services. Therefore, it is imperative to specify the community context in which the promotion of health behaviour and self-care is to take place.

This list of dimensions pretends not to be complete. Several important dimensions are still lacking in a complete description of self-care: the roles of lay and professional; the outcomes and efficacy of the various forms of health related behaviour; cultural affinity; innovation. Each dimension affects the scope of available procedures for improving health behaviour and self-care in late life. Despite the lack of completeness the above-mentioned dimensions clearly indicate the complexity of this area of interest and the importance of conceptualising the phenomenon carefully prior to choice of strategy in health education and clinical practice, and prior to formulation of recommendations for practice and research.

REFERENCES

Abrahams, J.P., Wallach, H.F., and Divens, S. (1979) "Behavioral Improvements in Long-Term Geriatric Patients during an Age-Integrated Psychosocial Rehabilitation Program." J. Am. Geriatr. Soc. XXVII, pp. 218-21

Aeldrekommissionen (1980) Aldersforandringer - aeldrepolitikkens forudsaetninger (Age-Related Changes - the Basis of Elderly Policy). Copenhagen

Aeldrekommissionen (1981) De aeldres vilkaar (The Living Conditions of the Elderly). Copenhagen

Almind, G., Freer, C.B., Muir Gray, J.A., and Warshaw, G. (1983) The Contribution of the Primary Care Doctor to the Medical Care of the Elderly in the Community. Institute of Gerontology, University of Michigan, and Institute of Social Medicine, University of Copenhagen

Amann, A. (ed.) (1980) Open Care for the Elderly in Seven European Countries. Oxford: Pergamonn Press

Baric, L. (1980) "Formal Health Education and the Prevention of Coronary Heart Disease." In European Monographs in Health Education Research 1, Scottish Health Education Unit, Edinburgh, pp. 35-185

Barney, J.L. and Neukom, J.E. (1979) "Use of Arthritis Care by the Elderly." The Gerontologist. 19, pp. 548-54

Bloom, S.W. (1963) The Doctor and his Patient. New York: Russell Sage Foundation

Bloom, S.W., Speedling, E.J. (1981) "Strategies of Power and Dependence in Doctor-Patient Exchange." In: Haug M.R. (ed). Elderly Patients and Their Doctors. New York: Springer Publishing Company, pp. 157-70

Botwinick, J. (1977) "Intellectual Abilities." In: Birren J.E., Schaie K.W. (eds.). Handbook of the Psychology of Aging. New York: Van Nostrand Reinhold Company, pp. 580-605

Butler, R.N. and Gertman, J.S., Oberlander, D.L., Schindler, L. (1979-80) "Self-Care, Self-Help, and the Elderly." International Journal of Aging and Human Development, 10, pp. 95-117

Byrne, D.G. and White, H.M. (1979) "Severity of Illness and Illness Behaviour: A Comparative Study of Coronary Care Patients." J. Psychosomatic Research. 23, pp. 57-61

Chapman, C.R., Sola, A.E., and Bonica, J.J. (1979) "Illness Behavior and Depression Compared in Pain Center and Private Patients." Pain. 6, pp. 1-7

Cicirelli, V.G. (1980) "Relationship of Family Background to Locus of Control in the Elderly." J. Gerontology. 35, pp. 108-14

Coe, R.M. (1981) "The Sick Role Revisited." In: Haug M.R. (ed.) Elderly Patients and Their Doctors. New York: Springer Publishing Company, pp. 22-33

Cummings, E. and Henry, W.E. (1961) Growing Old. New York: Basic Books

Dean, K. (1980) Analysis of the Relationships Between Social and Demographic Factors and Self-Care Patterns in the Danish Population (Ph.D. Dissertation). University of Minnesota

Dean, K. and Holstein, B.E. (1983) "Sygdomsadfaerd blandt aeldre I: Beslutningen om at reagere på sygdomstegn" (Illness Behaviour among the Elderly, I: The Decision to React to Signs of Illness). Ugeskr. Laeger. 145, pp. 593-6

Dean, K. and Holstein, B.E. (1983) "Sygdomsadfaerd blandt aeldre II: Selvbehandling og soegning af hjaelp" (Illness Behaviour among the Elderly, II: Self-Treatment and Seeking Advice). Ugeskr. Laeger. 145, pp. 687-9

Dean, K. (1984) Influence of Health Beliefs on Lifestyles: What do we Know? European Monographs in Health Education Research. 6, pp. 127-51

DeFriese, G.H. and Woomert, A. (1981) "Recent Developments in Self-Care and the Elderly in the United States. "Presentation to the International Research Colloquium in Self-Care and the Elderly, Institute of Gerontology, University of Michigan, Ann Arbor

Dooghe, G., Vanderleyden, L., and VanLoon, F. (1980) "Social Adjustment of the Elderly Residing in Institutional Homes: A Multivariate Analysis." International Journal of Aging and Human Development. 11, pp. 163-76

Fabrega, H. (1973) "Toward a Model of Illness Behavior." Medical Care XI No. 6, pp. 470-84

Fisseni, H.-J. "Unterschiedliche Lebensraumstrukturen: unterschiedliche Alternsstile." (Different Ways of Living: Different Ages). Z. Gerontologie 1982, 15, 272-9

From-Hansen, P. (1982) "Kliniske aldersforandringer" (Clinical Age-related Changes). In: Magnussen G., Pallesen A.E., Viidik A. (eds.). Den normale aldring II. Biologi og fysiologi. Copenhagen: Arkiv for praktisk laegegerning, pp. 32-48

Gatherer, A. & al. (1979) Is Health Education Effective? London: The Health Education Council

Haug, M.R. (ed.) (1981) Elderly Patients and Their Doctors. New York: Springer Publishing Company

Haug, M.R., Belgrave, L.L., and Gratton, B. (1984) "Mental Health and the Elderly: Factors in Stability and Change Over Time." J. Health Soc. Behav. 25, pp. 100-115

Heikkinen, E. (1982) Den normale aldring. Hvad er normal aldring, og hvordan undersøges den?

(Normal Aging: What is it and how is it examined?) In: Magnussen G., Pallesen A.E., Viidik A. (eds.) Den normale aldring II, Biologi og fysiologi. Copenhagen: Arkiv for praktisk laegegerning, pp. 216-30

Hickey, T. (1980) Health and Aging. Monterey: Brooks/Cole Publishing Company

Kasl, S.V. and Cobb S. (1966) "Health Behavior, Illness Behavior and Sick-Role Behavior: I. Health and Illness Behavior." Arch. Environ. Health. 12, pp. 246-66

Kasl, S.V. (1974) The Health Belief Model and Behavior Related to Chronic Illness. Health Education Monographs. No. 2, pp. 433-54

Katz, A.H. and Bender, E.I. (1976) The Strength in Us: Self-Help Groups in the Modern World. New York: Franklin Watts

Kuypers, J.A., Bengtson, V.L. (1973) "Social Breakdown and Competence: A Model of Normal Aging." Human Development. 16, pp. 181-201

Levin, L.S., Katz, A.H., and Holst, E. (1976) Self-Care. Lay Initiatives in Health. New York: Prodist

Lieberman, M.A. and Borman, L.D. (1979) Self-Help Groups ·for Coping with Crisis. San Francisco: Jossey-Bass Publishers

Litman, T. (1974) "Health Care and the Family: a Behavioral Overview." Soc. Sci. Med. 8, p. 495

Maddox, G.L. (1981) "Assessing the Functional Status of Older Patients: Its Significance for Therapeutic Management." In: Haug M.R. (ed.) Elderly Patients and Their Doctors. op. cit. 55-69

McDonald, R.J. and Suchy, I. (1980) Der Einfluss subjektiver Beschwerden auf Leistung und Befindlichkeit im Alter. (The Influence of Subjective Pain on Efficiency and Condition According to Aging) Z. Gerontologie, 13, pp. 346-58

Mechanic, D. (1962) "The Concept of Illness Behavior." J. Chron. Dis. 15, pp. 189-194

Mechanic, D. (1968) Medical Sociology. A Selective View. New York: The Free Press

Menaghan, E. (1982) "Measuring Coping Effectiveness: A Panel Analysis of Marital Problems and Coping Efforts." J. Health Soc. Behav. 23, pp. 220-34

Morgan, T.J. & al. (1984) "Old Age and Environmental Docility: The Roles of Health, Support and Personality." J. Gerontology. 39, pp. 240-2

Mossey, J.M. and Shapiro, E. (1982) "Self-Rated Health: A Predictor of Mortality Among the Elderly." Am. J. Public Health. 72, pp. 800-8

Neugarten, B.L., Havighurst, R.J., and Tobin, S.S. (1968) "Personality and Patterns of Ageing." In: Neugarten B.L. (ed.) Middle Age and Ageing. Chicago: University of Chicago Press, pp. 173-77

Neugarten, B. (1977) "Personality and Aging." In: Birren J.E., Schaie K.W. (eds.) Handbook of the Psychology of Ageing. New York: Van Nostrand Reinhold Company, pp. 626-49

Parsons, T. (1951) The Social System. New York: The Free Press

Pearlin, L.I. and Schooler, C. (1978) "The Structure of Coping." J. Hlth. Soc. Behav. 19, pp. 2-21

Robinson, D. (1980) "The Self-Help Component of Primary Health Care." Soc. Sci. Med. 14 A, pp. 415-21

Rosenstock, I.M. (1966) "Why People Use Health Services." Millbank Memorial Fund Quarterly. 44 (2), pp. 94-127

Rotter, J.B. (1966) Generalized Expectancies for Internal versus External Control of Reinforcement. Psychological Monographs: General and Applied, 80 No. 1, pp. 1-28

Schaie, K.W. (1977) "Quasi-Experimental Research Designs in the Psychology of Aging." In: Birren J.E., Schaie K.W. (eds.) Handbook of the Psychology of Aging. New York: Van Nostrand Reinhold company, pp. 39-58

Schmitz-Schertzer, R., Zimmerman, E.J., and Rudinger, G. (1983) Krisen im Alter. Ein Versuch einer multivariaten Analyse von Bevältigungsstrategien in Krisen. (Crises of Aging. A Multivariate Test Analysis of Strategies for Coping in Crises). Z. Gerontologie. 16, pp. 115-20

Shanas, E. (1981) "The Viewpoint of a Gerontologist." In: Haug M.R. (ed.) Elderly Patients and Their Doctors. op. cit. pp. 37-41

Suchman, E.A. (1965) "Stages of Illness and Medical Care." J. Hlth. Hum. Behav. 6, pp. 114-28

Svanborg, A. & al. (1980) H 70. "Hälsoundersökning av 70-aaringer i Göteborg" (H 70: The Health Examination of 70-Year-Old People in Gothenburg). Läkartidningen. 77, pp. 3729-86

Svanborg, A., Bergstrom, G., and Mellström, D. (1982) Epidemiological Studies on Social and Medical Conditions of the Elderly. Copenhagen: WHO Regional Office for Europe

Szasz, T. and Hollender, M.H. (1956) "A Contribution to the Philosophy of Medicine: The Basic Models of the Doctor-Patient Relationship." Archives of Internal Medicine. 97, pp. 585-92

Thompson, L.W., Gallagher, D., Nies, G., and Epstein, D. (1983) "Evaluation of the Effectiveness of Professionals and Nonprofessionals as Instructors of Coping with Depression Classes for Elderly." The Gerontologist 23, pp. 390-6.

Viney, L.L. and Westbrook, M.T. (1983) "Coping with Chronic Illness: The Mediating Role of Biographic and Illness-Related Factors." Journal of Psycho-somatic Research. 26, pp. 585-605

Wan, T.H. and Odell, B.G. (1981) "Factors Affecting the Use of Social and Health Services among the Elderly." Aging and Society

Wang, V.L., Terry, P., Flynn, B.S., Williamson, J.W., Green, L.W., and Faden, R. (1977) "Evaluation of Continuing Medical Education for Chronic Obstructive Pulmonary Diseases." J. Med. Educ. 54, pp.803-11

Ward, R.A., Sherman, S.R., and LaGory, M. (1984) "Informal Networks and Knowledge of Services for Older Persons." J. Gerontology. 39, pp. 216-23

WHO (1984) The Uses of Epidemiology in the Study of the Elderly. Technical Report Series 706, Geneva

Williams, T.F. (1981) "The Physicians Viewpoint." In: Haug M.R. (ed.) Elderly Patients and Their Doctors op. cit., pp. 42-46

Chapter 4

SELF-CARE BEHAVIOUR: IMPLICATIONS FOR AGING

Kathryn Dean

INTRODUCTION

A basic assumption of most research, planning and
programme development related to health is that
professional services are the most important, even
an exclusive health care resource. This assumption
ignores lay resources, resulting in a failure to
develop and effectively use them. Self-care behaviour is one of the most important factors contributing to the maintenance of health, and to its
restoration after the onset of illness or disease
(Belloc 1972, Belloc and Breslow 1973, Dean 1981,
Levin and Idler 1983, USDHEW 1979). Therefore,
self-care is a major determinant of physical and
psychological well-being and functional capacity.
     The health related behaviour of individuals,
defined predominantly as use of professional services, has been studies in recent years as though it
were static, formed by factors which each contribute
a relative, but fixed proportion of causative
influence. Health beliefs -- especially generalised
beliefs such as the value of health, vulnerability
to illness, and benefit of treatment -- together
with an array of demographic and social variables
and variables representing the illness experience
have been examined extensively in an attempt to
explain the use of medical services using statistical regression techniques. The conclusion of analyses of this sort is that need, often measured as
seriousness of symptoms or disability days, accounts
for most of the variation in illness-related use of
medical services. The concept of need has not been
critically examined in these atheoretical discussions of behaviour. The interactions, chains of
influence, and hidden relationships among the
variables are ignored in most regression analyses of

58

this type. Additionally, the bulk of health-related behaviour remains unstudied when the use of professional services is the subject of research investigation.

Self-care is shaped by complex dynamic processes which cannot be understood by examining behaviour in static analytic models. Individual motivation and the stimulus quality of the environment represent two major areas of influence. It is important to identify the processes shaping the interactions of variables representing these areas of influence. A major research and policy issue in relation to the subject of self-care is the relative influence of individual motivation and environmental stimulus on the self-care behaviour of old people. This chapter will maintain that environmental factors, only one of which is direct environmental stimulus, are the major determinants of motivation for self-care. Individual motivation and environmental influences are not separate independent influences, but rather form a chain of causation. In this model, motivation does not mean simply the will or intention to practise health protective preventive or treatment behaviours. Motivation refers to the set of perceptions, beliefs and attitudes that affect behaviour by creating an understanding of what is possible, effective or appropriate.

This chapter will focus on components of self-care behaviour which generally have been neglected in research concerned with health and illness behaviour, and about which, therefore, little is known. Because the available data are extremely limited, the discussion will rely heavily on findings from Danish studies of self-care behaviour. Information regarding the methodology and characteristics of the samples for the two Danish self-care studies discussed in the chapter is included in the appendix. The reason for discussing self-care in this volume, is of course, to relate the subject to aging. The latter sections of the chapter will discuss the meaning of age differences in self-care behaviour and the implications of these differences for health in old age.

Empirical findings regarding components of self-care which have been studied more extensively, e.g. decisions to seek professional care and medication behaviour are examined in detail in subsequent chapters of the monograph and will be mentioned in this chapter only when pertinent to the discussion. Only the self-care behaviour of individuals will be considered. Other forms of lay behaviour e.g. are provided by family members, in extended social networks, in mutual aid groups, and in interactions with professional caregivers are also important health care resources. Some of these forms of lay care are considered in subsequent chapters.

INDIVIDUAL SELF-CARE BEHAVIOUR

Evidence of the importance of individual self-care behaviour in the maintenance of health and the control of chronic disease is accumulating (Belloc 1973, USDHEW 1979). Late life health and behaviour related to health are influenced by self-care over the life course. Increases in morbidity and mortality with age in population groups are generally due to chronic rather than acute conditions. The effects of behaviour and life-style begin to accumulate early in life, contributing to the onset and course of chronic conditions (Riley and Bond 1983). The number, severity, and progression of chronic diseases rather than biological aging may determine health in old age. Statistical evidence indicates that an improved state of health at all ages may continue to expand life and functional capacity (Manton 1982). The self-care behaviour of individuals over the life course, therefore, must be recognised as a basic factor shaping the health of individuals as they grow older and, in turn, general health and functional capacity within elderly populations.

Valid and reliable information regarding self-care behaviour and the factors which shape and maintain health-enhancing self-care should be a priority subject of health research. Yet little is known about either the range of self-care behaviour or the combination of factors and processes determining its development. Serious methodological and conceptual weakness limit the usefulness of the sparse information which is available.

Most information on the subject of self-care has been extracted from data collected for other purposes. As mentioned before, investigations of lay health and illness behaviour have generally defined these subjects in terms of utilisation of professional services. Even the few investigations focused directly on self-care have often conceptualised the subject narrowly, as the use of "home remedies" in the form of mechanical appliances and/or dietary, herbal, or chemical substances. Such limited concepts may exclude some of the most beneficial forms of self-care, e.g. stress containment behaviours or responses to illness directed toward perceived causes of symptoms. Study of the tendency to do nothing to preserve health or treat symptoms also is excluded by narrowly defining the subject in what might be characterised as lay versions of professional treatment models. Just as major components of self-care were excluded in studies of health and illness behaviour which focused on utilisation behaviour, those studies which now define self-care in terms of a dichotomy, i.e. self-care vs. professional care, cannot examine the continuum of care and the interacting processes which shape particular choices or behavioural combinations.

Serious methodological problems which limit the usefulness of the existing information for building a body of knowledge regarding self-care relate to sampling procedures and statistical models used in the analysis of the data. Many investigations have been conducted on convenience samples. Few investigators have collected data using random sampling procedures to obtain population samples of sufficient size for a valid analysis of the interactions among potentially important demographic, social, and psychological factors. Statistical regression models, sometimes inappropriate to the data to be analysed, often have dominated the data analysis. Complex interactions and chains of influence have generally been ignored in health research. Still, useful information, either direct or implicit, regarding self-care and aging has been obtained.

What is Self-care Behaviour ?

While individual self-care forms the basis for health maintenance and care in illness, patterns of self-care are learned and reinforced in family and extended networks. Whether or not health practices and treatment decisions are made and carried out by individuals alone, they are developed in the context of family socialisation and support. Self-care is thus a social phenomenon. It is shaped by complex sociocultural conditions and processes and, in turn, influences the social situation. For example, since self-care is the basic component of care obtained in families and extended social networks, in self-help groups, in alternative care and in professional medical treatments, it determines the point of entry into professional health care systems as well as compliance with professional directives (Dean 1983). The following definition includes the continuum of individual self-care behaviour undertaken to preserve or promote health and to restore health or well-being during episodes of illness:

> Self-care involves the range of activities individuals undertake to enhance health, prevent disease, evaluate symptoms and restore health. These activities are undertaken by lay people on their own behalf, either separately or in participation with professionals. Self-care includes decisions to do nothing, self-determined actions to promote health or treat illness, and decisions to seek advice in lay, professional and alternative care networks, as well as evaluation of and decisions regarding action based on that advice. (1)

Old People's Potential for Self-care

Most old people live at home and function well with continued capacity for effective self-care. While the incidence and prevalence of health complaints do increase with age, correlations between chronological age and functional capacity are small (WHO 1980, Neugarten 1982). Furthermore, problems of declining function or disability associated with old age may arise from a preventable loss of function. Until at least 75-80 years, age is a poor predictor of the health of individuals.

A summary of available data on the functional status of aging persons in developed countries was included in a status report prepared for the World Health Organization Preparatory Conference for the United Nations World Assembly on the Elderly (WHO 1980). The report noted that:

1. Only approximately 4-6 percent of persons over 65 years of age are institutionalised.
2. Of those living in the community 8-14 percent have been found to be bedfast or house-bound due to functional impairment.
3. A comparative study of mobility and the capacity for self-care among the elderly populations of Great Britain, the United States, and Denmark found that 53-64 percent of the aged had no impairment.
4. A United States study of social, economic, physical, and mental conditions and the

capacity for self care of persons over 65 years of age found that 60 percent had no functional impairment on any dimension, while 14-17 percent were significantly and multiply impaired.

The conclusion regarding functional capacity reached in the report was the presence of a high level of functional competence until at least age 80 in the elderly populations of the developed world.

A prospective longitudinal study of a 70-year-old Swedish cohort found that only three percent of the 70 year olds suffer from impairment or disease requiring institutionalisation (Svanborg 1977). The results of a battery of psychological tests of vocabulary ability, logical reasoning, sensory-motor speed and coordination, immediate memory ability and memory of figures did not indicate any significant reduction in cognitive function among 70 year olds with the exception of reduction in sensory-motor speed. Furthermore, the capacity for increase in intellectual function remains until advanced old age (Baltes and Willis 1979). Thus, it is possible for psychological expansion to parallel physiological decline in old age. Attempts are now being made to allow for expansion of function as well as decline in definitions of aging. A definition of aging which recognises the positive potential of effective self-care at any age and appropriate for our consideration of the subject is:

Aging refers to the regular changes that occur in mature, genetically representative organisms living under representative environmental con- ditions as they advance in chronological age (Birren and Renner 1980).

The Problem of Maintaining Fitness while Growing Older

Unfortunately, dominant social forces militate against rather than enhance, self-health maintenance in old people. As documented repeatedly throughout this monograph, cultural stereotypes, professional providers of care, the content and organisation of health and social services and even the literature on aging encourages a negative cycle of reduced functioning among the elderly.

The scientific literature and the health systems of advanced industrial societies reflect a scientific technological treatment model which apparently has a more pervasive influence on the delivery of health care services to elderly people than differences in cultural concepts of health and disease and the wide variations in the organisation and delivery of services. The theoretical constructions of various disciplines combined with the still-dominant biological determinism in concepts of aging are major forces promoting and reinforcing a pathological model of old age. Professionals as well as the general public continue to adhere to the stereotypical notion of aging as inevitable biological decline (Riley 1983).

Professional constructs such as "disengagement" theory and "dependency ratios" create expectations about growing old which are projected onto and internalised by aging individuals. The non-productivity implied in the concept of dependency ratios suggests that the non-productivity is explained by individual incapacity rather than societal forces (WHO 1980, p.3).

Illsley alluded to this development in noting the similar trends of language, problem statements, and conclusions running through the presentations of a 1983 Oxford symposium on self-care and aging (2). Even with the intention of challenging the stereotypes of the pathological model of aging described by Johnson (Chapter 2) and armed with the data to do so, our professional concepts, jargon, and styles create the danger of only shifting the description and emphasis, while maintaining the image of a universal old person.

Increases in the frequency of illness and disability with age in populations, hide variations within which individual difference is the important factor (Neugarten 1982). Part of the problem arises from the specialised attention focused on the mortality, morbidity, and medical care needs of old people. With the commendable purpose of developing appropriate policies and services for the elderly, study of old people or of age differences in health and behaviour have had serious unintended consequences for our understanding of aging and the health care needs of old people. Kasl and Berkman have described the problem as follows:

> The fundamental problem is that we create a presumption of uniqueness - that the processes under observation are special to the targeted population subgroup - and we collect evidence that grows and accumulates in spendid isolation from similar data on the rest of the popu-

lation. Such intellectual and conceptual isolation at best leads to duplication of effort;
at worst, it leads to misinterpretation of data
and to adoption of distorted or misleading
theoretical positions (Kasl and Berkman 1977,
p.346).

It is now recognised that many of the mistaken
conclusions regarding biological aging processes
arise from interpretations and conclusions drawn
from analyses of cross-sectional data (Riley 1983).
Age differences in health status and functional
capacity found in cross-sectional data can only
suggest hypotheses regarding underlying causal
factors and processes. Rapidly expanding bodies of
literature in several health fields show that
biological changes as well as physical and psychological illnesses which may be more frequently seen
among older people are related to complex behavioural, psychological and social processes (Kasl and
Berkman 1981, Riley and Bond 1983, USDHEW 1977).

The functional capacity of old people is
consistently underestimated. When function is reduced, the stimulus provided by the environment may
be a limiting factor (WHO 1981). Deprived environ-
ments have negative effects on both motivation and
individual fitness. The deleterious effects which
result are easily confused with the process of
aging, and like negative stereotypes may be internalised by older people, creating negative self-
images and reduced expectations regarding functional
capacity and life satisfaction.

Self-reported decline in memory and energy
reduction among older people have been related to
the internalisation of cultural stereotypes (Fiske
1980). Older age also has been associated with
beliefs that good health is a matter of fate or
chance (Cicerelli 1980, Dean 1984) and with strong
beliefs in the capacity of medical science to
protect health (Dean 1984). Twenty-three percent of
a random sample of the adult population from two
geographic areas of Denmark (cf. Appendix, Study B)
had high scores on the scale of faith in medical
care to protect health; 54 percent of persons in
their seventies fell in the high score category on
this measure compared to only six percent of persons
in their twenties. Thus a vast difference existed in
the beliefs of old and young people regarding the
role of medical care in protecting health in this
sample.

In a three generation U.S. study of the family

as the basic unit of health care, the members of the senior generation were most likely to have thought about their health during the prior year. The senior generation, however, reported fewer health check-ups and manifested a serious lack of knowledge regarding health matters and home health care. While a majority of the younger generations thought ill family members had a right to be cared for at home, members of the oldest generation felt uncertain and a majority thought they would relinquish such responsibility to a hospital (Litman 1971).

Evidence that old people tend to accept negative stereotypes of aging was found in a review of research findings conducted by Riley and Foner (1968). They found that old people tended to accept disabilities as inevitable and irreversible, seeking palliative rather than preventive or corrective treatment (Riley and Bond 1983). A tendency for older people more often to choose palliative self-care responses rather than behaviours directed toward the cause of symptoms also was found in a Danish investigation of self-care responses to commonly experienced symptoms (cf. Appendix, Study A). For example, older persons, more often took medicines and/or used a heating pad to treat lumbar pain, while younger persons more frequently reported responses which might be characterised as secondary prevention such as exercise and the avoidance of stooping movements. The relationship between age and self-care response was most striking in relation to depression. There was a sharp rise with age in the proportions of persons who consulted physicians and took medicines for depression. Younger people, in contrast, more often discussed underlying problems with someone in their personal network or changed their activities rather than taking medicines or contacting physicians when depressed (Dean, Holst, and Wagner 1983).

Methods of coping with problems of everyday living, tension, and stress-producing life situations may be an important determinant of self-care behaviour. The above findings along with findings in the coping literature led to an exploration of stress reduction behaviour in a subsequent Danish self-care investigation (cf. Appendix, Study B). Consistent with findings mentioned above, the data suggests that many old people may have less active and preventive coping styles (Dean, unpublished data). Furthermore, the data suggests that habits of responding to tension and stress are related to both morbidity experience and self-care responses to episodes of illness.

A passive and pessimistic approach toward old age may inhibit or preclude active problem solving and efforts to achieve more satisfying situations. An active approach to creating environmental opportunity and/or reducing stress, many range from behaviour to expand functional capacity and seek social interaction to obtaining help in situations of neglect or abuse of basic rights and needs.

Information is also an important variable shaping self-care behaviour. Awareness of the existence and functions of agencies providing coping and development services was the dominant factor explaining their use in a Canadian investigation, while self-rated health, chronic conditions, and functional health were relatively unimportant. At the same time, however, older people were less aware of the service options available to them (Snider 1980).

There is evidence that when the importance of a behaviour is known, expecially if it has particular relevance, old people practise effective self-health maintenance. For example, the elderly are more likely to participate in blood pressure screening. Furthermore, old people are more likely to be in treatment for detected high blood pressure than younger people, and their likelihood of having blood pressure controlled when in treatment is greater. Thus old people are generally more successful at having high blood pressure detected and controlled (Kasl and Berkmann 1977).

In summary, while we know very little about health-enhancing behaviour, aging individuals face considerable obstacles unrelated to biological aging which may affect their self-health maintenance. These obstacles are often manifest as reduced motivation to remain fit. The level of motivation arises from beliefs, perceptions and expectations regarding the possible and by opportunities for action, both of which are shaped by the cultural and social structural factors that form their environment.

Self-care Behaviour in Illness

Little is known with certainty about the content and determinants of self-care responses to illness. With the growing recognition of the scope and importance of self-care, the focus of research has shifted somewhat. The spectrum of self-care in illness, analytic studies of alternative types of behavioural

67

responses to illness as well as the role of families
and other networks in health care have recently
become subjects of research investigations. At this
time, however, most of the available information
regarding individual behaviour in illness must be
obtained from studies of medication behaviour and
the use of professional services. Both subjects are
discussed at length in subsequent chapters and will
be mentioned in this chapter only when relevant to
the discussion of other topics. Two components of
self-care, decisions to do nothing about symptoms of
illness and non-medication self-treatment, have been
almost totally neglected in studies of lay behaviour
during illness.

Decisions to do nothing

Findings regarding the tendency to do nothing about
symptoms are rarely reported. Only occasionally have
investigators recognised that doing nothing about
symptoms or "letting nature take its course" are
self-care responses (Alpert & al. 1967, Dean 1981,
Haug and Lavin 1982, p. 3). Generally, this subject
has been discussed in relation to illness behaviour
with either a direct or implied criticism of people
who "delay" in seeking medical care. The subject has
seldom been included in empirical analyses of the
continuum of care in illness. Consequently, virtually no information is available regarding situations
where evaluation of symptoms by lay people result in
decisions that the best response is no treatment.
The course of illness in such situations has not
been investigated.

Self-care responses to common illness conditions have been studied in both Denmark and the
United States. Data were collected from a random
sample of the adult Danish population (cf. Appendix,
Study A) in order to study behavioural reactions to
six common illness conditions: "colds," lumbar pain,
skin rash, depression, influenza and chest pain. The
proportions of persons who took no action to care
for the six conditions ranged from seven percent who
did nothing to treat influenza to 29 percent who did
nothing about chest pain (Dean, Holst, and Wagner
1983).

When the six conditions were considered together in statistical analyses of alternative forms
of self-care responses, age differences in the
tendency to do nothing about symptoms did not
emerge. However, this was due to the fact that
combining different types of illness episodes masked

age differences in behaviour. Younger persons significantly more often did nothing about skin rash and chest pain, while a significantly larger proportion of older people reported no response to depression. This suggests that failure to control for the type of illness episode may distort or suppress findings regarding age differences in behavioural responses to certain illnesses.

Two variables exerted significant independent influence on the tendency to do nothing about common illness conditions. A variable strongly related to doing nothing about symptoms was reliance on doctors for counsel of non-medical problems. That is, persons who reported that they do not discuss their personal problems with their doctors more often did nothing to treat common symptoms.

Perceived health status was the second variable included in the investigation which exerted independent influence on the tendency to do nothing about common conditions. The influence of perceived health status on this response, however, was found only for women. Women who reported excellent or good health more often did nothing about the six conditions than those who characterised their health as fair or poor. Perceived health status was not a significant factor in the no action responses of men.

There were indirect influences of age on this form of response to common illness which point to be importance of underlying factors in the social situation. Older people were overrepresented in three groups who more often discussed their personal problems with their doctors. People living on disability or retirement pensions, persons who perceived themselves to be in poor health, and women more often discussed non-medical problems with their doctors. The combination of the three factors created a strong predictor. Said another way, older women living on pensions who characterised their health as relatively poor most often discussed their personal problems with their doctors. The latter variable thus represents a combination of factors which influenced whether or not common symptoms were treated.

Apparently women living on pensions who consider themselves to be in poor health either have more non-medical problems or fewer social resources on which to rely for support, which influences whether or not common problems are treated and, more specifically, which leads them to consult their doctors regarding these common problems about which many people do nothing and most people do not contact doctors. The use of medicines for these common symptoms also was independently related to the tendency to discuss non-medical problems with physicians, suggesting that this pattern of consulting doctors leads to greater use of medicine.

These relationships were explored in greater depth in a subsequent Danish study of self-care responses to illness (cf. Appendix, study B). In an investigation of behavioural reactions to all symptoms reported for a six-month period in Denmark, 37 percent of the conditions were found not to have been treated in any way. Neither the type of symptoms nor perceived health status were related to the tendency to do nothing about episodes of illness. The finding that persons who do not discuss personal problems with physicians more often do nothing about symptoms was replicated in this study, as were the relationships between discussing personal problems with the doctor and both physician consultation and use of medicines to treat illness.

As in the prior Danish investigation of self-care responses to common symptoms, the illness episodes of people who do not discuss their non-medical problems with physicians were less often treated, while those of persons who said they do seek support for non-medical problems from physicians more often decided to consult the doctor and took medicines when ill. These relationships were independent of the type of symptoms or the perceived seriousness of the illness episode. An exploration of the possibility that social network and/or social support variables may be involved in these relationships, revealed that persons who discuss non-medical problems with doctors did more often report insufficient or non-supportive social relationships.

Another variable which represents options for care and support in the personal life situation exerted independent influence on decisions to take no action in response to illness. Forty-two percent of the illness episodes reported by persons with no one to assume their usual responsibilities when they are ill were not treated, while this was the case for only 29 percent of the illnesses reported by persons who had someone in their personal social network who would take over their responsibilities when they were ill.

However, the perceived seriousness of the individual illness episodes, a variable representing the personal experience of illness, exerted the greatest influence on whether or not treatment resulted. There was also an independent gender effect of the tendency to do nothing about illness. A larger proportion of the illness episodes reported by men were not treated than was the case for women. A final variable which had an important influence on whether or not illness episodes were treated was the stress reduction behaviour reported by the respondents.

The tendency to do nothing about illness episodes varied considerably according to people's usual habits of coping with stress. More than one response was sometimes given to the question used to obtain information on this variable. Each respondent, however, was asked to indicate their most usual and frequent behavioural reaction to feeling stressed. The findings are based on typical behavioural reactions to stress. Those respondents who reported that they spend more time working or deliberately try to forget the problems underlying their feelings of stress along with those who said they discuss the problems underlying their stress with someone in their personal social network more often did nothing to treat illness. Likewise, those respondents who said they drink alcohol or practice some particular relaxing behaviour (e.g. reading, working in the garden, etc.) when stressed, proportionality more often said they did nothing about their symptom episodes. On the other hand, those persons who said they respond to stress by taking medicine, seeing their doctor or resting considerably more often treated their illnesses and/or sought treatment from professional caregivers. Furthermore, the effect of this variable is yet more extensive. Indirect effect of habits of stress reduction on the tendency to do nothing about symptoms were found in a relationship between stress reduction behaviour and perceptions regarding the seriousness of the illness episodes.

A different approach to examining reliance on physicians was used in a U.S. investigation (Lavin and Haug 1981). Attitudes toward patients rights and the challenge of physician authority were variables used to study reliance in an analysis conducted on data collected from a U.S. sample to study utilisation behaviour (nationwide sample of 1,509 non-institutionalised adults, 18 years of age or older). In a secondary analysis of the data, the dependent variable was defined as "self-care behaviour indexed by reported failure to contact a physician for certain common physical symptoms." While it is not possible to determine the proportion of illness episodes which were not treated at all, of relevance here was the finding that the most effective predictor of the tendency toward professional consultation was the level of dependence on physicians.

A subsequent analysis of the U.S. data found age differences in the influence of dependent attitudes toward physicians on consultation behaviour. Among people over 60 years of age, a lower level of behavioural challenge to physician authority was an important variable related to the tendency to consult physicians for non-serious common illnesses, while this variable did not play an important role in the consultation behaviour of the group of people under 60 years of age (Haug and Lavin 1983).

The tendency not to seek medical help for "serious common conditions" (defined as serious or not by a panel of physicians) was related to stronger belief in the patient's right to decision-making among persons both under and over the age of 60. This belief variable exerted more influence in the younger group, however. Similarly, while less belief in physician's authority was related to decisions among younger people not to consult doctors when ill, it was not a significant factor in the decisions of the group over 60 years of age.

Generally, younger more knowledgeable people were more skeptical of the efficacy of medicine, and the state of health did not affect these findings. Challenging physician behaviour, however, did not necessarily correspond with challenging attitudes. Past experience of medical error, health condition, and low belief in physician competence were the best predictors of behavioural challenges to physician authority (Haug and Lavin 1983).

The U.S. findings that older people more often believed that physicians should determine care decisions (see also Haug in this volume) is consistent with the greater faith in medical care among older people found in the Danish population. In both instances, greater reliance on medical care was related to physician consultation regardless of the nature of the illness episode.

Three groups of older people were studied in another U.S. investigation of responses to commonly experienced symptoms (Brody & al. 1983). The findings reported here are based on samples of people with normal mental functioning (N=51) and histories of diagnosed functional mental disturbances (N=46). The data collected in interviews indicated that nothing was done about 20 percent of frequently experienced symptoms reported by the sample members for four 24-hour periods. Although it is not possible to tell from this study the proportion of total symptoms for which no action was taken, the 20 percent is undoubtedly an understatement for two reasons. Firstly, only frequently experienced symptoms were examined in the analyses of the self-care responses. Secondly, symptoms which had been reported in a baseline interview using a 20-symptom checklist were found often not to have been reported in the 24-hour logs which obtained information about remedial actions. The unreported symptoms included shortness of breach, swelling of feet and ankles, leg cramps, frequent coughing, and forgetfulness. The fact that these commonly experienced symptoms were not reported in the logs suggests that they may be taken for granted rather than being recognised and treated as illness. Also possible is that self-treatment of these chronic conditions has been integrated into daily routines to such an extent that it is no longer spontaneously identified as symptom response.

The finding that nothing is done about many chronically experienced symptoms was also reported in a Scottish investigation (Bell & al. 1977). The results of these studies are consistent with those of the Danish investigations discussed earlier which found that the tendency to do nothing about symptoms was not limited only to acute and rapidly passing conditions. This may also be the case for medically-defined serious symptoms. In the U.S. study conducted by Lavin and Haug (1981), 55 percent of the sample members failed to contact a doctor for symptom episodes for which a panel of physicians considered a medical contact appropriate. This proportion, while diverging from the 69 percent not consulting for symptom episodes which the physician panel characterised as not serious enough for a medical contact, is far from the behaviour judged as appropriate by the medical panel. It is apparent that physicians and lay people often have different assessments of the appropriateness or necessity of medical contacts for illness.

It can readily be seen that the tendency to do nothing about symptoms is a complex behavioural response shaped by variables representing personal perceptions and aspects of the social situation. It is noteworthy that although certain types of symptoms may receive selective attention in specific age groups, e.g. skin conditions among younger people, no direct age differences independent of factors in the social situation were found in the tendency to treat illness episodes.

Non-medication Self-treatment

The use of medication is widely recognised as a dominant form of behavioural response to illness (Anderson 1975, Dean 1981, Dunnell and Cartwright 1972). Yet for all forms of self-medication there are other forms of behaviour which produce the same results (McEwen 1975). Non-medication self-treatments include alterations in diet, exercise, fresh air, relaxation techniques, and many other individualised forms of self-care. Some form of non-medication self-treatment probably is involved in the vast majority of self-care during illness. Research neglect rather than the infrequency of non-medical self-treatment accounts for our limited knowledge on this subject.

In Denmark, one or more non-medication self-treatment was reported for 76 percent of 3,100 common illness episodes (cf. Appendix, Study A). Over 80 percent of the persons with "colds" or influenza either increased their vitamin or fluid intake, dressed in warmer clothes, remained in bed, stayed at home, maintained normal routines with increased rest, or practised their own specific self-treatment. Eighty-three percent of persons reporting lumbar pain practised avoidance behaviours, some form of exercise, obtained massage, used a heating pad and/or obtained more rest. The most frequent non-medication responses to depression were discussing the underlying problems with someone in the personal network and, paradoxically, attempting to forget the underlying problems. Self-treatment of chest pain most often involved reductions in: 1. the pace of activities, 2. smoking and/or 3. the consumption of coffee or tea. Additional responses to chest pain included finding new ways to relax and exercise. Skin rash was the condition for which the self-treatment responses, frequently involving baths or salves, were least often non-medication treatments (Dean & al. 1983).

The U.S. investigation of responses to commonly experienced symptoms in groups of older people (Brody & al. 1983) revealed that frequently reported treatments for pain and digestive problems included the application of heat or cold, positioning of the affected body part, rest, sleep, and decreased activity. For other types of symptoms, increased social or leisure activity, dietary treatment, decreased activity, rest and problem-solving were more frequent responses to symptoms.

As mentioned above, limiting the concept of self-care to mechanical, chemical or dietary treatments may exclude some of its most beneficial forms (Dean, forthcoming). For example, rest and interrupting the normal routine when ill may be an especially beneficial form of self-care. A prospective U.S. study of 6,928 adults showed a pattern of greater mortality among persons with no disability days in comparison to those who reported one to three sick days during the year (Berkmann 1975). The greater mortality of persons with no sick days was independent of age, sex, "objective," and subjective health status and health habits.

Another form of potentially important non-medication self-treatment may involve forms of social interaction. A category of social activities accounted for 53 percent of "non-medical" responses recorded in a diary study of self-care conducted in Canada (Freer 1980). Findings from investigations of self-care responses to illness in Denmark suggest that behavioural responses to illness may involve complex patterns of social contact and social support. For example, the tendency to discuss non-medical problems with physicians is positively related to professional consultation and use of medicine for illness episodes and negatively related to decisions not to treat symptoms. These findings suggest that an absence of social support in the life situation may lead some people to seek professional help and use medicine for illness episodes that otherwise are not treated or that are cared for by non-medication self-treatment.

With the exception of a small negative correlation between age and bed-rest, no direct statistically significant age differences were found in non-medication self-treatment in the Danish investigation of self-care responses to all illness episodes reported for a six-month retrospective time period (cf. Appendix, study B). Most of the variance in illness responses was accounted for by the type of symptoms and the perceived seriousness of the illness episodes. Important exceptions were the influence of 1. the tendency to discuss non-medical problems with physicians on professional consultation and the use of prescription medication and 2. variables which represent stressful life situations on the tendency to remain in bed when ill.

People who discuss non-medical problems with

physicians not only contacted their doctors more often for episodes of illness, but took more prescription medicines than people who do not seek support from doctors for non-medical problems. This finding was not dependent on the type of symptoms experienced or the perceived seriousness of the illness episode. That is to say, for various types of acute and chronic illness conditions and whether or not the illness episodes for which consultation took place were considered serious, persons who said that they discuss their personal problems with physicians took more prescription medicines.

The second major exception to the influence on self-care responses of variables other than ones representing the illness experience is the impact of stressful situations. Both stressful life problems and reported difficulty in handling the daily routine were related to remaining in bed when ill. The greater tendency to remain in bed with illnesses occurring during stressful periods was independent of the type of symptoms and of the perceived seriousness of the illness episode. It should be noted that the effects of the stress variables were specific to remaining in bed rather than to remaining at home. Stressful situations apparently increase the discomfort of all types of illnesses, causing them to be more debilitating.

THE EFFECTS OF AGE ON SELF-CARE

Does aging influence self-care? This has been the assumption, implicit if not explicit, in many discussions of age differences in health and illness behaviour. Yet, evidence indicates that this is not the case as Austin and Loeb (1982) point out, the impression that old people in the United States as a group use health care services more than younger people is created by averaging the high health care costs of those most sick and disabled across the entire aged population. In this monograph, Ford presents evidence that, rather than increasing with age, individual patterns of contacting doctors are relatively stable over time. Evidence indicates that the use of non-prescription medication is not related to age (Dean 1981, Dunnell and Cartwright 1972). In subsequent chapters, Anderson and Cartwright with British data and Eve with U.S. data document the polypharmacy that readily accounts for age differences in the use of prescription medications. No independent age differences were found in the tendency not to treat common illnesses in Denmark. However, evidence of age differences is found in the tendency to choose palliative treatment responses rather than care directed toward possible causes of symptoms (Riley and Foner 1968, Dean & al. 1983). · Age was one of the major explanatory variables in use of medications and professional consultation for six commonly experienced illness conditions in an exploratory study of self-care behaviour in the adult Danish population. Specifically, a complex interaction between older age and female gender, along with perceived health status, discussion of non-medical problems with physicians, and employment status predicted the use of medication and professional consultation for the common symptoms of illness.

The investigation in Denmark of behavioural responses to all types of illness episodes found that age was not independently related to decisions to do nothing about symptoms or non-medication self-treatments. Nor were age differences found in the use of non-prescription medicines to treat the illness episodes. Professional consultation and the use of prescription medicine for episodes of illness occurred somewhat more frequently among older people, although the bivariate correlations were not large (gamma=.14, p=.000 and gamma=15, p=.000 for professional consultation and use of prescription medicine respectively).

The variable which was the important immediate determinant of the self-care responses to illness and, therefore, accounted for most of the statistical variance was the perceived seriousness of the illness episodes. Perceptions of the seriousness of illness episodes were related to doing nothing about illness ($\gamma = .34$, p=.000), remaining at home (γ=.35, p=.000), bed-rest (γ=.34, p=.000), use of prescription medicine (γ=.38, p=.000), and professional consultation (γ=60, p=.000). It is not surprising that variables representing the experience of illness explain illness behaviour. The important research task is to identify and understand the variables shaping the experience of illness. This problem is neglected in most studies of utilisation of professional services where variables representing the illness experience are analysed as parallel to social and psychological variables. Since they account for most of the variance in utilisation in regression procedures, social situational and attitudinal variables are often discounted as relatively unimportant (Mechanic 1978). The type of symptoms may be largely independent of factors in the social environment, but perceptions of the seriousness of the symptoms are shaped by social and psychological variables. Thus, variation due to social factors is already included in measures of the seriousness of reported symptoms (Mechanic 1978, Dean -- unpublished data).

This chapter cannot fully discuss the findings of all investigations of self-care behaviour in Denmark. Briefly, however, the conclusions may be drawn that episodes of illness, regardles of the type of symptoms, are not simple biological occurrences. Illness and reactions it elicits are shaped by complex interactions among social situational and attitudinal variables. Episodes of illness which were experienced as serious were reported more often by persons who:

1. were divorced or widowed;
2. considered themselves in relatively poor health;
3. responded to feeling stressed by taking medicine or trying to forget their problems;
4. were older;
5. expressed strong faith in the capacity of medical science to preserve or restore health;
6. expressed strong faith in the benefit of pharmaceuticals.

The effects of age, operating through perceptions of illness, apparently exerted less influence on self-care responses than marital status, perceived health status, and the ways people cope with stress. This impression is not entirely correct, however, for while aging itself does not cause these differences, the causal factors are themselves directly associated with age. That is, age exerted both small direct and considerable indirect effects on perceptions regarding the seriousness of illness episodes. Factors which have little or nothing to do with chronological age per se, but arise from the social structural, cultural, or personal life situation shape self-care through the experience of illness. The influence of age in the behavioural model of self-care in illness arising from the findings can be expressed as the following chain of influence:

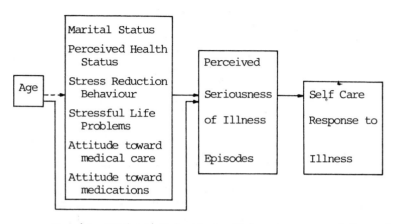

It is emphasised that this is a model and, thus, is simplified, a model for testing in subsequent investigations. Absent are the complex interactions and feedback loops involved in the process of change over time.

SELF-CARE AND AGING

Considerable challenge has been directed in recent years towards concepts of aging which posit relationships of inevitable decline and pathology with advancing age (Baltes and Willis 1977, Kasl and Berkman 1981, Manton 1982, McCrae 1982, Neugarten 1982, Riley 1976, Riley and Bond 1983). Neugarten (1984) has emphasised that a priori assumptions cannot be made about the health, capacity, or circumstances of old people. She considers the tendency to create a social category of age not only as useless, but also as detrimental to old people. The findings presented in this chapter are consistent with these conclusions. Although factors directly related to self-care behaviour are more often found in the older age groups, age itself exerts little direct influence. Furthermore, the factors associated with age vary among older people as well as across age groups.

Nevertheless, age differences do exist in illness and -- perhaps principally via the way illness is experienced -- in self-care responses to illness. Research findings suggest both cohort effects and effects of growing old in advanced technological societies. Riley (1976) points out the meaninglessness of using age categories per se as an analytic variable.

> In itself, age is a continuous measure; when the population of a country is arranged by chronological age, from newly born infants to the oldest people alive, age is a continuum. Hence, partitions of the population by age acquire meaning as age strata only as they index socially significant aspects of people and roles. (p. 191)

Cohort effects may be responsible for the age differences in attitudes toward medical care and medications as well as differences in stress reduction behaviour. Persons born around the turn of the century received their primary education and socialisation during the period of rapid advances in biological sciences and medicine. Expert medical opinion was not questioned. Younger people were educated during a period of growing recognition of the limits of medicine and the importance of social factors and individual behaviour for health.

The stereotypes and concepts of health and aging which developed during the past century permeated the cultural systems and institutions of the developed world. When concepts of aging lead people to expect decline and limit their sense of influence over their own health, a consequence may be passive and palliative health maintenance and treatment approaches. The likelihood of health enhancing daily routines may be reduced.

Great faith in medical care couples with a passive and pessimistic approach to health may preclude the type of interactions and exchange of information with professional caregivers which optimises the benefits of treatment regimes.

The implications of passive and palliative self-care behaviour for health and functional capacity in old age are many. Among the more relevant findings from the Danish self-care research in regard to self-care and aging are the inter-actions among age, habits of stress reduction and self-care responses to illness. Persons who respond-ed to feeling stressed by taking medicine or trying to forget problems more often characterised their illness episodes as serious, while those who said they respond to stress by discussing the problems underlying their stress with someone in their personal network reported fewer serious illness episodes. At the same time, proportionately fewer persons in the older age groups reported social responses to feeling stressed. Older people more often said they took medicine or contacted the doctor when stressed. If habits of coping with stress do affect the morbidity experience then there may be considerable long term health implications. The dangerous drug interactions which may result from frequent use of medications for both symptoms of illness and feelings of stress can have serious health consequences for old people. In addition to the possibility of direct negative effects on health and/or accidents which may be caused by drug reactions, passive and palliative responses to symptoms substitute for self-care approaches which can enhance fitness over time and contribute to secondary prevention of disability.

Whether or not internalised stereotypes regarding aging and passive/palliative attitudes toward health are cohort effects, they are shaped by the health, educational and cultural institutions of society. They are learned in formal education and from images in the popular media. They are reinforced in professional consultations, in family relationships, and in occupational settings. Thus, concepts and stereotypes of aging are a major aspect of the stimulus quality of the environment.

The life situations of many older people are apparently mirrored in the Danish findings regarding marital status and perceived health status. The findings regarding marital status more than suggest sadness and loneliness at the loss of a mate, divorced and widowed people more often had lower incomes, lived alone, were members of lower social class groups, and had less contact with friends. Similarly, persons who characterised their health as only fair or poor more often had difficulty getting through the daily routine and were more often members of the lower social class groups.

Thus, these factors directly or indirectly affect how illness is experienced and the response behaviours which result. Some of these factors arise from loss or change which occur more frequently because of advancing age, but others derive solely from social conditions which increase the problems and stress in the life situations of old people.

Important policy relevant research questions regarding health and aging relate to the effects of self-care on the incidence, severity, and progression of chronic disease and functional capacity. At the same time we must learn more about the factors and processes which shape self-care behaviour. Meanwhile, there are important policy and programme relevant implications in what is already known. Concepts and stereotypes of aging which negatively affect old people's perceptions of their potential as well as their opportunities for promoting their health can only be changed by broad-based public and professional educational efforts. Textbooks and other educational materials need to be examined and, when appropriate, changed. Removing errors is probably not sufficient to address the problem of long-term socialisation in expectation of automatic decline and disability with age. Countervailing concepts and images must be systematically introduced in all areas of education and the public media.

Health and social programmes must recognise that the social contact and support are important aspects of health maintenance. Persons coping with loss have greater support needs. The range and interface of health and social services available can significantly enhance the health maintenance and illness related self-care of old people.

NOTES

(1) This definition is based on an earlier one developed for a discussion of lay care in illness for a special issue of Social Science and Medicine (Dean, forthcoming) and in the work of Levin and Idler (1981, 1983) as well as a definition developed in a WHO working conference on Health Education and Self-Care, Geneva, 21-25 November, 1983. (WHO 1984A).

(2) Raymond Illsley chaired the 1983 international meeting referred to in Chapter 1.

Appendix

OVERVIEW OF THE RESEARCH METHODS USED TO STUDY SELF-CARE BEHAVIOUR IN DENMARK

Social survey methods have been used to study self-care behaviour in the Danish population. The two investigations mentioned in this chapter were concerned only with behavioural reactions to illness. Health maintenance components of self-care were not included in these studies.

STUDY A

A national survey was conducted to obtain baseline data to describe self-care responses to illness and to study a range of variables that might influence the behavioural reactions. A sample of common health problems was selected for the collection of symptom response data by means of a self-administered, mail questionnaire (Dean & al. 1983). Criteria used for selecting the study conditions were incidence in the general population, conditions common to the entire study population, symptoms that although commonly experienced are debilitating to an extent that the study of alternative responses is meaningful, general recognisability of the conditions in the lay population, and conditions that are essentially either alone or as part of a larger syndrome). Based on these selection criteria, the six conditions chosen were cold, skin rash, lumbar pain, influenza, depression, and chest pain.

No assumption was made about the appropriateness of the response. Self-care responses vary from a decision to take no action to a decision to consult a health-care provider immediately. Therefore, in this conceptualisation of self-care, professional consultation is one of a range of self-determined behaviours rather than a behaviour that is opposed to or contrasted with self-treatment. Consulting a physician is one option that individuals sometimes select in the process of evaluating their symptoms.

The survey instrument constructed on the basis of a pilot study utilised predominantly close-ended questions. Open-ended questions were used only to obtain detailed information regarding particular behavioural responses. For example, when a medication response was indicated, the respondent was asked what medication had been taken. Those persons who experienced the conditions during the six months prior to receiving the questionnaire reported their actual behavioural responses to the symptoms. In the event that a condition was experienced more than once, the respondents were asked to report their behavioural responses to the most recently experienced episode.

The questions requesting socio-demographic information were based on questions that have been used in the research instruments for the Danish Statistical Bureau, assuming that the respondents would be more receptive to and would answer more accurately questions with which they were familiar. The social status classification is one used in studies conducted by the Danish Social Research Institute. Based on educational attainment, occupation, and the number of subordinates supervised at the workplace, the index was constructed on the basis of an empirical investigation of the status ascribed to various categories by the general population.

The Sample

The study population of the self-care behaviour project consisted of Danish citizens between 18 and 78 years of age who resided in Denmark in the winter of 1978. The selection of illness conditions for which the morbidity experiences were relevant to the entire study population necessitated the exclusion of children from the study. Also, because persons of very advanced age would provide less valid data, the most elderly segment of the population was excluded. Finally, all non-Danish residents of Denmark were excluded from the study population to reduce the effects of cultural differences.

The characteristics of the study samples in relation to population are seen in Table 4.1. A somewhat greater representation of older people in the original sample compensated for the fact that they more frequently failed to return completed questionnaires. The sample for Study A, as expected in survey studies using self-administered postal questionnaires, contained an educational bias. The sample was representative of the sex, age, and marital status distributions of the Danish population.

Statistical Methods

Because the response data in the investigation were symptom-specific, summary scores were developed for each person based on the number of times a particular type of response was reported in relation to the number of symptoms. The scores were calculated for four types of self care responses: decision to take no action, non-medication, self-treatment, use of medicine, and decision to seek professional help.

The BMDP programme for log-linear analysis of multivariate frequency tables was used to examine the importance of the independent variables in relation to the four types of behavioural responses to common illness conditions. Symptom-specific information that clarifies or modifies the findings for the summary measures is lost in this procedure. Therefore, both the findings of the multivariate analysis and instances in which symptom specific self-care practices deviate from the findings for the summary measures have been reported (Dean & al. 1983, Dean and Holst 1981, Dean and Holstein 1983).

STUDY B

The data for Study B were collected by in-depth interviews with a geographic subsample of the survey respondents from Study A. Information was obtained regarding all illness episodes reported for the six months prior to the interviews. The time frame and problems regarding the retrospective nature of the morbidity data have been discussed elsewhere in detail (Dean 1980). In short, given available information regarding the limitations of retrospective data (NCHS 1977) in relation to the purposes of this project, a six-month retrospective study period was selected. Since the purpose of the study was not to measure morbidity, but to understand illness behaviour, the primary concern was to strike a balance between the problem of memory failure and that of obtaining data on a sufficient number of illness episodes for the analysis of comlex interactions among factors.

The interviews schedules obtained information on 140 items concerned with the social situations, perceived stress, life habits, and attitudes of the respondents. In order to minimise interviewer and coding bias closed-ended questions were constructed for most items of information. It was possible to select items for some attitudinal variables from previously tested scales. Data were collected for the same range of self care responses to illness as in Study A. A treatment form was completed for each illness episode reported by the respondents.

The Sample

The interviews were conducted with respondents from Study A living in two confined geographical areas. In order to represent major levels of urbanisation, we chose the northeast areas of Zealand including the capital city and its suburbs, and the northeast area of the peninsula of Jutland, which includes the largest provincial city, small towns, and rural communities. This selection assured representation of principal residential divisions, but small towns, and farming areas, as seen in Table 4.1, were underrepresented.

Additional effects of this constraint are that

Table 4.1: Characteristics of the Samples from Phases One and Two of the Danish Self-care Project

	National Population (18-78 years old) (N = 3,569,063) %	National Sample (18-78 years old) (N = 1462) %	Area Sub-Sample (20-80 years old) (N = 450) %
Sex			
Female	51	52	55
Male	49	48	45
Age*			
18-27	21	18	21
28-37	22	19	24
38-47	16	15	19
48-57	16	14	17
58-67	15	19	12
68-78	11	10	8
Civil Status			
Single	23	22	17
Married	65	64	68
Separated/Divorced	6	6	8
Widowed	7	5	5
No information	-	2	2

Table 4.1 (cont'd)

	National Population (18-78 years old) (N = 3,569,063) %	National Sample (18-78 years old) (N = 1462) %	Area Sub-Sample (20-80 years old) (N = 450) %
Education			
Basic school	43	40	41
Training programme	51	45	45
College or university	6	9	10
No information	-	6	4
Residential Community			
Capital city and suburbs	23	29	51
Cities over 2000	46	41	35
Towns and countryside	31	30	14

* The 1980 subsample is two years older, i.e. 20-80 years.

the interview study sample contains slightly greater proportions of women, younger persons, and married or separated/divorced persons in relation to single persons than the Study A sample did. The most serious effect is the educational bias resulting from a sample based on persons responding to a mailed questionnaire.

Statistical Methods

The statistical task faced in the analysis of the Study B data was to sort out the relationships among many complex variables to distinguish those variables exerting direct influence from those exerting indirect influence on the self-care responses to illness. Two special problems had to be overcome in proceeding with the analysis. Firstly, the number of variables included in the investigation was too great to analyse at one time. The second problem was related to the doubtful validity of p-values calculated for tables with 4-5 or more dimensions.

To deal with the first problem, a programme for screening the structure of the data was developed. The screening of the data involved three steps:

1. All marginal relationships were determined by using simple chi square test in two-dimensional contingency tables.
2. In all situations where marginal interactions among three variables were indicated, the conditional independence of each combination of two of the three variables given, the third was tested.
3. The third step of the screening procedure involved the generation of log linear graphic base models of the structure of the data by eliminating all variables which were marginally or conditionally independent.

The second problem, concerned with the correctness of p-values calculated for large multiple contingency tables, remained. An alternative is to calculate exact p-values. By simulating a large number of contingency tables which have the same constant sufficient margins as the observed table, statistical tests with their associated p-values can be calculated for each relationship in the model. As this method also opens the possibility of using the information available on ordered variables which the log-linear procedure wastes, it was utilised even though it is quite time consuming. Hypothesis testing and sub-analyses then proceeded on the basis of the findings of the screening procedures (Edwards and Kreiner, forthcoming; Darroch 1980, Bishop & al. 1975).

REFERENCES

Aeldrekommissionens 1 delrapport (1980) Aldersforandringer - aeldrepolitikkens forudsaetninger (Age-Related Changes - The Basis of Elderly Policy). Copenhagen, Stougaard Jensen

Aeldrekommissionens 2 delrapport (1981) De aeldres vilkaar (The Living Conditions of the Elderly). Copenhagen, Stougaard Jensen

Alpert, J., Kasa, J., and Haggerty, R. (1967) "A Mon h of Illness and Health Care among Low Income Families." Publ. Hlth. Rep., 820:705

Anderson, J., Buck, C., Danaher, K., and Fry, J. (1977) "Users and Non-users of Doctors: Implications for Self Care." Journal of the Royal College of General Practitioners, 27, p. 155

Anderson, J. (ed.) (1975) Self-Medication. Lancaster, England: MTP Press Limited.

Austin, C. and Loeb, M. (1982) "Why Age is Relevant in Social Policy and Practice." In: Neugarten, B. (ed.), Age or Need? Sage Publications, Beverly Hills/London/New Delhi, pp. 263-287

Baltes, P. and Willis, I. (1977) "Toward Psychological Theories of Aging and Development." In: Birren, J. and Schaie, K. (eds.), Handbook of the Psychology of Aging, Van Nostrand Reinhold, New York, pp. 128-154

Belgrave, L. and Gratton, B. (1984) "Mental Health and the Elderly: Factors in Stability and Change Over Time." Journal of Health and Social Behavior, 25:100

Bell, J., Black, I., McEwen, J., and Pearson, J. (1977) Patterns of Illness. A Comparative Study in a New Town. Report to Scottish Home and Health Dept.

Belloc, N. (1973) "Relationship of Health Practices and Mortality." Preventive Medicine, 2, pp. 67-81

Belloc, N. and Breslow, L. (1972) "Relationship of Physical Health Status and Health Practices." Preventive Medicine, 1, pp. 409-421

Berkman, P. (1975) "Survival and a Modicum of Indulgence in the Sick Role." Med. Care, 13, p. 85

Birren, J. and Renner, V. (1980) "Concepts and Issues of Mental Health and Aging." In: Birren, J. and Sloane, R. (eds.), Handbook of Mental Health and Aging, Prentice-Hall, Inc., New Jessey, pp. 3-33

Bishop, Y., Fienberg, S., and Holland, P. (1975) Discrete Multivariate Analysis: Theory and Practice. Cambridge, MA: The MIT Press

Brody, E., Klebon, M., and Moles, E. (1983) "What Older People Do About their Day-to-day Mental and Physical Health Symptoms." Journal of the American Geriatric Society. 31, p. 489

Cassel, J. (1976) "The Contribution of the Social Environment to Host Resistance." Am. J. Epidem., 104:107

Cicerelli, V. (1980) "Relationship of Family Background Variables to Locus of Control in the Elderly." Journal of Gerontology. 35:108

Darroch, J. & al. (1980) "Markov Fields and Log-linear Interaction Model for Contingency Tables." Annals of Statistics, 8, pp. 522-530

Dean, K. (1983) "Self Care: What People Do for Themselves." In: Hatch, S. and Kickbusch, T. (eds.) Self-help and Health in Europe. World Health Organization, Regional Office for Europe, Copenhagen, Denmark

Dean, K. (1984) "Use of Non-Prescription Medicines to Treat Illness Episodes." Journal of Social and Administrative Pharmacy. Suppl. 1.

Dean, K. "Lay Care in Illness." Soc. Sci. Med. (forthcoming)

Dean, K. and Holstein, B.E. (1983) "Sygdomsadfaerd blandt aeldre" (Self-care among the Elderly) Ugeskr. laeger 145, pp. 687-690

Dean, K. (1984) "Influence of Health Beliefs on Lifestyles: What Do We Know?" European Monographs in Health Education Research, pp. 127-151

Dean, K., Holst, E., and Wagner, M. (1983) "Self-care of Common Illness in Denmark." In: Med. Care. 21:1012

Dean, K. (1981) "Self-care Responses to Illness: A Selected Review." Soc. Sci. Med., 151:673

Dean, K. and Holst, E. (1981) "Sygdomsadfaerd" (Self-care Behaviour) Ugeskr. laeger, 143, pp. 3571-9

Dean, K. (1980) Analysis of the Relationships between Social and Demographic Factors and Self-care Patterns in the Danish Population. (Unpublished dissertation, University of Minnesota)

Dean, K. Unpublished data, Institute of Social Medicine, University of Copenhagen

Dunnell, K. and Cartwright, A. (1972) Medicine Takers, Prescribers and Hoarders. London, Routledge and Kegan Paul

Edwards, D. and Kreiner, S. (1983) "The Analysis of Contingency Tables by Graphical Models" Biometrika, 70, pp. 553-565

Fiske, M. (1980) "Tasks and Crises of the Second Half of Life: The Interrelationship of Commitment, Coping and Adaptation." In: Birren, J. and Sloane, R. (eds.) Handbook of Mental Health and Aging, Prentice Hall, Inc., New Jersey, pp. 337-373

Fleming, G., Giachello, A., Andersen, R., and Andrade P. (1984) "Self-Care: Substitute, Supplement or Stimulus for Formal Medical Care Services?" Medical Care, 22:950

Freer, C. (1980) "Self-Care: A Health Diary Study." Med. Care, 18:853

Giachello, A., Fleming, G., and Andersen, R. (1982) Self-Care Practices in the United States. Research Project Report. Center for Health Administration Studies, University of Chicago

Grimsmo, A. (1984) Fra aa bli syk - til aa bli pasient (From Being Ill to Becoming a Patient) Statens Institutt for folkehelse, Oslo

Hattinga Verschure, J. (ed.) (1980) Changes in Caring for Health. Uitgeversmaatschappij De tydstroomm, Lochem

Haug, M. and Lavin, B. (Aug. 1982) "Self-Care and the Elderly: An Empirical Assessment." Paper presented at the 10th World Congress of the International Sociological Association, Mexico City

Haug, M. (1983) Consumerism in Medicine: Challenging Physician Authority. Sage Publication, Beverly Hills/London/New Delhi

Illsley, R. (1981) "Problems of Dependency Groups: The Care of the Elderly, the Handicapped and the Chronically Ill." Social Science and Medicine, 15A:327

Kasl, S.V. and Berkman, L.F. (1977) "Some Psychosocial Influences on the Health Status of the Elderly: The perspective of social epidemiology." In: McGaugh, J.L. and Keisler, S.B. (eds.) Aging: Biology and Behavior. New York: Academic Press, pp. 345-388

Kutza, E. and Zweibel, N. (1982) "Age as a Criterion for Focusing Public Programs" In: Neugarten, B. (ed.) Age or Need? Sage Publications, Beverly Hills/London/New Delhi, pp. 55-100

Lavin, B. and Haug, M. (Aug. 1981) "Public Utilization of Self-Care: An Empirical Assessment." Paper presented at the American Sociological Assoc., Toronto

Levin, L. and Idler, E. (1983) "Self-Care in Health." Ann. Rev. Public Health, 4, pp. 181-201

Levin, L. and Idler, E. (1981) The Hidden Health Care System, Ballinger Publishing Co., Cambridge

Levin, L. Katz, A., and Holst, E. (1976) Self-Care, Prodist, New York

Litman, T. (1974) "Health Care and the Family: A Behavioral Overview." Social Science and Medicine, 8:495

Litman, T. (1971) "Health Care and the Family: A Three Generation Analysis." Medical Care, 9:67

Mechanic, D. (1979) "Correlates of Physician Utilization; Why Do Major Multivariate Studies of Physician Utilization Find Trivial Psychosocial and Organizational Effects?" J. Health Soc. Behav. 29:387

Mechanic, D. (1980) "Health and Illness Behavior." In: Last, J.M. (ed.) Maxcy-Rosenau Preventive Medicine and Public Health, 11th ed. New York: Appleton-Century-Crafts

Maddox, G. and Wiley, J. "Scope, Concepts and Methods in the Study of Aging." In: Benstock, R. and Shanos, E. (eds.) Handbook of Aging and the Social Sciences. New York: Van Nostrand

Manton, K. (1982) "Changing Concepts of Morbidity and Mortality in the Elderly Population." Health and Society, 60:2

McCrae, R. (1982) "Age Differences in the Use of Coping Mechanisms." Journal of Gerontology, 37:454

McEwen, J. (1975) "Self-Medication in the Context of Self-care: A Review." In: Anderson, J. (ed.) Self-Medication. Lancaster, England: MTP Press Limited

Menaghan, E. (1982) "Measuring Coping Effectiveness: A Panel Analysis of Marital Problems and Coping Efforts." Journal of Health and Social Behavior, 23:220

Nelson, D. (1982) "Alternative Images of Old Age as the Bases for Policy." In: Newgarten, B. (ed.) Age or Need? Sage Publications, Beverly Hills/ London/New Delhi, pp. 131-170

Neugarten, B. (1982) "Policy for the 1980s: Age or Need Entitlement?" In: Neugarten, B. (ed.) Age or Need? Sage Publications, Beverly Hills/ London/New Delhi, pp. 19-55

Riley, M.W. (1976) "Age Strata in Social Systems." In: Binstock, R. and Shanas, E. (eds.) Handbook of Aging and the Social Sciences. Van Nostrand Reinhold, New York, p. 191

Riley, M.W. and Bond, K. (1983) "Beyond Ageism: Postponing the Onset of Disability." In: Riley, M.W., Hess, B., and Bond, K. (eds.) Aging in Society: Selected Reviews of Recent Research. Lawrence Erlbaum Assoc., pp. 243-252

Riley, M.W. and Foner, A. (1968) Aging and Society I: An Inventory of Research Findings. Russell Sage, New York

Snider, E. (1980) "Awareness and Use of Health Services by the Elderly." Medical Care, 18:1177

Svanborg, A. (1977) "The Gerontological and Geriatric Population Study in Göteborg, Sweden." Acta Medica Scandinavica, Suppl. 611, pp. 5-37

U.S. Department of Health, Education and Welfare (1979) Healthy People: The Surgeon General's Report on Health Promotion and Disease Prevention. Background Papers. Washington: Govt. Printing Office

Viney, L. and Westbrook, M. (1982) "Coping with Chronic Illness: The Mediating Role of Biographic and Illness-Related Factors." Journal of Psychosomatic Research, 26:595

World Health Organization (1980) "The Well-being of the World's Aging Citizens, A Status Report." Secretariat paper, IRP/ADR101/10, WHO, Regional Office for Europe, Copenhagen, Denmark.

World Health Organization (1981) Report of WHO Preparatory Conference for United Nations World Assembly on Aging. Mexico City, 8-11 December 1980, IRP/ADR!=!, 3986B. WHO, Regional Office for Europe, Copenhagen, Denmark

World Health Organization (1984) Health Education in Self-Care: Possibilities and Limitations. Report of a Scientific Consultation. Geneva, 21-25 November 1983. R984,HED/84.1

Chapter 5

PREVENTIVE HEALTH BEHAVIOUR AND HEALTH MAINTENANCE PRACTICES OF OLDER ADULTS

William Rakowski

I. INTRODUCTION

Prevention and health promotion have established a dominating presence in professional and popular literature. This chapter will discuss conceptual concerns and psychosocial elements of preventive health behaviour and health maintenance practices among persons aged 65 years and older, with a particular focus on older adults' health-related perceptions and on the family support context of later life. Preventive and health maintenance behaviours are treated as one component of the broader domain of self-care activities. The discussion will not attempt to prove that benefits can be expected to occur for society or for the older individual through public policy directed either at particular types of preventive practices or, even more specifically, at particular psycho-social variables believed to facilitate performance of those practices. In fact, multiple (and perhaps competing) criteria against which to assess benefits will be outlined.

Nor can this paper cover the entire area of prevention, as a broader subject relevant to the later decades of life. Coverage under third-party reimbursement, for example, may encourage or discourage preventive practices, quite apart from research on psychological and social strategies to achieve health promotion goals. In addition, many preventive strategies can be introduced through governmental legislation and subsequent enforcement of regulations (e.g., fluoridated water, environmental safety standards, user taxes on unhealthy substances, building codes, consumer product content and material requirements). Socio-economic policies may, therefore, help to create a preventive environment, independently of any active behavioural efforts by older individuals and their social support networks. Policies and resource allocation directed at promoting an individual's performance of specific good health practices are clearly on the frontiers of prevention and older adulthood. As a result, it is not yet evident how initiatives at the level of the person and the family to foster preventive and health maintenance behaviours are best incorporated into a larger public policy on prevention.

The Concept of Preventive and Health Maintenance Behaviour

Concepts such as prevention and health maintenance in the context of older adulthood present an especially interesting challenge of determining boundaries for discussion. In a strict sense we might adopt the definition of "health behaviour" which was proposed originally by Kasl and Cobb to include, "... any activity undertaken by a person believing himself to be healthy, for the purpose of preventing disease or detecting it in an asymptomatic stage" (1966, p. 246). Given the prevalence of chronic illness and impairment in later adulthood, however, large numbers of older adults do not have the luxury of being able to believe that they are as completely healthy as this definition implies. The definition of prevention must, therefore, be extended to include activities whose primary objective is to control an older individual's existing "at risk" health status to the fullest extent possible. This perspective was in fact adopted in the often-quoted report of the United States' Surgeon General (Filner & Williams, 1979, pp. 367-386), where the theme of health promotion for the elderly was discussed from the framework of services which would reduce unnecessary functional dependency and institutionalisation.

The terms "preventive" and "health maintenance" behaviour are used in this paper to encompass activities of two types, with the understanding that an individual may have both purposes in mind when he or she engages in the behaviour. The term preventive refers to activities intended by the individual to reduce his or her risk of developing a serious illness condition. The term health maintenance refers to activities which are intended to continue and, if possible, improve one's current level of health for as long a time as possible. Health maintenance is probably slightly broader in its connotations. For example, the use of a seat belt and obtaining a regular dental examination might be more usually labelled as preventive measures to avoid specific problems, while a programme of regular physical activity and discussion of health matters with family or friends may have a more general purpose of "keeping fit" or improving vigour. Health maintenance may also be a term with greater acceptability for persons having existing illness conditions, for whom a term such as "preventive health activities" might imply an unrealistic goal. Use of the two terms, therefore, provides a measure of flexibility, while retaining the broad range of appropriate target behaviours that is necessary when discussing prevention.

The Scope of Preventive/Health Maintenance Behaviour

The potential range of preventive and health maintenance behaviours and, by inference, the scope of the monumental task facing researchers and policy makers needs to be clearly delineated. What data will be acceptable enough to warrant the conferring of "legitimacy" on behaviour? The list of preventive practices is potentially as open-ended as is the definition of optimum health. Priorities of behaviour have yet to be established; nor is a comprehensive list of practices available as a basis for setting priorities.

Drawing from apparent consensus and certain specific sources (e.g., Harris & Guten 1979, Langlie 1977, U.S. Dept. of H.H.S. 1980 b, U.S. Dept. of H.E.W. July, 1979), several types of behaviour appear to qualify for consideration as being preventive and/or health maintaining in nature:

> Moderation in the use of alcohol;
> Limited use of tobacco;
> Obtaining regular medical examinations (with tests appropriate for one's sex);
> Obtaining immunisations as necessary;
> Obtaining regular dental examinations;
> Obtaining regular eye examinations;
> Performing self-exams at appropriate intervals;
> Monitoring of dietary intake (e.g. nutrients, calories, fat, salt, sugar, caffeine, fibre, trace minerals);
> Monitoring of weight;
> Maintaining an adequate sleep pattern;
> Participation in physical activity/exercise on

a regular basis;
Informed use of over-the-counter medications;
Informed use of vitamin supplements;
Not using medications prescribed for other persons;
Following an appropriate schedule of meals;
Responding to organised health screening outreach efforts;
Destroying old or unused medications; Checking expiration dates;
Seeking information on illness problems and health issues of aging;
Maintaining an appropriate balance of work and relaxation activities;
Dressing appropriately for weather conditions;
Taking proper care of feet and toe nails;
Using seat belts when a driver and a passenger;
Avoiding settings known to pose environmental hazards of pollution or other contamination;
Performing appropriate personal hygiene practices;
Using dental floss and/or denture care materials;
Engaging in activities considered to promote a "positive outlook on life";
Staying abreast of new information about health and health care;
Participating in health education activities;
Rearranging furniture and other household items to accomodate to physical/sensory changes; checking for safety hazards;
Keeping a first-aid kit and smoke detector in the dwelling; and
Having a repertoire of strategies for the management of stress producing life-events.

The definition of what constitutes an appropriate level or type of any of these behaviours often will require a technical knowledge of particular topics (e.g., nutrition, physiology, pharmacy, medicine). Also, specification of these appropriate levels will undoubtedly be dependent on our state-of-the-art judgments of what constitutes a healthy level of given behaviour and how best to achieve it. This double qualification of caution should be taken seriously both by professionals who proscribe or endorse activities and by older adults who ultimately are decision-makers and consumers acting from informed self-interest.

Conceptual Considerations

Preventive and health maintenance behaviours share a common objective of promoting individual well-being. To date, however, basic differences among these activities, themselves, have not been discussed. Since the list of preventive behaviours which might be created is so open-ended, conceptual distinctions along which to organise behaviour must exist to assist not only research but also debates and resource allocation decisions for particular preventive practices. The following distinctions are intended to help that process along.

Penetration and Reorganisation. One useful distinction might be made in the depth of penetration or integration which different preventive/maintenance activities have into an individual's daily routine. Some activities, such as medical and dental exams, are rather discrete in nature, usually occurring at only a few points during the year, with each visit covering a relatively brief period of time. Others, such as sleep patterns, dietary monitoring, and maintaining a work/relaxation balance, are much more continuous, and might require day-to-day attention. Strategies and facilitative variables that work for short periods may not be as effective over prolonged periods, as suggested by the rates of "relapse" noted in risk reduction programmes (Matarazzo 1982).

A related characteristic is the extent of reorganisation or intrusiveness which initiating new behaviour would require in an individual's normal pattern of activities. Low penetration behaviour should not be assumed to have low demands for reorganisation, especially when we propose a behaviour package to achieve risk reduction. Again, we will be well-advised to consider the relatively short versus long-term time span involved. Although we often use the term health behaviour, our discussions and health promotion objectives implicitly involve health-related activity patterns and attitudes.

Accessibility. Another distinction is that of the ease of access to give assistance with preventive and health maintenance behaviours by family members, friends, and professionals. For example, while the destruction of old medications and even the decision whether or not to respond to screening or health education programme outreach can be relatively discrete events in time, they may be much less accessible than are medical and dental visits. As for the older person, it may also be especially important to consider family members' perceptions of having to "go out of their way" in order to carry out the activity.

Prevention vs. Abuse. It has seemed more common to find literature emphasising substance abuse, misuse, or other inappropriate health behaviours of older adults, as opposed to literature which has identified behaviours performed explicitly for preventive purposes. A third conceptual question is whether a preventive orientation is indicated simply by the absence of whatever we define as being indicative of abuse or misuse. Is the "profile" of the preventive older person just a mirror image of the non-preventive older person? For purposes of research, is it also important to determine whether or not the individual possesses a preventive intent for his actions? Determination of the intention of a mode of behaviour will be helpful to better understand the preventive orientation of older persons.

The "Preventive" Older Adult
Two essential questions must eventually be answered, namely: Which preventive and health maintenance behaviours are actually of greatest benefit and "worth" encouraging in the older population? And what set of behaviours should we employ as a standard for identifying preventively-oriented older persons? A multi-behavioural classification of older individuals on a continuum reflecting a high to low preventive orientation might be used as a predictor variable, an outcome measure to evaluate intervention programmes, or a criterion for eligibility to receive services. It is likely that our research will move toward the determination of weights or relative values for each item of behaviour in a preventive/maintenance package.

As noted in another paper (Rakowski 1983), however, there can be at least six distinct "courts" in which the benefits of health promotion efforts with older adults can be judged. Each of these courts of evaluation are appropriate, therefore, as a potential standard for determining the weights to apply to behaviours such as those listed earlier. They include:

1. The "court of cost containment: Which preventive/health maintenance behaviours are best able to help control the rate of growth of health care expenditures with older adults?

2. The "court" of survivorship: Which preventive/health maintenance behaviours result in greatest reductions of mortality?

3. The "court" of morbidity: Which preventive/health maintenance behaviours produce the greatest improvement in standard indicators of impairment (e.g., days of activity limitation, days of hospital usage, disease incidence rates)?

4. The "court" of the quality of life: Which behaviours are best able to improve and maintain the older adult's quality of life, as reflected by standard psychological and social indicators (e.g., morale, life satisfaction, social network size, future outlook)?

5. The "court" of behavioural change: From a pragmatic standpoint, which preventive/maintenance behaviours are the most amenable to influence over the short and/or long term?

6. The "court" of productivity: For those older persons still employed or employable, which preventive/maintenance behaviours are most beneficial for continued job performance?

For better or worse, the behaviours found to be important across these six "courts" of evaluation need not have extensive overlap. Moreover, if the same preventive/maintenance behaviours do not contribute comparably in each area, our specification of the behavioural hierarchy comprising a preventive life-style can have corresponding variability. As a result also, political and value judgments about which court deserves priority emphasis may have a large influence on which preventive/health maintenance behaviours are considered to be most worthy of promotion among older adults.

II. BACKGROUND DATA ON PREVENTIVE ACTIVITIES

Favourable Evidence

The current status of aggregate data, however limited, on behaviours which suggest a preventive or health maintenance orientation among older adults presents us with a somewhat mixed picture. Research by Breslow and associates in Alameda County, California, has found older adults located along the entire spectrum of their composite index of good health practices (Belloc & Breslow 1972), as has a national probability survey of the United States' population which extended the sampling base of Breslow & al. (National Center for Health Statistics, 4 November 1980). In addition, activities such as health fairs, lecture series on health topics, and health education workshops apparently are able to attract ample numbers of elderly persons. On the one hand, various sources have suggested that older adults show acceptable rates of commonly accepted favourable health practices. For example:

1. General medical examinations: National surveys have indicated that older adults have comparatively high rates of making general medical examination and preventive care office visits (National Center for Health Statistics, 1 April 1981; Haug 1979; Lairson & Swint 1978), in particular for hypertension, eye examinations, and inoculations. At least among women, these higher rates may be most pronounced for persons aged 65-74 (National Center for Health Statistics, Aug. 1981).

2. Use of alcohol: It appears that persons aged 65 and over are more likely to report abstinence from alcohol and less frequent consumption of relatively large amounts of alcohol at any one sitting (National Center for Health Statistics, 4 November 1980; Mishara & Kastenbaum 1980; National Institute on Alcohol Abuse and Alcoholism, 31 Dec. 1982).

3. Smoking: Use of tobacco for smoking appears to be less frequent among older adults, who report a greater proportion of persons never having smoked and a lower prevalence of current smokers (National Center for Health Statistics, 4 Nov. 1980; U.S. Dept.

of H.H.S. 1980 a). Status as a former smoker is less obviously associated with age, although the number of cigarettes smoked per day by elderly current smokers may be less than for any other age group (U.S. Dept. of H.H.S. 1980 a).

At least on the aggregate level, such data could give us reason for optimism. However, it is reasonable to expect that persons who have engaged in a set of distinctly unfavourable health practices are at least slightly more likely to have died prior to age 65 (Belloc 1973; Breslow & Engstrom 1980). We should not too quickly, therefore, draw the inference that the aging process is accompanied by an attitudinal and behavioural trend toward greater health consciousness. In this regard, optimists might point to certain demographic trends which promise a more favourable disposition toward health maintenance behaviour among successive cohorts future elderly. For instance:

1. The general educational level of the population aged 65 and over is gradually improving, though most notably for the Anglo population. The basic assumption (and hope) is that more extensive formal education will promote greater familiarity with the arguments in favour of health maintenance and better access to the necessary resources to follow through with such motivations. It is also assumed that better formal education will produce a population of older adults with higher expectations of the health care system, which in turn will be translated into a demand for preventive-oriented services.

2. The income status of older adults is not as objectively abject now as in previous years. Although it is certainly possible to argue with government definitions of the poverty level, and recent changes instituted in the United States Social Security System have generated lively debate, the income position of recent and hopefully future cohorts of older adults seems to be more secure. Reimbursement by Medicare and third-party insurance carriers for older adults' membership in Health Maintenance Organisations may eventually dovetail with economic trends of income status to help

make preventive care an affordable "luxury" to larger numbers of the older population.

3. Small but steady gains in life-expectancy have occurred over the past decades. Expressions of interest in issues related to "the elderly" used to denote a focus on persons aged 65 and over. It seems more common now for policy discussions pertinent to aging to imply a focus on the frail or at-risk elderly -- usually viewed as including persons primarily aged 75 and over. Even in gerontological circles, discussions are now more often heard advocating need as opposed simply to age as the criterion of eligibility for services. Coupled with a clear trend among the media to highlight active and seemingly "youthful" older adults, it appears likely that greater numbers of persons already "old" by legislative definition and persons aged 40-65 will be exposed to the possibility of maintained health and well-being into very late life.

Contradictory Indications

Although points such as those noted above hold promise for observing high rates of behavioural practices considered to be preventive and health maintaining in nature among older adults, other data could raise some questions:

1. Pap smear: Despite the age-associated prevalence of death from malignant neoplasm of the cervix, the rate of office visits for Pap smear tests appears to decrease with successive age groups (National Center for Health Statistics, August 1981; National Center for Health Statistics, March 1977; Celetano, Shapiro, & Weisman 1982; Kleinman & Kopstein 1981). Correspondingly, women aged 65 and above have reported the highest rates of never having had a Pap smear, and having had no smear within the past five years.

2. Breast examination: Rates of breast examination by a doctor appear lowest among women aged 65 and above (30.5% stated in 1973 that they had never had one). Moreover, in 1973, 29.7% of the National Health Interview Survey aged female sample reported

never having had either a breast examination or a Pap smear and only 48% had had
both (National Center for Health Statistics, March 1977; Celetano, Shapiro, &
Weisman 1982). However, for neither Pap
smears nor breast examination, is it known
whether the lower rates are due more to the
women's failure to request the exam, or the
clinician's failure to conduct it during a
standard visit.

3. Dental visits: The low rate of dental
visits among older adults is widely known
(Andersen & Anderson 1979; Kiyak 1981). In
1973 an estimated 49 percent, and in 1978,
44.3 percent of persons aged 65 and over
had not seen a dentist in five years or
more (U.S. Dept. of H.H.S. 1980 a).

4. Nutrition: Older adults appear to be at
greater risk of having inadequate dietary
intake, characterised by a lower than
desired level of nutrients, yet greater
prevalence of obesity (Davis & Randall
1983; Posner 1979).

Will we ever know the "true" status of
preventive and health maintenance behaviour by older
adults? Will it be easier to determine precisely the
extent of favourable practices or to document the
prevalence (or reduction) of unfavourable or harmful
practices? Will it be easier to document the extent
of temporally limited behaviours with less penetration in an older person's daily routine, simply
because such activities are more readily recognised
and counted? Will there always be a need to improve
the health behaviours of older adults, and to better
understand the processes which underlie such behaviour? It is hard to imagine either a social system
or a gathering of scientists in which the answer to
this latter question would be anything other than
"Yes." Therefore, the search for antecedents of
health maintenance behaviour will be a long and
continuing process. The comments which follow will
examine some areas which may prove fruitful.

III. INTERVENING AND FACILITATIVE FACTORS

A. Health Beliefs and Perceptions
The chains of causation among the health beliefs and
health maintaining behaviours of older adults have

certainly not been documented to satisfy the criteria of scientific scope, precision, or methodological rigour. It quickly becomes evident that a definite need exists for prospective investigations, of representative random samples of older adults, which compare a full range of potential predictors (health perceptions, family support, demographic, personality traits, and coping skills), for several behavioural measures. In the absence of such projects, the health perception literature does hint at some interesting avenues for inquiry, which have not yet been investigated in relation to preventive and health maintenance behaviour.

Prior Behaviour and Health Beliefs

In a retrospective study of swine flu inoculation in a one-county area, Rundall and Wheeler (1979) found that perceived susceptibility to the disease and perceived danger from the immunization were most important in a multivariate analysis for distinguishing among utilisers and non-utilisers of the programme. Utilisers tended to report greater susceptibility and less expected danger; overall R^2 was .34, including the other potential predictors. In univariate analyses, support was also found for the variable of perceived efficacy of the immunisation. Of comparable importance, however, was the finding that number of visits to the physician during the previous year was the only non-belief variable in the multivariate analyses associated with having received the immunisation.

Swine flu inoculation was also the topic of a retrospective report by Aho (1979) on a largely Black and Portuguese sample randomly recruited through two senior centers. Having received the inoculation was associated with 1. planning to receive future flu shots and other shots; 2. stronger belief in the protection afforded by the shot; 3. greater perceived safety of the inoculation; 4. less uncertainty about the future likelihood of contracting flu; 5. having previously received other flu shots; and 6. a larger proportion of friends and relatives who had received the shot. Interestingly, neither the Rundall/Wheeler nor Aho studies found support for importance of the perceived severity of the flu, if it were contracted.

Although not looking strictly at behaviours which were preventive in nature, a secondary analysis by Coulton and Frost (1982) may also be informative. Using data from the Cleveland General

Accounting Office (GAO) study and adopting the Anderson and Newman (1973) model of need, predisposing, and enabling factors, Coulton and Frost found that perceived need was predictive of medical care ambulatory visits, use of mental and personal care services, and recreation service usage over the following year. Again, however, prior use of social and health service was important, perhaps unexpectedly so, entailing 18 percent additional variance for ambulatory care use (more than all other predictors combined), and eight percent for recreational services.

Some attention might also be given to knowledge of available preventive and health maintenance services. Even though knowledge is not a guarantee of usage, lack of knowledge would seem to be an almost certain guarantee of non-usage, at least on personal initiative. Snider (1980) investigated a selective set of predictors of knowledge of preventive and health maintenance service availability among 405 elderly residents of Edmonton, Canada. Health beliefs were not among the set of predictors. From among those predictors used, more extensive educational background and greater extent of prior agency use were the most strongly associated variables with service knowledge. The visibility of prior usage is again conspicuous and suggests that established patterns of behaviour may play an especially important role in any attempt to encourage preventive and health maintenance activities. Consequently, the relation between prior usage and current health perceptions is very likely to be an especially significant area for study.

Self-Rated Health

Among the more frequently cited statistics in the literature is that at any given time about 85 percent of the population aged 65 and over are estimated to have at least one chronic condition. At the same time, older adults are commonly observed to persevere in the face of notable impairments and seem to hold favourable assessments of their health relative to age peers (Minkler 1978). There are even some suggestions that persons who survive to be among the "old-old" hold at least as positive views of their health status and maybe even more favourable views) as do younger elderly (Ferraro 1980; Linn & Linn 1980). Do such positive self-health judgments tend to promote preventive behaviour? Or does a belief that one is doing "about as well as can be expected for someone my age" act to subtly inhibit health maintenance behaviour? Are continuous activities with high penetration harder to influence than discrete activities?

A related issue is whether perceptions of poor health can serve as an effective motivator for prompting the individual to engage in activities which might help to prevent further deterioration. In this arena, the potentially motivating effects of beliefs may be fighting an uphill battle. Correlates of poor self-health ratings among the elderly have included objective indices of physical impairment (Ferraro 1980; Fillenbaum 1979; Markides & Martin 1979; Linn & Linn 1980; Linn, Linn, & Knopka 1978; Tissue 1972); lower income (Cantor & Mayer 1976; Ferraro 1980; Graney & Zimmerman 1979-81; Minkler 1978); less formal education (Ferraro 1980; Graney & Zimmerman 1979); membership in non-Anglo ethnic groups (Cantor 1979; Cantor & Mayer 1976; Carp & Kataoka 1976; Linn, Hunter, & Linn 1980; shorter future outlook (Rakowski 1979); and lower morale or life-satisfaction (Graney & Zimmerman 1979; Larson 1978). At least on the surface these several correlated factors would seem to present a formi-dable package, with strong potential for thwarting even the best of motivations to maintain health status.

Irreversibility of Aging

It has often been asserted, though less often documented in data, that older adults are more likely to attribute symptoms to normal and irrevers-ible "aging," to under-report symptoms, and to anticipate decrement as an expected part of the aging process (Brody & Kleban 1981, 1983; Kart 1981; Litman 1971). Uncomfortable and only semi-humorous comments by older adults and even persons in middle-age regarding presumed signs of memory loss attest to the potential depth and concern generated by such an outlook. Again, however, it is not yet possible to determine the conditions under which this expectation promotes or inhibits preventive health behaviour (e.g., in combination with low internal health locus of control). Brody and Kleban (1981, 1983) have noted the only modest proportion of symptom experiences which were brought to the attention of health professionals or others, leading one to question whether a tendency to gloss over the reporting of symptoms is paralleled by comparable lack of action on a day-to-day basis. German,

Shapiro, Chase, and Vollmer (1978) noted that among elderly in disadvantaged sections of Baltimore, serious illness conditions received treatment, while the less serious tended not to be under treatment, except in the geographic area where an HMO had been initiated. Again, the reasons for such an occurrence deserve study.

Congruence of Perceptions

Several studies, cited above, have examined the correspondence between relatively objective medical /physical indices and older adults' self-rated health. Another set of studies have looked at the congruence of ratings between older persons' and health care providers' (usually doctors) judgments of the patient's health status (Maddox & Douglass 1973; LaRue, Jarvik, & al. 1979; Linn, Linn, & Knopka 1980; Linn, Hunter, & Linn 1980; Linn, Linn, & Stein 1982; Rakowski, Hickey, & Dengiz, in preparation). Although congruence of perceptions has been observed at statistically significant levels, rates of agreement suggest the situation is still one where the "cup" may be viewed as being half empty or half full (e.g.., Graney & Zimmerman 1979; Rakowski, Hickey, & Dengiz, in preparation). In addition, most studies have focused on ratings of present health, have used only a single question, and have often used a dichtomous scale for the patients' and providers' rating (which will tend to maximise the estimate of congruence). Congruence has less often been the primaty focus of investigation.

The absence of extremely high rates of congruence should not be surprising since patients are more likely to place their health and treatment in a broader personal context, with an emphasis on maintenance of functional activities of living, while medical professionals more often focus on identification of pathology and dysfunction. However, the consensus among several reports that a high potential for non-agreement exists begs the question of whether there are impacts associated with either the personal health behaviour of the older person or on the behavioural predispositions of the provider. Although the influence may be quite subtle (e.g., non-verbal cues, shorter appointment time, less thorough questioning, less complete symptom reporting), we can not afford to investigate older adults' health perceptions outside of the interpersonal context with the provider in which they exist.

108

Locus of Control

A recent review of literature on the construct of
health locus of control presented both the progress
made to date and several questions yet to be
resolved (Wallston & Wallston 1982). Although the
empirical evidence is not uniform, the locus of
control construct continues to have strong intuitive
appeal and generates a large body of research. The
introduction of a multidimensional approach to locus
of control generally (Levenson 1973, 1981) and in
relation to health perceptions (Wallston & Wallston
1982) seems especially promising, since it will now
be possible to develop typologies of individuals
which allow for seemingly contradictory beliefs
(e.g., high internal and high powerful other loci of
control). The nature of chronic conditions as often
progressive and irreversible, their extension into
the forseeable future, possible trends in late life
future perspective (to be discussed later), and
beliefs about what constitutes "normal" physical
aging appear to create an especially ripe context
for examining the relevance of perceived control
among older adults.

Dimensions of Health Perceptions

We need to adopt a broader perspective on the
assessment of health-related perceptions. For the
most part, it seems that investigators have been
satisfied to obtain a single rating of perceived
health status, on a 4- or 5-point scale. Factor-
analytic efforts such as that by Mancini and Quinn
(1981) should be commended and replicated. In our
previously noted study of congruence (Rakowski,
Hickey, & Dengiz, in preparation), and in a project
currently underway, we have included 15 questions
pertaining to perceived health and treatment status.
The objective of using multiple questions should not
simply be to statistically derive health-related
factors in which several items are considered to
represent a single underlying dimension. There may
also be great utility in investigating what this
writer prefers to call "ripple effects" of perceived
illness problems across health-related domains.

One of the essential tasks of coping with
chronic illness appears to be the determination of
how far the roots of a problem extend into other
areas of life. The present writer (Rakowski & Dengiz
1984), and Mancini and Quinn (1981) have both
observed the correlations among several health-

related perceptions when more than one item was employed. The use of a single summary score derived from the items of a factor may too easily mask the individual's experience of multiple effects in the health domain (e.g., expected near future health, locus of control over future health, expected difficulty following treatment or keeping appointments). In combination with potential effects on life satisfaction (Larson 1978) and/or social contacts, the experience of far-reaching roots or ripples may indeed be a salient one, with implications for the perception of activities intended to be preventive or health maintaining.

Future Time Perspective
Discussions of preventive and health maintenance behaviour in later life should also consider the future orientation and future time perspective of the older person, and better understand how a future perspective is involved in health-related perceptions. There is little doubt as to the importance of future outlook as a general characteristic of personality throughout the lifespan (Gorman & Wessman 1977; Kastenbaum 1977, 1982; Markson 1973; Rakowski 1979). There also appears to be consensus that time perspective can adopt a qualitatively different tenor in later adulthood, characterised by what Kastenbaum called a "foreshortened future perspective." The future now comes to have a realised limit. Moreover, as Markson (1973) noted, the absence of a string of normative life-events and rites-of-passage in late life implies that it is increasingly left to the individual to structure the content and time-table of future events. The connotations are by no means intended to be inevitably pessimistic.

In such a context, however, an understanding of the nature of arguments used to encourage preventive and health maintenance behaviour is important. One prime element of reasoning emphasises the long-term future gains which become more probable as a result of risk-minimising and health enhancement activities. Periods of years often are spanned in the space of a relatively few written or spoken words. Reliance seems to be placed on what Bortner and Hultsch (1974; Hultsch & Bortner 1974) termed the "normative expected life cycle." For younger adults at least, the analogy is that of a personal rainbow, spanning decades, the proverbial "pot" at the end being made more rich through better health and

vigour, and perhaps by postponement of the anticipated decrements of aging. An implicit understanding
and acceptance of this normative process by potential consumers of advice seems to underlie much of
the publicity given to health promotion efforts.

In this writer's jugment, based on the literature and my own work (Rakowski 1979, 1982; Rakowski
& Hickey 1981; Rakowski & Dengiz 1984), it will be
important to know how older adults perceive the time
frame of expected benefits, relative to any given
preventive or health maintenance activity and their
own anticipated futures. For example: How long is it
expected to be before benefits will be felt? How
long can these benefits be expected to last? How
great an investment of personal resources, including
physical and mental energy, is expected to be
necessary in order to see benefits initially and to
maintain them over time? The statistical "promise"
of better health or reduced risk can be expected to
have only limited success with many subgroups of
elderly, who may have existing difficulty meeting
basic needs for adequate food, shelter, and transportation.

Summary Comments (III. A.). The role played by
health beliefs in the preventive and health maintenance behaviour or older adults can only be determined with greater empirical precision over the coming
years. A subsequent section of this paper will
return to the area of beliefs, to offer a broader
framework around which research might be organised.
It should be noted that a reasonably comprehensive
set of "potentially relevant" health beliefs for
older adults have not yet even been specified with
some measure of consensual validation among authors,
let alone been the subject of systematic study to
determine relative importance. The well-known Health
Belief Model (Becker 1974; Becker & Maiman 1975;
Becker, Haefner, & al. 1977), and a model proposed
by the present writer (Rakowski & Hickey 1980)
provide at least two places to begin. However, they
should not be viewed as complete inventories. The
arena of individual's "common sense" ideas of
illness (Lau & Hartman 1983; Leventhal & Hirschman
1982) may be a fruitful area of study with older
persons. Along a similar line of thought, we should
recognise that perception-oriented models of health
behaviour tend to adopt a subtle assumption that
individuals have the luxury of time to thoroughly
deliberate their potential actions. The process of

deliberation, including the component of actual or perceived available time needs to be given serious attention.

B. Social Supports: Family and Friends

Family Support and Preventive/Health Maintenance Behaviour

There is little doubt that marital and parent/child relationships continue to be of central importance into later life. Having a family support network appears to be a better state of affairs than not having one. Davis and Randall (1983) have summarised literature on food habits of the elderly, noting that older persons who live alone, compared to those living with someone else, have been observed to have less adequate dietary intake and less variety in their diets, to eat fewer foods requiring preparation, and to be more likely to skip the evening meal. They also note that the social context of eating is likely to improve food habits. Similarly, misuse or abuse of alcohol can be related to changes in family status which unfavourably affect social support (Mishara & Kastenbaum 1980; NIAAA, 31 Dec. 1982). Brand and Smith (1974) reported that the lowest post-hospital compliance and the highest rate of readmission occurred for the non-married. There is also the well-known role of the family as a line of defense against placement in a long term care institution (Brody, Poulshock, & Masciocchi 1978; Branch & Jette 1982; Shanas & Sussman 1981).

However, research has tended to concentrate on family support during crises and periods of chronic illness, to look at unhealthy practices of older persons rather than specifically at preventive ones, and to emphasise the need for programmes to assist family care givers in managing stressors. Discussions of familial influence on preventive and health maintenance behaviours may, therefore, need to be centered around the potential for effectiveness, rather than on documented effects. Based on the gerontological family literature, certain themes do appear with some frequency, and give promise for a favourable influence:

1. Most persons aged 65 and over have at least one living child, and contact of some type is reported on a regular basis (Shanas 1979; 1980). The normative pattern is more

one of a "modified extended family," rather than the "isolated nuclear family" (Sussman & Burchinal 1962).

2. Younger generations, despite feeling a "squeeze" from both ends of the generational spectrum, tend to believe in assisting their parents and in-laws when an apparent need arises (Brody 1981). Shanas and Sussman (1981) have referred to this sense of responsibility as "the almost subconscious need to respond to kith and kin" (1981, p. 228).

3. Complementary to those feelings, older adults tend to turn to family members first, rather than to community service agencies (Brody 1981; Cantor & Mayer 1978; Stoller & Earl 1983; Stanford 1978; Valle & Mendoza 1978).

4. The historical trend toward four- and five-generation family networks is continuing (Shanas 1980). Johnson and Bursk (1976) have referred to a "psychologically extended family," as a parallel to the modified extended family of residential proximity and contact. Might such a psychologically extended family contribute to a broader base of support for its older members, both through sheer numbers and also through the obvious evidence of a lineage, with at least some degree of responsibility for the welfare of the older generations?

5. At least one family member (child, spouse, daughter-in-law, sibling) usually takes on primary care-giving responsibility, despite the necessary personal sacrifices and stresses which result (Blenkner 1965; Shanas & Sussman 1981; Silverstone & Hyman 1982).

Therefore, for those older persons -- healthy or ill -- who still have living members from their family of orientation or procreation, a context of concern about health status is very likely to exist. Hayes-Bautista's (1979) description of "coaches and arbitrators" to facilitate access to services is no less true for older adults. On the other hand, there are also good reasons to temper any excessive enthusiasm for the reliance that can be placed on the family support network:

1. Older adults themselves are reluctant to bother other family members (Brody & Kleban

1981). It is not hard to imagine situations in which potential benefits of family support would be attenuated by the older adult's reluctance to ask for help, especially if help were necessary on a daily basis or had just been requested in the very recent past.

2. Qualitative reports of family experience in care-giving provide ample enumeration of dynamics which can work against achieving adequate communication (Farkas 1980; Hausman 1979), even given the best of intentions. The communication necessary to plan for health-related matters is difficult to achieve and maintain. In fact, it may be useful for gerontologists to examine seriously what particular factors "should" in theory start and keep family members in active communication. The list may be surprisingly short. It is entirely possible that the presses found in day-to-day activity actually work against thorough communication. The impression which one receives from the literature (and from informal discussion with older adults) is the existence of a continuing balance among a desire for personal independence, a recognised need for assistance, a preference for help from one's family, and a desire not to be a burden.

3. Related closely to communication is the issue of congruence of perceptions among older adults and family members. Some current data (Cicerelli 1981; Rakowski & Hickey 1983; Reifler, Cox, & Hanley 1981) suggest that a high potential exists for perspectives on health and treatment to differ among care-givers and care-receivers. As with the question of patient /provider congruence, the family "cup" may be viewed as being half empty or half full depending upon one's emphasis on congruence or lack of congruence. The importance of non-agreement remains an empirical issue, since the literature has not yet investigated whether observed differences represent strong disagreement or would be easily resolved. It seems reasonable, however, to hypothesise that a lack of congruence on the perceived need or potential usefulness of preventive care will

attenuate any favourable influence by the family.

4. Despite the apparent effectiveness of family education and support groups for care-givers of impaired older adults, we do not yet have evidence of a trickle-down effect to the older persons receiving assistance (Clark & Rakowski 1983). Even if a trickle-down does occur, we will need to document whether prevention and health maintenance activities are a component of the effect.

5. We must not fall into the trap of too quickly idealising the family status of older adults or the family's potential for effectiveness (Ward 1978; Litman 1971; Nydegger 1983; Treas 1977). This caution against idealisation extends to our view of ethnic group elderly, whose family networks may not have the potential for supportiveness that they are often presumed to possess (Carp & Kataoka 1976; Cheung, Cho, & al. 1980; Newton 1980). Much of the enthusiasm which one finds in the literature continues to be a reaction against pessimistic overtones which accompanied the "isolated nuclear family" concept, and its structuralist-functionalist implication that generational interaction and support were outdated. The pioneering research of Sussman (1953, 1954) initiated a countercurrent of efforts to disprove the nuclear family proposition, through a focus on variables such as residential proximity, exchange of services, and frequency of visits with one's adult children. In more recent years, such reports have been a reaction against the stereotypic view that older adults were virtually dumped into nursing homes by selfish and callous relatives.

6. Even though it is usual for someone to serve as the responsible family member, "the family" may boil down to only one or perhaps a small subset of persons. Unfavourable experiences in other care-giving situations or the lack of support from one's spouse can short-circuit "the family's" ability to provide assistance (Shanas & Sussman 1981). The family support literature is extremely clear on one key

> point -- patterns of interaction among members in the context of assistance to parents or other older members will reflect styles of interpersonal interaction established years before.
>
> 7. Although not yet a demonstrated problem, we will at some point have to deal with the definition of "family member" as it has been affected by divorce and remarriage trends over recent years. The legal issue of grandparents' visitation rights has in fact already become highly salient. The impacts on size of social networks and availability of helpers has still to be determined.

A Recommendation for Study

The above noted pro's and con's of family support are sufficient to prohibit many broad generalisations about what the family can be counted on or expected to do. Therefore, an examination of family effectiveness from the perspective of their capability for penetration into an older member's daily activities may be useful. Such a concept could then be used as a complement to the accessibility aspect of individual preventive/maintenance behaviour, as discussed earlier. In addition, the concept of family penetration capability would be closely related to discussions of person-environment fit in the general gerontological literature (Lawton & Nahemow 1973). Hypotheses regarding the effectiveness of the family could then be developed based upon the degree of fit or match between: 1. the depth of penetration which the target health behaviours have in the individual's daily routine; 2. the accessibility of the behaviour to family involvement, all else being equal; and 3. the family's actual capacity to have access to those behaviours.

Perhaps the most simple dimension, and probably the least useful for determining family capability, would be the number of preventive and health maintenance behaviours which can be assisted. Another dimension would be the discrete as opposed to continuous nature of the preventive or maintenance behaviours being assisted. That is, can the family provide assistance primarily for events that are one-time (e.g., drive to doctor or dentist office, call county health department for information on food nutrients), and/or for activities which may occur much more regularly, perhaps daily (e.g., monitor alcohol or tobacco use, help with relaxation training, monitor food intake)?

The frequency with which assistance can be given may constitute a third aspect of penetration. For example, an individual family member may have low frequency of assistance but with an activity that requires continuous involvement, while another might assist frequently, but only with discrete activities. At issue again is the short- versus long-term nature of the involvement, since an initial pattern of assistance may not be the one which is most feasible over the long run.

The speed with which help can be delivered is rarely analysed in the literature. However, it would seem that delay in the family's ability to give assistance (whether due to distance, conflicting schedules, discrepant perceptions, or competing demands on care-givers) is an important aspect of penetration. Even using these basic dimensions, it may be possible to classify families on their "potential for penetration". An interesting question will be how to integrate the older adult care-receiver into evaluation of the family's potential supportive role. Such a capacity might be short-circuited at the outset by an older adult who is unwilling to accept help, whether overall or in selected circumstances. Controls might also be incorporated for the congruence of perceptions; characteristics of the family environment, and the number of family members who are available to help, insofar as respite from responsibility is possible.

IV. THE PSYCHOLOGY OF HEALTH AND PSYCHOLOGY OF ILLNESS IN LATE LIFE

Research on individual variables or categories of variables will, of course, give necessary and beneficial insights for understanding older adults' preventive and health maintenance behaviours. Most persons are familiar with the conceptual approach of Anderson and Newman (1973) and with the development and refinement of the Health Belief Model (Rosenstock 1966; Becker 1974; Becker & Maiman 1975). In addition, the present writer has collaborated in an effort to integrate a temporal perspective with personal and family health perceptions into a stage- or process-oriented model of late life health behaviour (Rakowski & Hickey 1980). Despite the utility of these and other model frameworks (e.g.,

Fabrega 1973; Igun 1979; Langlie 1979; Suchman 1965), an even broader perspective may have to be adopted in order to guide the interpretation of data, the integration of results from several studies, the development of additional model frameworks, and the design of intervention programs.

In this regard, a distinction between a "psychology of health" and a "psychology of illness" in late life may be helpful. Prevention and health maintenance imply a positive mind-set, one which recognises irreversible impairment if it exists, but still attempts to maximise capabilities. The purposes of establishing a distinction between perceptions of "healthiness" and "unhealthiness" would be:

1. To prevent using the term "health rating" as a subtle euphemism for how sick an individual believes himself to be;
2. To avoid treating health and illness as the two end-points of a single continuum, as if one were the exact and quantitative mirror-image of the other; and
3. To encourage researchers to think in terms of a continuing balance between health and illness perceptions, a balance which appears to be present in the context of chronic impairment.

The nature of many chronic illnesses does not permit a clear definition of oneself as either "sick" or "well." For example, Segall (1976) and Kassebaum and Bauman (1965) have discussed ways in which chronic illness should be viewed as constituting more of an at-risk role rather than as a traditional sick role. Chronic conditions present the individual with the recurrent need to decide whether (or in what ways) he is "really" healthy or unhealthy, perhaps due to acute exacerbations, a change in environmental or social supports which make an impairment more or less evident, and/or an actual deterioration in physical health status.

Literature on coping with chronic illness amply testifies to the significance of the task of "normalising" one's life-style, in order to work with and around any limitations (e.g., Strauss & Glasser 1975; Bregman 1980). A review of numerous reports by this writer yielded the following list of basic questions and tasks faced by the individual:

1. Questions to be answered:

    How much can I really do now? What are my limits? How far do the roots of my problem

extend?
What kind of health trajectory am I on?
What comes next?
Am I still the person I used to be before
the illness?
Which impairments or losses do I deal with
first?
How much about my condition should I
explain to others?
What caused my condition or illness?

2. Tasks faced by the person with chronic
impairment:

Monitor stability and changes in health
status;
Evaluate the importance of any changes for
better or worse;
Separate feelings toward the illness from
feelings toward oneself;
Teach/organise others on how to deal with
the impairment;
Anticipate the future of the condition and
health status; adjust to any uncertainty;
Set priorities for important activities to
maintain, if time must be saved due to
slower pace;
Replace or find alternatives for what has
been lost or given up;
Learn through experience how to deal with
the condition (implies trial-and-error and
creativity);
Evaluate advice from family and friends;
Evaluate the course of any treatments or
therapies;
Maintain motivation to carry out tasks;
View the setting as a challenge, not as a
threat;
Work through "relationships" established
with a machine or prosthetic device;
Maintain sexual identity;
Find a source for emotional release; and
Learn how to talk with health and social
service personnel.

The resolution to many of these issues clearly
implies the need to achieve a balance between
feelings of good- and ill-health. However, both
perceptions can be comparably strong. Therefore, it
may be important to investigate the conditions under
which the balance shifts, with consequent effects on
preventive health behaviour, in addition to simply
correlating individual health and illness indices

with behavioural measures. A parallel set of tasks which might be faced by family care-givers of impaired older members has been abstracted by the present writer (Clark & Rakowski 1983). The literature amply testifies to the delicate balancing act which family members must perform, having strong feelings of responsibility for older relatives' health status, while recognising obvious limitations. In addition, the literature on health professional education often notes the attitudinal and value conflicts engendered by contact with chronically impaired patients/clients. It seems likely, therefore, that the perspectives on prevention held by all of the major parties involved (person, family, provider) might be approached from separate health and illness conceptions.

V. CONCLUDING COMMENTS

One of the subtle threads which runs through the gerontological literature reflects the time-honoured theme of, "Those that have are those that get." There can be few, if any, guarantees that the "good life" or "success" will accompany anyone's chronological aging. If I had to cast my lot, however, with the objective of putting the odds in my favour, I would choose a life-style and personal history characterised by: excellent health, high income, a physically active life-style, extensive formal education, a satisfying marriage which continued for as long as I lived, a flexible personality, and an active informal support network. To the extent that these variables help to define "those that have" throughout earlier decades of life, I would feel that much better prepared to deal with whatever might occur in my old age and have a maximum chance of being one of "those that get" for as long as possible.

Public policy on prevention and health maintenance for later adulthood can not realistically present a blank check to researchers and practitioners, since the objectives of health promotion are open-ended. Yet it would seem that the force of societal trends will require that some policy and resource allocation decisions be made. Preventive and health maintenance behaviours represent knowledge, skills, and habits which individuals must work at achieving, refining, and maintaining, no mattter what age of life. They are among the traits that people must have the resources to "get," rather than "having" simply as a function of inheritance, birth, or luck-of-the-draw. In my opinion, with or without formal societal interventions, there is a risk that succesfully pursuing preventive and health maintenance behaviours will be the luxury of "those older people that have" other advantages of life.

Should such a statement be viewed as unnecessarily skeptical or pessimistic, let us again consider our definition of what constitutes a "preventive/maintenance behaviour," but with an orientation toward the future. It is not beyond the realm of possibility that in our professional judgment, the use of personal microcomputers to plug into a nationwide "Prevention Information Resource Bank" would someday constitute an appropriate activity, and a laudable objective for public policy to foster. On a less ambitious level, perhaps we would advocate for interactive cable television to be used as a home-based preventive behaviour resource. Which older adults would be best prepared to use such tools and, therefore, be at the "cutting edge" of their age group's involvement in prevention? I believe the answer of "those who have the past experience and current resources" would be pretty much on target.

The discussion in this paper has dealt with health perceptions, future outlook, family support and other social support. I have also tried to identify some generic conceptual issues pertinent to specifying characteristics of preventive/maintenance behaviours, to studying the potential effectiveness of the family and other social supports, and to the study of health and illness perceptions. Somewhere in the maze of statistical results and associations, we may find the combinations of antecedent/consequent variables which define "those older people who have" adequate personal and social support resources to be successful in prevention and health maintenance. It will then be up to us to decide how best to assist older persons who do not have those resources.

REFERENCES

Aho, W.R. (1979) "Participation of Senior Citizens in the Swine Flu Inoculation Program: An Analysis of Health Belief Model Variables in Preventive Health Behavior." Journal of Gerontology, 34, 201-208

Anderson, R., & Andersen, O.W. (1979) "Trends in the Use of Health Services." In: H.E. Freeman, S. Levine, & L.G. Reeder (Eds.), Handbook of Medical Sociology, Third Edition, Englewood Cliffs: Prentice-Hall

Anderson, R., & Newman, J.F. (1973) "Social and Individual Determinants of Medical Care Utilization in the United States." Milbank Memorial Fund Quarterly, 51, (Winter), 95-124

Becker, M.H. (Ed.) (1974) "The Health Belief Model and Personal Health Behavior." Health Education Monographs, 2

Becker, M.H., & Maiman, L.A. (1975) "Sociobehavioral Determinants of Compliance with Health and Medical Care Recommendations." Medical Care, 13, 10-24

Belloc, N.B. (1973) "Relationship of Health Practices and Mortality." Preventive Medicine, 2, 67-81

Belloc, N.B., & Breslow, L. (1972) "Relationship of Physical Health Status and Health Practices." Preventive Medicine, 1, 409-421

Blenkner, M. (1965) "Social Work and Family Relationships on Later Life with Some Thoughts on Filial Maturity." In: E. Shanas & G.F. Streib (Eds.), Social Structure and the Family. Englewood Cliffs: Prentice-Hall

Bortner, R.W., & Hultsch, D.F. (1974) "Patterns of Subjective Deprivation in Adulthood." Developmental Psychology, 10, 534-545

Branch, L.G., & Jette, A.M. (1982) "A Prospective Study of Long-term Care Institutionalization among the Aged." American Journal of Public Health, 72, 1373-1379

Brand, F.N., & Smith, R.T. (1974) "Medical Care and Compliance among the Elderly after Hospitalization." International Journal of Aging and Human Development, 5, 331-346

Bregman, A.M. (1980) "Living with Progressive Childhood Illness: Parental Management of Progressive Neuromuscular Disease." Social Work in Health Care, 5, 387-408

Breslow, L., & Enstrom, J.E. (1980) "Persistence of Health Habits and Their Relationship to Mortality." Preventive Medicine, 9, 469-483

Brody, E.M. (1981) "Women in the Middle and Family Help to Old People." The Gerontologist, 21, 471-480

Brody, E.M., & Kleban, M.H. (1981) "Physical and Mental Health Symptoms of Older People: Who Do They Tell?" Journal of the American Geriatrics Society, 29, 442-449

Brody, E.M., & Kleban, M.H. (1983) "Day-to-day Mental and Physical Health Symptoms of Older People: A Report on Health Logs." The Gerontologist, 23, 64-70

Brody, S.J., Poulshock, S.W., & Masciocchi, C.F. (1978) "The Family Caring Unit: A Major Consideration in the Long-term Support System." The Gerontologist, 18, 556-561

Cantor, M.H. (1979) "The Informal Support Network of New York's Inner City Elderly: Is Ethnicity a Factor?" In: D.E. Gelfand & A.J. Kutzik (Eds.), Ethnicity and Aging: Theory, Research, and Policy. New York: Springer

Cantor, M., & Mayer, M. (1976) "Health and the Inner City Elderly." The Gerontologist, 16 (1, part 1), 17-24

Cantor, M.H., & Mayer, M.J. (1978) "Factors in Differential Utilization of Services by Urban Elderly." Journal of Gerontological Social Work, 1, 47-61

Carp, F.M., & Kataoka, E. (1976) "Health Care Problems of the Elderly of San Francisco's Chinatown." The Gerontologist, 1 (1, part 1), 30-38

Celetano, D.D., Shapiro, S., & Weisman, C.S. (1982) "Cancer Prevention Screening Behaviour among Elderly Women." Preventive Medicine, 11, 454-463

Cheung, L.Y., Cho, E.R., Lum, D., Tang, T., & Yau, H.B. (1980) "The Chinese Elderly and Family Structure: Implications for Health Care." Public Health Reports, 95, 491-495

Cicerelli, V.G. (1981) Helping Elderly Parents: The Role of Adult Children. Boston: Auburn House

Clark, N.M., & Rakowski, W. (1983) "Family Caregivers of Older Adults: Improving Helping Skills." The Gerontologist, 23, 637-642

Coulton, C., & Frost, A.K. (1982) "Use of Social and Health Services by the Elderly." Journal of Health and Social Behavior, 23, 330-339

Davis, M.A., & Randall, E. (1983) "Social Change and Food Habits of the Elderly." In: M.W. Riley, B.B. Hess, & K. Bond (Eds.), Aging in Society: Selected Reviews of Recent Research. Hillsdale, N.J.: Lawrence Erlbaum Associates

Fabrega, H. (1973) "Toward a Model of Illness Behavior." Medical Care, 11, 470-484

Farkas, S.W. (1980) "Impact of Chronic Illness on the Patient's Spouse." Health and Social Work, 5, 39-46

Fengler, A.P., & Goodrich, N. (1979) "Wives of Elderly Disabled Men: The Hidden Patients." The Gerontologist, 19, 175-183

Ferraro, K.F. (1980) "Self-ratings of Health among the Old and the Old-old." Journal of Health and Social Behavior, 21, 377-382

Fillenbaum, G.G. (1979) "Social Context and Self-assessments of Health among the Elderly." Journal of Health and Social Behavior, 20, 45-51

Filner, B. & Williams, T.F. (1979) "Health Promotion for the Elderly: Reducing Functional Dependency." In: Healthy People -- The Surgeon General's Report on Health Promotion and Disease Prevention, Background Papers, 1979. DHEW Publication No. (PHS) 79-55071. Public Health Service, Washington, D.C.: U.S. Government Printing Office, July 1979

German, P.S., Shapiro, S., Chase, G.A., & Vollmer, M.H. (1978) "Health Care of the Elderly in Medically Disadvantaged Populations." The Gerontologist, 18, 547-555

Gorman, B.S., & Wessman, A.E. (Eds.) (1977) The Personal Experience of Time. New York: Plenum

Graney, M.J., & Zimmerman, R.M. (1980-1981) "Causes and Consequences of Health Self-report Variations among Older People." International Journal of Aging and Human Development, 12, 291-300

Harris, D.M., & Guten, S. (1979) "Health-protective Behavior: An Exploratory Study." Journal of Health and Social Behavior, 20, 17-29

Haug, M. (1979) "Age and Medical Care Patterns." Paper Presented at the 1979 annual meeting of the Gerontological Society of America, Washington, D.C., November

Hausman, C.P. (1979) "Short-term Counseling Groups for People with Elderly Parents." The Gerontologist, 19, 102-107

Hultsch, D.F., & Bortner, R.W. (1974) "Personal Time Perspective in Adulthood: A Time Sequential Study." Developmental Psychology, 10, 534-545

Igun, U.A. (1979) "Stages in Health-seeking: A Descriptive Model." Social Science and Medicine, 13A, 445-456

Johnson, E.S., & Bursk, B.J. (1977) "Relationships between the Elderly and their Adult Children." The Gerontologist, 177, 90-96

Kart, C. (1981) "Experiencing Symptoms: Attribution and Misattribution of Illness among the Aged." In: M. Haug (Ed.), Elderly Patients and their Doctors. New York: Springer

Kasl, S.V., & Cobb, S. (1966) "Health Behavior, Illness Behavior and Sick Role Behavior: I. Health and Illness Behavior." Archives of Environmental Health, 12, 246-266

Kastenbaum, R.J. (1977) "Memories of Tomorrow: On the Interpenetration of Time and Later Life." In: B.S. Gorman & A.E. Wessman (Eds.), The Personal Experience of Time. New York: Plenum

Kastenbaum. R.J. (1982) "Time Course and Time Perspective in Later Life." Chap. 4 in, C. Eisdorfer (Ed.), Annual Review of Gerontology and Geriatrics: Volume 3, 1982. New York: Springer

Kassebaum, G.G., & Bauman, B.O. (1965) "Dimensions of the Sick Role in Chronic Illness." Journal of Health and Human Behavior, 6, 16-27

Kleinman, J.C., & Kopstein, A. (1981) "Who Is Being Screened for Cervical Cancer?" American Journal of Public Health, 71(1), 73-76

Lairson, D.R., & Swint, J.M. (1978) "A Multivariate Analysis of the Likelihood and Volumne of Preventive Visit Demand in a Prepaid Group Practice." Medical Care, 16, 730-739

Langlie, J.K. (1977) "Social Networks, Health Beliefs, and Preventive Health Behavior." Journal of Health and Social Behavior, 18, 244-260

Larson, R. (1978) "Thirty Years of Research on the Subjective Well-being of Older Americans." Journal of Gerontology, 33, 109-129

LaRue, A., Bank, L., Jarvik, L., & Hetland, M. (1979) "Health in Old Age: How Do Physicians' Ratings and Self-ratings Compare?" Journal of Gerontology, 34, 687-691

Lau, R.R., & Hartman, K.A. "Common-sense Representations of Common Illness." Health Psychology, 2, 167-185

Lawton, M.P., & Nahemow, L. (1973) "Ecology and the Aging Process." In: C. Eisdorfer & M.P. Lawton (Eds.), The Psychology of Adult Development and Aging. Washington, D.C.: American Psychological Association

Levenson, H. (1973) "Multidimensional Locus of Control in Psychiatric Patients." Journal of Consulting and Clinical Psychology, 41, 397-404

Levenson, H. (1981) "Differentiating among Internality, Powerful Others, and Chance." In: H. Lefcourt (Ed.), Research with the Locus of Control Construct (Vol. 1). New York: Academic Press

Leventhal, H., & Hirschman, R.S. (1982) "Social Psychology and Prevention." In: G.S. Sanders & J. Suls (Eds.), Social Psychology of Health and Illness. Hillsdale, N.J.: Lawrence Erlbaum Associates

Linn, M.W., Hunter, K.I., & Linn, B.S. (1980) "Self-assessed Health, Impairment and Disability in Anglo, Black, and Cuban Elderly." Medical Care, 18, 282-288

Linn, B.S., & Linn, M.W. (1980) "Objective and Self-assessed Health in the Old and Very Old." Social Science and Medicine, 14, 311-315

Linn, B.S., Linn, M.W., & Knopka, F. (1978) "The Very Old Patient in Ambulatory Care." Medical Care, 16, 604-610

Linn, M.W., Linn, B.S., & Stein, S.R. (1982) "Satisfaction with Ambulatory Care and Compliance in Older Patients." Medical Care, 20, 606-614

Litman, T.J. (1971) "Health Care and the Family: A Three Generational Analysis." Medical Care, 9, 67-81

Maddox, G., & Douglass, E. (1973) "Self-assessment of Health: A Longitudinal Study of Elderly Subjects." Journal of Health and Social Behavior, 14, 87-93

Markson, E.W. (1973) "Readjustment to Time in Old Age: A Life Cycle Approach." Psychiatry, 36, 37-48

Mancini, J.A., & Quinn, W.H. (1981) "Dimensions of Health and Their Importance for Morale in Old Age: A Multivariate Examination." Journal of Community Health, 118-128

Markides, K.S., & Martin, H.W. (1979) "Predicting Self-related Health among the Aged." Research on Aging, 1, 97-112

Matarazzo, J.D. (1982) "Behavioral Health's Challenge to Academic, Scientific, and Professional Psychology." American Psychologist, 37, 1-14

Minkler, M. (1978) "Health Attitudes and Beliefs of the Urban Elderly." Public Health Reports, 93, 426-432. 8, 147-165

Mishara, B.L., & Kastenbaum, R. (1980) Alcohol and Old Age. New York: Grune & Stratton

National Center for Health Statistics, U.S. Department of H.H.S (1980) Advancedata, Number 64, November 4, 1980; HHS Publication No. 81-1250

National Center for Health Statistics, U.S. Department of H.H.S. (1981) Advancedata, Number 69, April 1, 1981; HHS Publication No. (PHS) 81-1250

National Center for Health Statistics, U.S. Department of H.E.W. (1977) Vital and Health Statistics. Series 10, Number 110, March 1977, DHEW Publication No. (HRA) 77-1538

National Center for Health Statistics, U.S. Department of H.H.S. (1981) Vital and Health Statistics. Series 13, Number 59, August 1981, DHHS Publication No. (PHS) 81-1720

National Institute on Alcohol Abuse and Alcoholism (1982) NIAAA Information and Feature Service. December 31, 1982

Newton, F. C-R. (1980) "Issues in Research and Service Delivery among Mexican-American Elderly: A Concise Statement with Recommendations." The Gerontologist, 20, 208-213

Nydegger, C.N. (1983) "Family Ties of the Aged in Cross-cultural Perspective." The Gerontologist, 23, 26-32

Posner, B.M. (1979) Nutrition and the Elderly. Lexington, Mass.: Lexington Books

Rakowski, W. (1979) "Future Time Perspective in Later Adulthood: Review and Research Directions." Experimental Aging Research, 5, 43-88

Rakowski, W. (1982) "Temporal Context and the Perceptions of Geriatric Patients." Social Science and Medicine, 16, 241-244

Rakowski, W. (1983) "Research Issues in Health Promotion with Older Adults." Paper presented at the annual meeting of the National Council on the Aging, Detroit, MI, March

Rakowski, W., & Dengiz, A.N. (1984) "A Health Belief Interview for Clinical Geriatrics." The Gerontologist, 24, 120-123

Rakowski, W., & Hickey, T. (1980) "Late Life Health Behavior: Integrating Health Beliefs and Temporal Perspectives." Research on Aging, 2, 283-308

Rakowski, W., & Hickey, T. (1981) "A Brief Lifegraph Technique for Work with Geriatric Patients." Journal of the American Geriatrics Society, 29, 373-378

Rakowski, W., & Hickey, T. (1983) "Geriatric Patients and Family Resource Persons: Examining Congruence of Health Beliefs and Temporal Perspective." Interdisciplinary Topics in Gerontology, vol. 17, 1-9

Rakowski, W., Hickey, T., & Dengiz, A.N. "Congruence of Health and Treatment Perceptions among Older Patients and Providers of Primary Care." Manuscript in preparation.

Reifler, B.V., Cox, G.B., & Hanley, R.J. (1981) "Problems of the Mentally Ill Elderly as Perceived by Patients, Families, and Clinicians." The Gerontologist, 21, 165-170

Rosenstock, I.M. (1966) "Why People Use Health Services." Milbank Memorial Fund Quarterly, 44 (part 2), 94-127

Rundall, T.G., & Wheeler, J.R.C. (1979) "Factors Associated with Utilization of the Swine Flu Vaccination Program among Senior Citizens in Tompkins County." Medical Care, 17, 191-200

Segall, A. (1976) "The Sick Role Concept: Understanding Illness Behavior." Journal of Health and Social Behavior, 17, 163-170

Shanas, E. (1979) "The Family as a Social Support System in Old Age." The Gerontologist, 19, 169-174

Shanas, E. (1980) "Older People and Their Families: The New Pioneers." Journal of Marriage and the Family, 42, 9-15

Shanas, E., & Sussman, M.B. (1981) "The Family in Later Life: Social Structure and Social Policy." In: R.W. Fogel, E. Hatfield, S.B. Kiesler, & E. Shanas (Eds.), Aging: Stability and Change in the Family. New York: Academic Press

Silverstone, B., & Hyman, H.K. (1982) You and Your Aging Parent. New York: Pantheon

Snider, E.L. (1980) "Factors Influencing Health Service Knowledge among the Elderly." Journal of Health and Social Behavior, 21, 371-377

Stanford, E.P. (1978) The Elder Black. San Diego: Campanile Press

Stoller, E.P., & Earl, L.L. (1983) "Help with Activities of Everyday Life: Sources of Support for the Noninstitutionalized Elderly." The Gerontologist, 23, 64-70

Strauss, A.L., & Glaser, B.G. (Eds.) (1975) Chronic Illness and the Quality of Life. St. Louis: C.V. Mosby

Suchman, E.A. (1965) "Stages of Illness and Medical Care." Journal of Health and Human Behavior, 6, 2-16

Sussman, M.B. (1953) "The Help Pattern in the Middle Class Family." American Sociological Review, 18, 22-28

Sussman, M.B. (1954) "Family Continuity: Selective Factors which Affect Relationships between Families as Generational Levels." Marriage and Family Living, 16, 112-120

Sussman, M.B., & Burchinal, L. (1962) "Kin Family Network: Unheralded Structure in Current Conceptualizations of Family Functioning." Marriage and Family Living, 24, 231-240

Tissue, T. (1972) "Another Look at Self-rated Health among the Elderly." Journal of Gerontology, 27, 91-94

Treas, J. (1977) "Family Support Systems for the Aged: Some Social and Demographic Considerations." The Gerontologist, 17, 486-491

U.S. Department of H.E.W. (1980) Health: United States 1979. Public Health Service, Office of Health Research, Statistics, and Technology; DHEW Publication No. (PHS) 80-1232

U.S. Department of H.E.W. (1979) Healthy People -- The Surgeon General's Report on Health Promotion and Disease Prevention, Background Papers, 1979. DHEW Publication No. (PHS) 79-55071. Public Health Service, Washington, D.C.: U.S. Government Printing Office, July

U.S. Department of H.H.S. (1980) Health: United States 1980. Public Health Service, Office of Health Research, Statistics, and Techology; DHHS Publication No. (PHS) 81-1232, December, 1980 (a)

U.S. Department of H.H.S. (1980) Promoting Health/ Preventing Disease: Objectives for the Nation. Public Health Service, Washington, D.C.: U.S. Government Printing Office, 1980 (b)

Valle, R., & Mendoza, L. (1978) The Elder Latino. San Diego: Campanile

Ward, R.A. (1978) "Limitations of the Family as a Supportive Institution in the Lives of the Aged." Family Coordinator, 27, 365-374

Wallston, K.A., & Wallston, B.S. (1982) "Who Is Responsible for Your Health? The Construct of Health Locus of Control." In: G.S. Sanders & J. Suls (Eds.), Social Psychology of Health and Illness. Hillsdale, N.J.: Lawrence Erlbaum Associates

Chapter 6

ILLNESS BEHAVIOUR IN THE ELDERLY

Graeme G. Ford

INTRODUCTION

In a recent article, Mechanic defines illness behaviour as:

> ... the manner in which persons monitor their bodies, define and interpret their symptoms, take remedial action and utilise the health-care system.
> (Mechanic 1982)

Put simply, the study of illness behaviour recognises the fact that even in societies with highly evolved systems of health care, the over-whelming majority of symptoms experienced are not presented for medical evaluation; the decision to seek medical aid is only one possible outcome in a complex process of assessment and decision-making which is shaped by culture, attitudes, folk medical knowledge, personal biography, influence from social networks, present goals and perceptions of the costs and benefits of entering the "sick role," as well as by the inherent ambiguity of most symptoms them-selves. Most medical decision-making is done by laymen and not by medical practitioners. The extent to which illness is "private business" has been documented over the last 30 years in a number of important population studies (Pearse and Crockel 1944, Wadsworth & al. 1971, Dunnell and Cartwright 1972, Hannay 1979) which have shown that, typically, only between 1/3 and 1/4 of reported illness episodes led to medical consultation and, further-more, that consultation is only loosely related to the medically defined severity or experience of discomfort of the symptoms.

130

From a medical point of view the recognition of the extent of lay illness behaviour represents a problem. There is a widespread frustration with "inappropriate" patterns of use of medical services; identified and treated illness is seen to be the tip of a vast "clinical iceberg" of untreated disease blocked from the practitioner by (from a narrowly medical point of view" "irrational" consultation patterns of patients, while at the same time doctors complain endlessly about the volume of consultation for clinically trivial, self-limiting or otherwise untreatable complaints (Dunnell and Cartwright 1972).

Much of the work by sociologists has accepted this medicalised "social problem" definition of illness behaviour and has concentrated on unravelling the complexities of variations in help-seeking behaviour, but others have argued for a sociology of health behaviour which takes a standpoint separate from that defined by medical interests. As West expresses it:

> ... This shift has involved a reformulation of the problem from one in which the task was viewed as the identification of social and psychological variables that impeded the (irrational) proto-patient from doing what he ought to do - consult the doctor - to another in which much greater attention is directed to the person as a conscious, reflective actor engaged in the process of making sense of various kinds of body changes within the framework of his own "lay knowledge."

Lay knowledge and the process of lay decision-making is seen as a part of an organised set of behaviour with its own internal logic, a logic which demands separate sociological analysis without which illness behaviour will necessarily remain un-interpretable and, from a purely medical viewpoint, irrational.

Because of this overlapping of practical and theoretical interest, there is a vast and growing body of literature on illness behaviour, but surprisingly few studies deal directly with the elderly. The neglect of age as a possible base for investigating illness behaviour is particularly surprising in view of the current high visibility of the elderly as a special group within the health field.

The following reviews the rather limited

information available on the illness behaviour of the elderly and outlines some of the sociological elements in the illness process. In the first section we aim to establish some basic facts in order to dispel some prevalent stereotypes and as a commentary on the medical image of the elderly as a "problem" group. The second section outlines some important sociological factors in explaining illness behaviour as a base from which to consider just how the illness behaviour of the elderly might differ from that of younger populations. Throughout, we concentrate on the non-institutionalised, mentally well-functioning elderly as institutionalised or confused old people raise issues beyond the scope of traditional illness behaviour research.

THE ELDERLY AS CONSULTERS: THE MEDICAL "PROBLEM"

If sociologists have not attended to age when researching illness behaviour, those who frame policies and deliver services for the elderly do necessarily apply implicit assumptions about illness behaviour amongst the elderly. The increasing demand for screening and surveillance of the old by gerontologists and those interested in the health care of the elderly clearly rests on a belief that the usual self-referral basis for medical care delivery is inappropriate for this group, that in some way the submerged "iceberg" of unidentified need is especially large and especially invidious. This assumption is partly borne out by screening exercises. There are certainly a considerable number of unidentified medical conditions among the elderly. However, this does not necessarily imply a vast reservoir of unnecessary suffering. A recent Oxford study identified an average of 2.6 conditions per elderly patient, one of which, on average, was unknown to the practitioner, and a high proportion of these conditions were amenable to some medical amelioration. The authors remark, though:

> ... Patients were well adapted in most cases to their problems so that the quality of life of these old people was relatively unimpaired. Only 10% were poorly adjusted to their problem. (Tulloch and Moore 1979)

The medical view seems to be framed by the particular nature of risk amongst the elderly as much as by clear evidence of widespread general medical neglect. There does seem to be a greater fragility in the system of functioning of the elderly and a greater likelihood of the emergence of what is sometimes described as "the Social Breakdown Syndrome" (Kuypers and Bengtson 1973). Undoubtedly, many old people do present to clinicians in distressing states of unnecessary collapse. Williamson has expressed something of the frustration and bafflement which confronts the clinician approaching the elderly with a set of medically defined expectations when he asks rhetorically:

> ... Why is it that many old people seem to behave in this rather irrational and obstinate fashion and fail to report significant disabilities to their doctors?
> (Williamson 1981)

He then proceeds to answer his own question in terms of a range of factors which he speculates will cause the elderly to underconsult. They include the tendency to ascribe remediable illness to the inevitable decline of old age, overdeference of the elderly towards their doctor, fear of the implication of accepting the definition of being ill with its connotations of incompetence, and the less severe implications for normal functioning posed by illness in the case of the elderly as compared with younger working age groups. All these are, of course, plausible but for the most part they are unsubstantiated by any solid research, and together, they contribute to the rather undifferentiated image held by many practitioners of the elderly as inexplicably irrational and inefficient utilisers of services and, as a consequence, a problem to themselves.

The Relationship of Health to Ageing - The Overall Picture

We now examine what we know about the illness and consultation behaviour of the elderly to see what we know about its distinctness from the younger adult population, to look for internal differentiation within the elderly, and to consider whether the medical stereotype of older people as inefficient services users can, in fact, be upheld.

A small number of rather incontrovertible facts about the elderly strongly shape our expectations. The elderly do make very heavy demands on the health services. Table 6.1 shows just how disproportionate these demands are. This is not, however, to demonstrate that many elderly people in the community receive large numbers of services. Table 6.1 also shows the penetration of services discovered by a recent population survey of the elderly in Aberdeen (1).

A second fact which is in the forefront of our minds when we think of the health of the elderly is the change in the nature of the health problems they experience. We all know that the elderly experience far more conditions of a longstanding chronic nature than do younger population groups, and we extrapolate from this changes in the nature of the demands they make on services from cure to care.

In Britain, The General Household Survey is a prime source of information on differences in the health and crude health seeking behaviour of different age groups within the population. Table 6.2 gives some of the basic trends. The proportion of the population suffering from chronic conditions can, indeed, be seen to rise steadily throughout the life-span until by the age of 75, 56 percent of men and 64 percent of women report some longstanding ailment. Evidence from other surveys, specifically of the elderly, suggests that the GHS figures may be a considerable underestimate. Using essentially the same questions, but with the additions of some more open-ended categories, the Aberdeen study found only 19 percent of those aged 60 to 75 who claimed to be entirely free from chronic illness and less than eight percent for those over 75 (Taylor and Ford 1983 a). This seems to be essentially in agreement with findings from a previous English study (Abrams 1978).

Not only does the overall incidence of chronic illness increase, but the proportion of individuals with multiple conditions rises. Again, in the Aberdeen sample, the proportion who suffered from four or more longstanding conditions rose from 17 percent in the younger half of the sample to 32 percent of the "old" elderly. Evidence from screening studies suggests that these self-reported figures do have a grounding in increases in underlying disease. Williamson & al., in their classic early study, found an average of 3.3 clinical conditions per old person. This compares with 2.3 diseases per person in a similar study of middle-aged respondents (South-East London Screening Study Group 1979). Equally important, the nature of the conditions differed somewhat. In the middle-aged sample 95 percent of conditions were considered to

Table 6.1: Service Usage by the Elderly

(a) Service Use by Elderly Persons

Percent over 65 in population (1)	14%
Percent of consultations due to 65 plus (2)	40%
Total bed days (3)	48%
Beds "blocked" by elderly (4)	36%

(1) Source: RG Scotland Annual Report, HMSO, 1980, Table N2.2
(2) Source: Trends in General Practice, 1977, RCGP, p. 50
(3) Figures for Edinburgh Royal Infirmary, 1976 - Kinnaird & al. "The provision of care for the elderly," p. 23
(4) Figures for Scotland: source fact sheet RCP conference "Appropriate Care for the Elderly," Edinburgh, 22 October 1980

(b) Ratio of Use by Persons Aged 75> to those Aged 65-74

Health Visitor	2.3
District Nurse	3.4
Chiropodist	5.3
Home Help	4.1
Meals-on-Wheels	2.7
Residential Care	6.5
Psychiatric Hospital	3.3
Other Hospitals	6.5
GP Consultations	1.2
GP Home Visits	1.7

Source: The Provision of Care for the Elderly, J. Kinnaird, Sir John Brotherson and J. Williamson (eds.), Churchill Livingstone, 1981, p. 10

(c) Percentage of Aberdeen Elderly Receiving Services

Home Help	10.5
Meals-on-Wheels	1.6
Regular Visits from *	
- GP	10.8
- Health Visitor/Nurse	18.4

* 3 or more times a year

Source: Aberdeen "Styles of Ageing" Survey, 1980

Table 6.2: Percentages with Chronic and Acute Illness and
Consultation Patterns

	Chronic Conditions	Acute Illness	Outpatients	Consultations (Av. No. per year)
MALES				
15-44	21	10	11	2.7
45-64	39	14	13	4.4
65-74	50	12	15	4.6
75+	56	17	13	5.2
FEMALES				
15-44	20	13	12	4.8
45-64	38	14	13	4.3
65-74	52	16	16	5.1
75+	64	22	16	8.0

Source: The General Household Survey, 1979, HMSO, Tables
7.1, 7.12, 7.13

be minor, while in the case of the elderly 8.5 percent were considered to be severe and 12.5 percent were either moderate or severe. The ageing effects seem clear if not perhaps dramatic. We can see from Table 6.2 that the trend is slight through adulthood and only shows a marked increase after 75. Consultation patterns generally follow the age-related increase in chronic and acute conditions. Interestingly, outpatient referrals show no increase with age; indeed, they fall significantly for elderly males. This may lend some weight to the idea that practitioners are even more pessimistic about the possibility of successful intervention with the elderly than are the elderly themselves (Haugh (ed.) 1981 - various contributions).

Differentiating Approaches to Illness and Ageing

Clearly, a slow but definite increase in illness is experienced by the elderly, both chronic and acute, with a consequent change in consulting behaviour, and the figures reveal sex differentials which persist pretty much unchanged throughout the life-span. But to what extent is this decline in health shared by all the elderly?

In a recent paper, Roos and Shapiro report on a Canadian study which investigates differentiation in service use by the elderly (Ross and Shapiro 1981). The study utilised the master register of the Manitoba Provincial Health Insurance Commission. As payments to physicians are conditional on returning claims for all patient contacts, the register represents an accurate source of information on Canadian service use. The basic aim was to discover whether the known high usage of services by the elderly arises from a heightened demand by old people in general or whether a minority of the elderly consume a disproportionately high share of services. They extracted consultation records on almost five thousand elderly individuals for two consecutive years. The variables which they considered were "number of ambulatory visits" and "total days in hospital." As might be expected, there were considerable variations in use; 1/5 of the sample never visited the doctor in the study period while, at the other extreme, eight percent of the sample accounted for 35 percent of all visits. The pattern for hospital use was more differentiated still, with 4/5 of the sample reporting not hospital treatment and three percent using a massive 47 percent of all hospital days. Ten percent, in fact, accounted for 78 percent of all hospitalisation.

More interestingly, they were able to investigate consistency over time. The correlation between visits in year one and in year two was 0.64, indicating a high degree of stability in patterns of use. Less than nine percent of those who had been high users (7 or more annual visits) initially were low users (2 or less visits) in year two, and only eight percent of low users moved into the high user category. The pattern for hospitalisation was less clear-cut; 83 percent of those with no hospital experience in year one had none in year two while of those in the high use group, approximately half required no treatment in the second year. On the other hand, 1/4 of those who were very high users in the period remained high users. What seems to be suggested is an irreducible core of high hospital users with a large pool at risk of hospitalisation at some time. (Thirty-two percent had some hospital experience in the two years of the study.) Hospitalisation, even for considerable periods of time, is followed by return to the category of non-user for most people. Physician contact did not change with age to any significant degree but hospitalisation showed a large age effect. Those 85+ had three times as many days in hospital as did those aged from 65 to 69. The authors conclude

> ... The elderly are not, as has often been assumed, high users of ambulatory care and hospital days. Instead, a small proportion of elderly persons use a great deal of health care and account for a disproportionately large share of service utilisation. (2)

This bifurcation is very much the pattern revealed by previous studies of younger samples; indeed, some earlier work suggests a positive polarisation in old age with the proportion of very high and very low users both increasing (Densen & al. 1959).

Perhaps the most widespread assumption made about the elderly and their health behaviour concerns the tendency to misascribe symptoms of remediable illness to the inevitable decline into old age and to endure discomfort unnecessarily. At the same time the chronic nature of much of the disease experienced by this group is believed to exacerbate this tendency to underutilisation. Chronic conditions present symptoms continuously or episodically over a period of time and advances in the condition are likely to be slow and incremental.

Many studies have described the process of "normalisation" of chronic complaints, levels of symptomatology unacceptable to those free from such conditions become defined as the normal baseline of good health, warranting no medical actions. For both these reasons, the elderly are considered to be particularly prone to suffer ailments without seeking help.

The Canadian study dispelled some of the stereotypical images of the elderly as an undifferentiated group, but the analysis of use was not grounded in any investigation of underlying need. In a recent study in Glasgow, Hannay looked at what he calls "incongruous" consultation, both "trivial" presentation and the "clinical iceberg" of apparently serious needs which is not brought to the practitioner (Hannay 1979). Starting from a comprehensive symptom checklist, he looked at the relationship between symptom experience and consultation taking into account the patient's own estimate of the seriousness and painfulness of the symptoms. Symptoms identified as serious but not acted on contribute to the iceberg, while consultations for symptoms which are not felt to be serious are considered to be trivial. In a sample of 1,183, 88 percent had one or more symptoms in the two weeks preceding the interview, with an average of five per person. Approximately 1/3 of them led to consultation. Twenty-six percent of all symptoms fell within the definition of the clinical iceberg and a further 11 percent constituted trivial consultations. Hannay found that females are consistently more inclined to underconsult than males at all ages, but the effects of age are complex. Females are more likely to underconsult in the 30 to 45 age band than at any other time. In both males and females, the elderly are less likely to form part of the iceberg of unmet need than the middle aged. For trivia there is a pretty steady increase throughout the life span with elderly females especially likely to consult for non-serious conditions.

In Hannay's study the elderly are treated as an undifferentiated group but, as we have already seen, it is increasingly clear that age divisions within the elderly are in some directions more significant than differences between the elderly as a whole and younger age groups. Increasingly, it is suggested that we need to distinguish between the "young" old and the "old" old. The figures from the General Household Survey clearly reveal a substantial increase in reported illness for those over 75, and we can use the data from the Aberdeen survey to investigate the more detailed age differences within the elderly. Table 6.3 shows the mean number of symptoms reported in a period of a month, broken down by sex in five-year age bands. It also gives the ratio of symptoms to symptoms consulted over (3). The number of symptoms reported by both sexes climbs steadily with age. Considering the consultation ratios, we see that the familiar figure of one consultation for every three conditions holds for this elderly sample, and there appears to be no age change in this figure. There may be some tendency for females to underconsult in the mid-period, but in general, the tendency to consult for symptoms recorded is the same for both sexes, despite the higher overall level of symptoms experienced by females. Table 6.3 also presents data for chronic conditions identified and gives a consultation ratio for those over the preceding twelve months. There is a more evident age gradient than there was for acute conditions in numbers of conditions reported. The gain is not dramatic in extreme old age but rather constant throughout the age range. On average, the sample had contacted their doctors for one out of every two chronic conditions reported in the last year and, again, it is hard to detect any clear pattern by age. Females, again, report considerably higher levels of chronic illness at all ages, but there is no sex difference in the tendency to consult.

Most of the literature presupposes the emergence of illness out of generally good health, so it is interesting to use this data to examine what happens to consultation for acute symptoms in the presence of recognised longstanding illness. The argument is often heard that the elderly will tend to ignore many symptoms as they will have learned to tolerate generally poor health. We can see a very strong association between number of symptoms and chronic conditions. Of course, they are not mutually exclusive, but the symptom list consisted predominantly of the sorts of ailments, e.g. headaches, diarrhoea and so on, which are not usually ascribed to chronic conditions. Those with no chronic conditions report few symptoms and seem to form a health elite. Furthermore, those with few chronic conditions are less likely to consult over the symptoms they do have. In the presence of any chronic illness the number of chronic illnesses seems to make no difference to the tendency to

Table 6.3: Symptoms, Chronic Conditions and Consultation Ratios, by Sex and Age Band

(a)

Age	Symptoms		Consultation Ratio		Number	
	M	F	M	F	M	F
59-64	1.8	2.8	3.5	3.6	58	61
65-69	2.7	2.8	2.8	3.6	55	54
70-74	2.2	3.3	2.9	4.1	60	54
75-79	2.6	4.2	2.8	2.9	48	53
80-84	2.4	4.1	2.7	3.0	57	49
85+	2.2	2.7	3.6	3.2	35	35

(b)

Age	Chronic Conditions		Consultation Ratio		Number	
	M	F	M	F	M	F
59-64	1.6	2.0	1.6	2.3	58	61
65-69	1.9	2.1	2.1	2.1	55	54
70-74	1.7	2.9	2.5	1.8	60	54
75-79	2.0	3.6	1.7	1.8	48	53
80-84	2.4	3.0	1.8	1.6	57	49
85+	2.5	3.0	2.3	2.4	35	35

(c)

Chronic Conditions	Symptoms	Consultation Ratio	Number
0	0.8	5.5	95
1	1.8	3.4	126
2-3	3.0	3.0	255
4+	5.3	3.3	127

Source: Aberdeen "Styles of Ageing" Study, 1980

consult. If we further break down the analysis by age (not shown) we see that where few or no chronic conditions exist, the <u>very</u> elderly are less likely to attend to recent symptoms, but where there are a number of chronic conditions, they are more likely to seek help for symptoms.

Little support can be taken from the figures, then, for the idea of a general tendency towards declining attention to symptoms as a function of ageing or for "normalising" ill health in the presence of chronic illness. If anything, there is a suggestion that chronic ill health sensitises people to the need to attend to symptoms and that this may even increase in old age.

Neither are the elderly found to be pessimistic about their health. In the Aberdeen study the respondents were presented with a number of attitudinal items on health activism and optimism. They were found to exhibit a remarkably high level of both optimism and active orientation with no apparent age gradient. This finding has been universally upheld by studies using similar attitude items.

However, neither do the elderly ignore minor everyday aches and pains. Both Hannay in Britain and Haug in the USA found that the elderly showed a general inclination to present "trivial" conditions more than other age bands, and Cartwright and Anderson report that the elderly are less worried about consulting their doctors for trivial conditions than are younger age groups (Cartwright and Anderson 1981).

All the evidence presented so far suggests that the illness behaviour of the elderly shows strong continuity with that of the younger groups; changes are changes of degree rather than kind. Old people are every bit as varied in their illness experiences and service use. They show no clear tendency to underconsult, in contrast to the tendency of the population as a whole, and they appear to attend to the symptoms they have to roughly the same degree, whatever their age. Of course, figures like these must be treated cautiously, for there are considerable methodological difficulties. A general inclination may exist in older people to report fewer symptoms in an interview situation, and we must continually be aware that population surveys of the elderly lose more severe cases through institutionalisation and non-response. However, little objective support seems to exist for some of the popular stereotypes of illness behaviour of the elderly in the community.

The Remaining Problem

Having said this, we have to take note of the clinical experience which argues that when the elderly do become a problem, they do so in ways which can be especially difficult to deal with. They may pose unique problems which are particularly intractable, and they do make disproportionately large demands on the health services as a result.

We are unlikely to be able to explain the particular problem of the elderly in terms of their general illness behaviour. Rather, we should focus on the way in which the special problem of uncontainable illness and dependency arises out of the general population of the well functioning elderly. Attention would be directed as much towards the context in which the illness occurs as to the nature of the illness itself. Likely, elderly people become problems not just because of the overall increase in the incidence of illness or because of willful and irrational aspects of their response to illness (there is an element of "blaming the victim" here), but because of the depletions in their resources to cope with illness. These resources are of many different sorts, physical, psychological, social, and material -- and are distributed in a highly differentiated fashion amongst the elderly (Ford and Taylor 1983). Many can absorb quite high levels of illness and disability without any need to change their normal responses. Searching for explanations of the special problem of the elderly in ad hoc hypotheses about illness behaviour is fundamentally misdirected.

ILLNESS BEHAVIOUR: THE SOCIOLOGIST'S ACCOUNT

In this second section of our paper, we now turn our attention to the general explanation of illness behaviour within the sociological literature.

Studies of illness behaviour are legion; the space available is inadequate for a summary and evaluation of even a small fraction of all the explanatory models which have been proposed. What we attempt to do, then, is to use the literature selectively to build up a picture of our current state of knowledge of illness behaviour, relating our account, where possible, to the situation of the elderly. By doing this, we aim to explore the extent to which the illness behaviour of older people can be encompassed within a more general sociological perspective and at the same time reveal processes which might apply differently to ageing individuals within our general understanding of the illness process.

As we suggested in the introduction, sociologists delight in contrasting the "medical model" of illness and illness behaviour with a more sociological model which seeks to take the "patient's eye view." Of course, the medical model has little empirical reality, but is a useful abstraction which can serve to clarify some underlying orientations. Broadly, the "medical model" views illness as a relatively uncommon event, qualitatively different from a normal state called "good health." Symptoms, then, are experienced in a fairly straightforward and unequivocal fashion. A total identity of interest is seen between the symptomatic person and the medical profession. The sufferer holds the recovery of health as an absolute goal and acknowledges that the only route available is through the esoteric body of medical knowledge. The doctor is seen as the final arbiter as to whether legitimate "illness" exists and whether the individual is entitled to "go sick." In the presence of significant symptoms, the only rational course is immediate referral to competent medical authority. Many of these assumptions were built into Parsons' seminal work on the sick role (Parsons 1951), along with the additional observation that society made performance demands on individuals which were incompatible with significant degrees of sickness; hence, the individual not only had an interest in seeking cure, but an obligation, socially sanctioned, to do so. Acceptance of this set of assumptions directs attention towards a particular limited part of the total illness process, particularly to the decision to consult. A large part of the recent history of the study of illness behaviour consists of the relaxation of these "medical model" assumptions and the consequent extension of the material out of which to construct a more sociological explanation.

Recognition of the widespread nature of symptomatology, the relevance of the layman's own theories about his illness, the effect of social networks on consultation decisions, all draw attention to the pre-consultation phases in illness behaviour and to the illness work done by the lay public as a necessary constituent part of the response to symptoms; illness is no longer seen as exclusively doctors' business.

Multivariate Studies of Consultation

A large part of the literature on illness behaviour concentrates on explaining volume of consultation or utilisation of services factorially, by attributes of the individual involved, the symptoms, or the medical context.

Quite complex models have been evolved. The best known of these are associated with the Health Beliefs Model and with the work of Anderson and his colleagues (Rosenstock 1966, Anderson and Newman 1973, Becker 1979). The Health Beliefs Model treats consultation as a product of four fundamental aspects of health belief:

1. The individual's perception of suscepti-bility to a given illness;
2. The perceived seriousness of the illness;
3. Benefits expected to follow from health care use; and
4. Perceived cost and difficulties in health care use.

A rather broad and indefinite set of "enabling" factors have also been evolved including a range of socio-demographic variables and general health beliefs, and the importance of "cues" in initiating action is emphasised. Anderson, for his part, divides his explanatory variables into Predisposing factors, socio-demographic variables and health beliefs; Enabling factors, family resources and community resources; and Need factors, relating to objective health status and perceived health needs.

A large number of multivariate studies of illness behaviour have drawn variables in a rather atheoretical way from this base literature and a number of these studies deal directly with the elderly (Wan and Odell 1981, Stoller 1982, Coulton and Frost 1982).

The overwhelming finding seems to be the rather low explanatory power of the model. The variance explained ranges from nine to 13 percent in the studies mentioned. In most cases, the bulk of the explained variance is due to need factors, i.e. objective and subjective health measures, and the wide range of variables dealing with socio-demo-graphic, attitudinal, and other "sociological" factors as well as variables dealing with service availability seem to contribute almost nothing. One exception is in the study by Stoller. She dis-tinguished between the act of contacting a physician and the subsequent volume of visits. In neither case, could she explain more than a small part of the variance, but while the volume of visits was explained largely by need factors, in explaining initial contact need, enabling and predisposing factors all contributed to a significant extent. The overall explained variance, however, was only 13 percent. Mechanic confirms this pattern (Mechanic 1979). He reviews a wide range of survey-based multivariate studies and confirms that at best they seem to explain about 20 percent of the variance in service contact and use, with need factors apparently contributing most to the explanation. The apparent ineffectiveness of this approach may be partly due to specific methodological difficulties, but they do include, in various combinations, a large number of the variables which have been identified by more qualitative studies as being important. He concludes that:

> ... The determinants of help-seeking are part of a dynamic process involving responses and feedback from the environment and cannot be simply abstracted through general descriptors of the persons involved or their environments. In theory people with identical symptoms might behave differently depending on what is going on in their lives and on situational factors and this cannot be captured through cross-sectional study.

In an interesting recent study, Berkanovic and colleagues attempted to resolve some of the methodological weaknesses in the Health Beliefs Model (Berkanovic & al. 1981). Pointing out that at least part of the difficulty lies in the attempt to predict overall rates of usage rather than responses to specific illness experiences, they designed a study in which subjects were visited at six-weekly intervals over a period of twelve months. The dependent variable was the use or non-use of physician services for each illness episode reported. The independent variables were all those variables previously developed within the Health Beliefs model. In addition, a similar set of questions were developed relating to the specific symptoms experienced. In this study, they were able to explain an impressive 57 percent of the variance in physician use, substantially more than any of the studies reviewed by Mechanic. However, the overwhelming weight of explanation fell on those variables relating to the specific symptoms. In particular, the disability caused by the symptoms, the perceived seriousness of the symptom and the perceived efficacy of care are the most powerful predictors. The authors are disturbed by the lack of structural patterning in consultation; socio-demographic variables, patterns of services and general health attitudes contributed almost nothing to the model. They conclude, pessimistically, that they are able to demonstrate little more than that "... an individual is more likely to see the physician when he believes a physician might do him some good." (4)

The Need for a Process View of the Illness Episode

In distinction to the attribute-based models mentioned in the previous section, a number of writers have produced accounts of illness and consultation which treat illness as a temporal process consisting of a number of distinct stages, each of which must be negotiated prior to any medical contact being initiated (Suchman 1965, Fabrega 1973, Igun 1979). These models are diverse and complex. What they share is an appreciation of the uncertain outcome of any illness episode. Consultation is only one possible end point with many illness episodes being resolved without re-course to "professional" resources or, indeed, remaining unresolved. Figure 6.1 gives a minimal framework within which to consider any such illness episode. What the figure emphasises are the percep-tual and cognitive processes which necessarily precede the "medically rational" act of consultation and the pathways by which the episode can be resolved without any such contact being made. It is also implicit that while the episode is presented as a temporal flow, the speed of progress through each stage is highly variable, in some cases more or less instantaneous, while in others progress from stage to stage is more or less indefinitely protracted. Movement through these stages is itself a topic for enquiry.

The following section briefly develops the main sociological perspectives on the illness episode in its various phases. We then conclude with a brief consideration of the main ways in which the illness behaviour of the elderly has been held to differ from that of younger groups.

Figure 6.1: The Illness "Episode"

SELF LIMITING ILLNESS

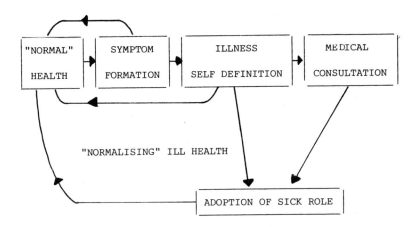

RECOVERY OR "NORMALISING" ILL HEALTH

"Normal Health" and Symptom Formation

We begin from the observation that health is a relative and subjective concept; furthermore, it is a concept of some complexity. Individuals are seen to define themselves as healthy in the presence of demonstrable clinical pathology and observable functional impairment. This would appear to be particularly true for the elderly who steadfastly maintain, in survey after survey, that they enjoy excellent health despite the presence of multiple chronic conditions.

Some of the relevant processes are biological. Individuals vary in their capacity to experience pain from symptomatic conditions and some evidence suggests that pain might be culturally modulated (Mechanic 1978:264). In addition, the relationship between disease and pain alters with age, specific conditions being less likely to manifest themselves through pain and associated unpleasant sensations. More illness in the elderly is asymptomatic or has unspecific symptomatology (Kart 1981). Not surprisingly, most clinical observations relate to serious conditions. Laboratory work shows fairly extensive sensory impairment with age (Hickey 1980), so by extrapolation we can expect that experience of minor symptoms on a day-to-day basis might be modified in the elderly, but exactly how remains unclear. Other factors, however, are social. Individuals in different social positions vary in the extent which they attend to "dis-ease." In a recent study of a group of lower-working-class middle-aged housewives in Aberdeen, the authors found that:

> ... The norms of what constituted good health were conspicuously low. Good health was being able to work, being healthy enough "for all practical purposes."
> (Blaxter and Paterson 1982)

There are two dimensions to this: On the one hand a cultural acceptance of illness as widespread and irremediable for "people like us," a cultural stoicism in the face of overwhelming odds. Beyond that, though, we have to realise that not all unpleasant bodily states are automatically defined as symptoms and ascribed to illness. The ascription of the label "symptom" implies that the subjectively perceived sign is associated in some way with a perception of abnormality or threat, with "proto-illness." If "aches and pains" are a widespread and normal state of existence for people with particular sets of life experiences then "aches and pains" are not symptoms and cannot suggest illness.

Williams has recently explored the meanings associated with health in a sample of elderly Aberdonians (Williams 1983). At one level, they show a close adherence to a lay version of the medical model of disease and illness. A valid claim to be ill must be accompanied by a legitimating disease. Good health, however, was not implied in any simple way by the absence of disease, neither was bad health necessarily implied by the presence of a clinical condition. A further key concept was supplied by the idea of strength and weakness. People were believed to have varying "reserves of strength" which also defined their state of health. Simple disease, which could be tied down to a specific location and a specific cause, e.g. arthritis of the knee, did not carry any general implications for the state of health. Indeed, the capacity to overcome specific illnesses serves to reinforce the reserve of strength and conforms good health. While illness might be thus isolated, there was a general tendency to construct a chain of interpretation which linked illness episodes bio-graphically. Illnesses, particularly those which could not be tied to a particular local cause, could over time define a "weakness" with the suscepti-bility to further illness. People found no difficul-ty in identifying ill health in the absence of specific symptoms where there was known to be a weakness or where the reserves of strength were "spent." More importantly, existence of a weakness modifies perception of specific symptoms. Apparently insignificant problems can be attended to as serious if they suggest a threat from a known weakness. This situation implies an awkward dilemma for the sufferer: Normal activity carries the threat of causing a flare-up in the weak spot while sick role behaviour is denied by the widespread sanctioning of hypochrondria; from the medical point of view it generates apparently inexplicable patterns of be-haviour.

Lay Theories of Disease: Illness Self Definition

The preceding account draws attention to one of the most obvious weaknesses in a large part of the traditional illness behaviour literature. Symptoms have generally been considered in isolation, evalu-ated and acted upon in terms of intrinsic qualities of seriousness and threat. Some important insights have been gained from this point of view. Factors which have been shown to affect consultation include the discomfort, unfamiliarity, seriousness (threat to life), disruptiveness (visibility and disruption to functioning), pain and damage (e.g. bleeding), attribution of responsibility (self-caused) and embarrassment caused by specific symptoms (Jones & al. 1981).

However, this ignores the way in which symptoms aggregate to illnesses and illnesses are embedded in personal biographies. Attempts to interpret symptoms in terms of lay theories and taxonomies seem to be fundamental to the illness behaviour process, both as a necessary diagnostic step which precedes the formulation of a course of action and also as a part of a general "search after meaning" (Blaxter 1983). How and whether a symptom can be incorporated in a lay disease model has widespread implications for the subsequent development of the illness episode. Robinson gives examples in his health diary based study which show how symptoms are accumulated and evaluated until they form a pattern which overall suggests a course of action or inaction (Robinson 1971). The attachment of a diagnostic label is often experienced as a relief as it terminates the search for new manifestations and symptoms and usually suggests a line of action. Robinson points out that the majority of episodes relating to health have a self-evident quality; they are readily related to past experiences or general health "knowledge." Once a label is found the course of action follows an acknowledged "recipe." The point, of course, is that the content of lay taxonomies and theories is a cultural product and varies across subcultures and time. Each successive generation will have theories and recipes which are the unique product of its historical experiences, and its behaviour will be consequently modified (Blaxter 1983) in ways which can only be fully understood by examining the nature of the particular lay theories held by that generation. At the other extreme, some symptoms seem so threatening, it would appear that they must short-circuit the interpretive process simply because they are unfamiliar and uninterpretable within existing knowledge. Actually, even in the presence of what appear to be severe and compelling symptoms, behaviour seems to be modified by lay diagnosis. Cowie studies 27 patients who had recently suffered a heart attack (Cowie 1976). Of these, only five correctly self-diagnosed the problem and sought medical help. Three more sought help because they had no idea what was wrong with them, and 16 initially applied an incorrect self diagnosis, usually indigestion. Eighteen of the patients engaged in self medication and delayed significantly in contacting their doctor, in a few cases for several months. Contact with the doctor occurred either when the symptoms were reinterpreted as a heart attack or when they grew too severe to be consistent with the original self diagnosis.

Responses to the Perception of Illness: Ignore, Consult or "Go Sick?"

Thus far, we have been documenting cognitive elements in the illness process. These may provide an adequate understanding in many cases where the subsequent action follows from the disease identification as a "recipe," but often further elements need to be considered.

Starting from the observation that non-consultation and delay are the norm rather than the exception, Zola was one of the first writers to reformulate the central question of illness behaviour studies away from the issue of non-consultation and to ask why people who habitually ignore symptoms do sometimes decide to consult (Zola 1966:1973). Studies of cancer patients show that people tolerate quite severe symptoms for long periods of time without seeking help, but ultimately most do, of course, consult. Zola felt that the severity of the symptom did not itself provide an answer. In terms of our model, and contrary to the "medical view," no natural and smooth progression occurs from symptom experience to consultation, marred only by the odd irrational obstacle; rather, powerful factors tend to impede and inhibit movement through the stages of the illness process. The overwhelming tendency, according to Zola, is to accommodate to illness; he argued that consultation occurred when accommodation broke down, and not as a result of intrinsic features of the symptoms or illness. He identified important "trigger" events which broke into the process of accommodation and precipitated help-seeking. He was able to show marked cultural differences in the extent to which these triggers influenced consultation.

To suggest that accommodation is a more natural response than seeking a cure may seem curious; after all, we all agree that illness is to be avoided and health is desirable. Two separate elements need to be considered. Alonzo begins from the fact that most symptoms and illness <u>are</u>, in fact, contained within everyday situations: In addition to ill people wanting to get well, a wide range of possibilities seem to exist for symptomatic and ailing individuals to avoid "becoming sick" (Alonzo 1979). Many social settings are quite elastic and can contain substantial quantities of illness. Thus, he directs attention away from the properties of individuals or of symptoms and focuses instead on properties of situations. Situations, of course, vary enormously in their capacity to withstand side involvement in illness and the extent to which illness can be contained is a function both of the severity and nature of the symptoms and the tightness and particular requirements of the situation. The point is that individuals move back and forward between situations with different demands all the time and have a multitude of options for living with a degree of illness short of entry to the sick role. People, he argues, take advantage of the looseness of situations to avoid going ill. From their point of view, the elderly are generally believed to face fewer "high involvement" situations (typically associated with work); as a result they can manifest higher levels of symptomatic illness than younger people without experiencing pressures to withdraw from the situation or seek the sick role. Old people may seek out or be channelled into undemanding situations and at the same time may be accorded "special license" within existing situations on account of their age.

The second factor concerns the relativity of the goal of good health. Traditional writing and certainly the medical profession proceed as if health and the avoidance of illness are the paramount human concern. They have confused health as a desirable end with health as an absolute end. In reality countless studies have shown that the pursuit of health is balanced against a wide range of often conflicting concerns. Going sick makes onerous demands and often the equation works out in favour of ignoring illness. Koos's working class respondent is by now legendary, but her observations bear repeating:

> ... I wish I really knew what you meant about being sick. Sometimes I felt so bad I could curl up and die but I had to go on because the kids had to be taken care of and besides we didn't have the money to spend for the doctor. How could I be sick?
> (Koos 1954)

In any illness episode, the costs of going ill are more or less constantly evaluated against the threat which seems to be posed by the illness. How the balance works out is a complex function of knowledge, pressures and priorities, and one which can change at any time as a result of really quite small changes in information available, or the context in which the individual finds himself.

A further element which has been identified as being important in the illness process is the influence of social networks. Suchman, in an early study in New York, found that 75 percent of the people in his sample of consulters had taken advice from kin or friends before deciding on a course of action. Friedson built the idea of lay consultation networks into a central element in his account of illness behaviour. In addition to the impact of cultural transmission of ideas about illness (Friedson 1971), Friedson argued that structural properties of the social network could affect the tendency to consult formal medical agencies. He argued that cohesive networks with a cultural standpoint different from that of the average medical practitioner might inhibit help-seeking. This would be especially true for working class or ethnically differentiated groups. Subsequent studies have generally upheld the association of strong networks with low service utilisation although the strength of the relationship has not often been seen to be strong. One recent study of the elderly, which focused on consultation with new services, where presumably the uncertainty and the influence of a network were at their greatest, confirmed that the majority of individuals discussed their problems with others before reaching a decision to contact the service. However, the implication of the extended network was questioned (Booth and Babchuk 1972). The number of available kin affected the decision to confer with anyone at all, but for those who did use lay consultations the majority discussed the condition with only one other person. There was a differentiation in function between the interaction between kin and friends. Friends provided largely instrumental advice while relatives provided expressive support. This is, of course, largely due to the fact that friends, being of a more nearly similar age, were more likely to have had direct experience of the relevant problem. The adult daughters, however, appeared to serve more often in the instrumental role when consulted by their mothers. Importantly:

... Respondents with the fewest interpersonal resources came from the lowest social strata and were elderly. Moreover, individuals in these two categories tended to postpone reaching health care decisions longer than other clients.

In this context, network influences seemed to promote rather than inhibit contacts.

In fact, these studies treat networks only from one point of view, as lay "doctors" to be consulted. They ignore the important fact that networks are venues for ongoing interactions where participants have interests and relationships extending beyond the immediate health problem. The closer the person involved is to the sufferer the less appropriate seems the technical, affectively neutral image of "consultation." Most sick role behaviour probably occurs without medical validation and is accomplished by negotiation with those most directly concerned. Robinson has presented a tentative but suggestive model for the sort of interpersonal processes involved (Robinson 1971). At any point in the development of an illness, both the sufferer and his "significant others" will have views on the legitimacy of sick role behaviour based on the balance between the costs (to all concerned) of going sick and the threat to the health of the sufferer of engaging in normal activities. This opens up, on the one hand, the possibility of disputed status, but on the other, our attention is directed to the possibility for magnanimity, for "exchange." The afflicted person can eschew his rights to go sick in return for moral and interpersonal credit. If two parties disagree on the status of the sick person and mutually perceive the disagreement, acceptance of the other's definition of the situation, tolerance of unjustified claims to the sick role or acceptance of unnecessary nurturance is viewed as a "gift" to the sufferer. The important thing is that the transaction confers identity and does so on both participants. A large number of different analytical situations exist and by taking this interactive interpretation we begin to understand the rich evaluative language which we knew surrounds illness behaviour. Negotiation over sickness serves to define people as "selfless," "soft," "over-anxious," "malingerer," and so on. Illness is seen as part of a broader set of activities, a constituent part of the "skilful game of exchange" actively manipulated by participants in the process of securing and maintaining social credit and identity. For the elderly in particular the maintenance of a viable identity seems to be a particularly difficult problem, and negotiations over illness behaviour may come to occupy a key role in interpersonal relations in the absence of other resources which make them valued exchange partners (Matthews 1979).

Clearly, the health behaviour of individuals is likely to be highly susceptible to changing patterns of close family interaction. We know little about how the health behaviour of any individual is affected by close conjunction of a spouse who may in turn exhibit high symptomatology or chronic illness. If we accept Robinson's analysis of illness behaviour as intrinsically manipulative and constitutive of broader identities, then it seems likely that variations in reactions will be strongly associated with the quality and nature of prior relationships. By extension, reference to a peer group who themselves show higher levels of illness and disability must in some ways affect one's own perception of health and health behaviour. Booth and Babchuk showed how important the peer group could be as a repository of instrumental health care knowledge (Booth and Babchuk 1972). But we know that the elderly consistently perceive their peers as experiencing worse health than they do themselves (Harris 1976) and define themselves as fortunate to enjoy such good health relative to those of similar ages, so again influences may be quite complicated.

After Consultation

What happens, then, when people do decide to consult a doctor? We run through the post-consultation phase of the illness episode only briefly. Although, of course, many of the same or similar elements affect the post consultation course of the illness as determined pre-consultation behaviour, affecting compliance, re-consultation and so forth, nevertheless the recourse to medical intervention and the entry of the doctor on the scene introduces a whole new set of issues and a vast new literature beyond the scope of the present paper.

Contact with the doctor introduces a new set of uncertainties. Apart from the difficulties inherent in diagnostic process itself, the patient can be seen as going to the consultation with a wider agenda than that often adopted by the doctor. The patient may seek symptom alleviation, comfort, explanation, and cure while doctors concentrate on diagnosis and cure. The consultation is a fragile achievement since the social interaction and technical communication which is achieved must often bridge a void created by cultural distance. The elderly are often seen as having particular problems in achieving an adequate consultation. The educational and cultural gulf is likely to be at its widest, and there is reason to believe that doctors in general find elderly patients unrewarding, as they present many intractable complaints of little medical interest (Williams 1981). After a diagnosis is achieved, the patient continues to monitor the progress of the disease and to evaluate the appropriateness of the treatment partly in terms of information given by the doctor, but largely still in terms of his pre-existing lay understanding of illness. New symptoms have to be evaluated as part of the expected development of the disease, as unexpected symptoms but still connected with the disease and casting doubt on the diagnosis, or as manifestations of a new and unconnected illness. From the doctor's point of view this lay interpretation may interfere with the course of the treatment, leading to non-compliance or drop-out. From the patient's point of view, it is an essential stage in assessing the efficacy of his overall plan to deal with his troublesome symptoms. Return to normal health is equally problematic. Exit from the sick role in many cases is just as uncertain as entry. When has a cure been achieved? In many cases, of course, cure is not achieved. Chronic illness raises questions of adjustment to the permanent presence of symptoms. Many studies have focused on coping with long-term disablement and with the normalisation of chronic illness, but few of them deal with the particular experience of the elderly where adjustment takes place in a situation of diminished bodily reserves and the constant spectre of decline into dependency.

Specific Theories about the Elderly
The elderly have sometimes been characterised as a group uniquely denied full integration into society, the first stage in life characterised by massive general role loss. Along with this comes social deregulation. Old age is seen as a period of normlessness, with few social demands and little guidance as to appropriate or required behaviour.

> ... Others have few expectations of them and provide no guide to appropriate activity ...

> Their lives become socially unstructured. This
> is a gross discontinuity for which they are not
> socialised and role loss deprives them of their
> very social identity.
> (Rosow 1973)

The implication is that they are freed on the
one hand from the fairly stringent demands for
health that work and other adult roles demand, freed
from the sanctioning of co-participants with strong
interests in their role performance, and at the same
time have the time available to attend to health
with few competing priorities. Actually, it is
probably unproductive to view the transition to old
age in quite such stark terms. While there is
movement out of roles with tight role performance
criteria, nevertheless there are role demands in
almost every publicly enacted situation and the
change is likely to be a matter of degree. As
suggested by Alonzo, we need to attend to the
specific properties of situations in which the
elderly find themselves. If, as Rosow suggests,
"role loss deprives them of their very identity,"
then at the very least, maintenance of the basic
proprieties of public situations is likely to become
a prime requirement for the construction of any
viable social identity -- particularly difficult in
the presence of chronic and disabling illness with
visible external impairment.

If the socially given role constraints of adult
life do, in fact, bear less heavily on elderly
populations, then in order to understand how
interpersonal and social demands affect health
behaviour, we may have to turn our attention to the
highly differentiated patterns of voluntaristic
life-style exhibited by the elderly (Taylor and Ford
1981). Health priorities are set by demands for
normal functioning and life-style seems to be a
crucial concept in gaining some insight into the
differential threat posed by changes in health
status. Life-styles define how and to what degree
specific threats can be "accommodated," to use
Zola's term, or whether they pose threats to normal
functioning with "trigger" help seeking.

The elderly may, in fact, be more differentiated in these respects than younger populations. The
elderly woman with an ailing and dependent husband
may be effectively placed in the position experienced by Koos's respondent, while the elderly isolated
widow is effectively removed from all performance
demands imposed by society.

It has been argued that age alters priorities, so that the maintenance of health might become an obsession or an irrelevance for the elderly. This is particularly so in recognition of the relatively short life span remaining and the reality of impending death. Ethnographic studies have emphasised the extent to which death is a constant concern for the very elderly (Matthews 1979, Hockschild 1973). And sociologists have pointed to the importance of understanding the elderly individuals' time orientation (Hendricks and Hendricks 1976). Still (1980) has shown that awareness of the nearness of death explains considerably more of the variation in activities in old people than does physical incapacity or age; he interprets this as a voluntary process of disengagement amongst those who perceive themselves as having a limited time horizon.

Rakowski and Hickey (1980) have recently proposed a model of health behaviour in late life which attempts to incorporate a temporal perspective. They believe that:

> ... Beliefs that the future is unimportant, that one has accomplished all that was intended in life, or that one is living on "borrowed" time are almost sure to have some impact on health behaviour. In the presence of restricted future expectations ... health beliefs may need to be relatively stronger in order to promote effective personal health care.

They develop a version of the Health Beliefs model reformulated from the traditional "content" emphasis and viewed from a process point of view. At each stage in the process, they suggest, we need to incorporate a time perspective as well as questions relating to integration in a family support structure. The model is too complex to allow a detailed description here, but repays closer examination.

Current generational differences in attitudes may also be important, and generations of the elderly are seen as having a particular set of attitudes and expectations which originate with particular historical experiences and which affect their attitudes towards health and use of services (Cain 1967, Moen 1978).

> ... Essentially I want to advance the hypothesis that those who are already past 65 in contemporary America represent a style of life and have needs and aspirations which are in

sharp contrast to the style and needs and aspirations of those who are now beginning to enter the old age category.
(Cain 1967)

In general, older cohorts are seen as having less education, having endured more arduous work conditions, having lived with privation in their earlier lives, and having been socialised in an ideology of individualism in such a way that their expectations and demands are reduced. Their perception of deprivation are relative both to their own past selves and to the cohort of peers who shared the same general past history. The implication which is drawn is, on the one hand, that current generations of old people make limited demands due to a lifetime pattern of experience which is relatively resistant to short-term influences and health educative movements. The imminence is also suggested of a coming generation of "new" elderly who, because they are better educated, more "liberal" in ideology, and have higher personal expectations, will initiate an entirely different and more extensive set of health service demands. Blaxter and Paterson document generational differences in their study contrasting middle-aged mothers with their own daughters.

... Many of the grandmothers paid lip service to the marvels of modern scientific medicine ... On the whole, however ... they often preferred, for themselves, to fall back upon "mind over matter" models of cure ... The younger generation, as might be expected, took modern scientific medicine much more for granted. For them, its benefits should be available.
(Blaxter and Paterson 1982)

The argument for cohort differences based on differing socio-historical experiences seems attractive. At the present level of knowledge and research, the problem may be in identifying exactly which historical phases experienced at which phase of their life cycle significant "breaks" occur. Cain sees a watershed at the end of the First World War with a distinct break or "historical hinge" between the cohort of the 1890s and that of the 1900s. The difficulty is that Blaxter's middle-aged grandmothers voice very much the sentiments of Cain's older cohort, but are born on average 30 to 40 years later. This, of course, is partly compounded by their lower working-class origins, but it suggests that we have to be alert to intra-cohort differences as well as to the need for a more detailed treatment which runs from an investigation of demonstrated cohort differences to an historically-informed attempt to ground these differences in historical experiences rather than extrapolating expected differences from a brief generalising social history of the relevant period. Cohort effects, though, would repay much more detailed and methodologically sophisticated investigation.

CONCLUSION

In the first section of this paper we marshalled evidence to counteract the view that the illness behaviour of the elderly is in some way fundamentally different from younger groups, although they clearly do form a special case in terms of their greater potential vulnerability to the consequences of illness. To deny that they differ fundamentally does not imply that there are no special factors to consider which affect the elderly differentially within our general understanding of the illness process. In the second and third sections, outlining one particularly sociological account of illness behaviour, we drew, where possible, on the rather limited number of studies of the elderly. Where this was not possible, we drew attention only to the most obvious ways in which the elderly might be affected by the processes discussed. It should be clear that an infinite number of specific hypotheses could be derived from the rich material available. The fact remains that at the present time little data exists to allow us to take a differentiated look at the illness behaviour of old people in any other than the crudest and most speculative way.

From a sociological point of view, what seems to be required is a clear appreciation of the illness episode as a complex <u>process</u> and an attempt to build integrated process models out of the currently rather disparate, if individually interesting, research findings available. Only when we have a more balanced and integrated general model will we be in a position to identify, other than speculatively, the particular pressures and dilemmas which bear on the elderly.

For the clinician and administrator, the problem is rather different. The contextual richness of the sociological account may have a function in dispelling misconceptions, in informing against generic imputations of "irrational" behaviour. However, as yet, the sociologist can offer little in the way of practical advice for the targeting of services. The recent growth of interest in identifying "Risk Groups" within the elderly denotes an increasing awareness of the need to distinguish between the general body of well-functioning elderly and sub-groups at heightened risk of socio-medical crisis. Unfortunately, as we have argued elsewhere (Taylor, Ford, and Barber 1983), little evidence exists that the ad hoc socio-demographic groups commonly identified as "Risk Group" actually provide much useful guidance in forming case identification strategies. Indeed, the limited success of the Health Beliefs tradition and, in particular, the findings of Berkanovic must cast some doubt on the possibilities of any approach resting on rather broad socio-demographic attributes of individuals.

Future progress would seem to depend, on the one hand, on refinement of our understanding of those aspects of socio-demographic and attitudinal factors which most contribute to risk or to inefficient service use, perhaps along the lines of the identification of essential patterns of resources and crucial resource deficits. On the other hand, future progress depends on a clarification of our model of illness process to the point where we can begin to identify common enduring or transient risk situations. By bringing these together, we might be able to make some progress towards predicting social breakdown and designing appropriate support and intervention strategies.

NOTES

(1) This is part of an ongoing longitudinal study of 619 elderly people in Aberdeen City; the initial survey was conducted in 1980. Roughly equal numbers were interviewed in five-year age/sex cohorts from age 65. Details of the sampling are in Taylor and Ford, 1983. Figures reported here have been reweighted to represent the true distribution in Aberdeen. In future references, this will be called "The Aberdeen Study."

(2) A subsequent nine-year follow-up by the authors, as yet unpublished, upholds this general pattern of stable differentiation over an extended period of time.

(3) These patterns have to be qualified by the understanding that we are looking at figures for an

elite of survivors; deaths and institutionalisation will remove a significant proportion, particularly at the higher age bands. Our figures are lower than those of Hannay, largely due to his inclusion of psychological symptoms and his utilisation of a rather longer symptom list.

(4) Given the retrospective nature of the data it might be more accurate to say that they are more likely to report a belief in the efficacy of treatment for those ailments for which they chose to consult.

REFERENCES

Abrams, M. (1978) Beyond Three Score Years and Ten, Age Concern, London

Alonzo, A.A. (1979) "Everyday Illness Behaviour: A Situational Approach to Health Status Deviations," Social Science and Medicine, 13

Anderson, R., and Newman, J. (1973) "Societal and Individual Determinants of Medical Care Utilisation in the United States," Milbank Memorial Fund Quarterly, 51

Banks, M., Beresford, S., Morrell, D., Walker, J., and Watkins, C. (1975) "Factors Influencing Demand for Primary Medical Care in Women Aged 20-44 Years: A Preliminary Report," International Journal of Epidemiology, 4

Becker, M.H. (1979) "Psychosocial Aspects of Health Related Behaviour," In H.E. Freeman & al. (eds.), Handbook of Medical Sociology, Prentice Hall

Berkanovic, E., Telesky, C., Reeder, S. (1981) "Structural and Social Psychological Factors in the Decision to Seek Medical Care for Symptoms," Medical Care, XIX, No. 7

Blaxter, M. (1983) "The Causes of Disease: Women Talking," Social Science and Medicine, 17, 2

Blaxter, M., and Paterson, E. (1982) Mothers and Daughters: A Three Generational Study of Health, Attitudes and Behaviour, Heinemann Educational Books, London

Booth, A., and Babchuk, N. (1972) "Seeking Health Care from New Resources," Journal of Health and Social Behaviour, 13

Cain, L.D. (1967) "Age Status and Generational Phenomenona: The New Old People in Contemporary America," Gerontologist, 7

Cartwright, A., and Anderson, R. (1981) General Practice Revisited: A Second Study of Patients and Their Doctors, Tavistock, London

Coulton, E. and Frost, A.K. (1982) "Use of Social and Health Services by the Elderly," Journal of Health and Social Behaviour, 23

Cowie, B. (1976) "The Cardiac Patient's Perception of His Heart Attack," Social Science and Medicine, 10

Densen, P.M., Shapiro, S., and Einhorn, M. (1959) "Concerning High and Low Utilisers of Services in a Medical Care Plan, and the Persistence of Utilisation Levels over a Three Year Period," Milbank Memorial Fund Quarterly, 37

Dingwall, R. (1976) Aspects of Illness, Martin Robertson, London

Dunnell, K., and Cartwright, A. (1972) Medicine Takers, Prescribers and Hoarders, Routledge and Kegan Paul, London

Fabrega, G. (1973) "Towards a Model of Illness Behaviour," Medical Care, 11

Ford, G., and Taylor, R. (1983-84) "Differential Ageing: An Exploratory Approach Using Cluster Analysis," International Journal of Ageing and Human Development, 18, 2

Freidson, E. (1971) Profession of Medicine, Dodd Mead & Co., New York

Hannay, D.R. (1981) The Symptom Iceberg: A Study of Community Health, Routledge and Kegan Paul, London

Louis Harris & Associates Inc. (1976) The Myth and Reality of Ageing in America, National Council on the Ageing, New York

Haug, M.R. (ed.) (1981) Elderly Patients and Their Doctors, Springer Pub. Co., New York

Haug, M.R. (1982) "Age and Medical Care Utilisation Patterns," Journal of Gerontology, 36, 1

Hendricks, C.D. and Hendricks, J. (1976) "Concepts of Time and Temporal Construction among the Aged with Implications for Research," In J.F. Gubrium (ed.), Time Roles and Self in Old Age, Human Sciences Press, New York

Hickey, T. (1980) Health and Ageing, Brooks/Cole Pub. Co., Monterey

Hochschild, A.R. (1973) The Unexpected Community, Prentice-Hall, New Jersey

Igun, U.A. (1979) "Stages in Health Seeking: A Descriptive Model," Social Science and Medicine, 13A

Jones, R.A., Wiese, H.J., Moore, R.W., and Haley, J.R. (1981) "On the Perceived Meaning of Symptoms," Medical Care, XIX, 7

Kart, C. (1981) "Experiencing Symptoms: Attribution and Misattribution of Illness among the Aged," In M.R. Haug (ed.), Elderly Patients and Their Doctors, Springer Pub. Co., New York

Koos, E.L. (1954) The Health of Regionville: What the People Thought and Did About It, Hefner Pub. Co., New York

Kuypers, J.A., and Bengtson, V.I. (1973) "Social Breakdown and Competence: A Model of Normal Ageing," Human Development, 16

Matthews, S.H. (1979) The Social World of Old Women: Management of Self-Identity, Sage Publications, London

Mechanic, D. (1978) Medical Sociology: Second Edition, Free Press, New York

Mechanic, D. (1979) "Correlates of Physician Utilisation: Why Do Major Multivariate Studies of Physician Utilisation Find Trivial Psychosocial and Organisational Effects?" Journal of Health and Social Behaviour, 20

Mechanic, D. (1982) "The Epidemiology of Illness Behaviour and its Relationship to Physical and Psychological Distress," In D. Mechanic (ed.), Symptoms, Illness Behaviour and Help Seeking, Prodist, New York

Moen, E. (1978) "The Reluctance of the Elderly to Accept Help," Social Problems, 25, 3

Parsons, T. (1951) The Social System, Free Press, New York

Pearse, I., and Crocker, L. (1944) The Peckham Experiment, Allen & Unwin, London

Rakowski, W., and Hickey, T. (1980) "Late Life Health Behaviour: Integrating Health Beliefs and Temporal Perspectives," Research in Ageing, 2, 3

Robinson, D. (1971) The Process of Becoming Ill, Routledge and Kegan Paul, London

Roos, N.P., and Shapiro, E. (1981) "The Manitoba Longitudinal Study on Ageing: Preliminary Findings on Health Care Utilisation by the Elderly," Medical Care, XIX, 6

Rosenstock, I.M. (1966) "Why People Use Health Services," Milbank Memorial Fund Quarterly, 44

Rosow, T. (1973) "The Social Context of the Ageing Self," Gerontologist, 13

South-East London Screening Study Group (1977) "A Controlled Trial of Multiphasic Screening in Middle Age: Results of the South-East London Screening Study," International Journal of Epidemiology, 6, 4

Still, J.S. (1980) "Disengagement Reconsidered: Awareness of Finitude," Gerontologist, 20, 3

Stoller, E.P. (1982) "Patterns of Physician Utilisation by the Elderly: A Multivariate Analysis," Medical Care, XX, 11

Suchmann, E.A. (1965) "Stages of Illness and Medical Care," Journal of Health and Human Behaviour, 6

Taylor, R., and Ford, G. (1981) "Lifestyle and Ageing," Ageing and Society, 1, 3

Taylor, R., and Ford, G. (1983) "Inequalities in Old Age: An Examination of Age, Sex and Class Differences in a Sample of Community Elderly", Ageing and Society, 3, 2

Taylor, R., Ford, G., and Barber, H. (1983) "The Elderly at Risk: A Critical Review of Problems and Progress in Screening and Case Finding," Research Perspectives on Ageing, 6, Age Concern, London

Tulloch, A.J., and Moore, V. (1979) "A Randomised Controlled Trial of Geriatric Screening and Surveillance in General Practice," Journal of the Royal College of General Practitioners, 29

Wadsworth, M., Butterfield, W.J.H., and Blaney, R. (1971) Health and Sickness: The Choice of Treatment, Tavistock, London

Wan, T.T.H., and Odell, B.G. (1981) "Factors Affecting the Use of Social Services among the Elderly," Ageing and Society, 1, 1

West, P.B. (1979) "Making Sense of Epilepsy," In D.J. Osborne, M.M. Grunberg, and J.R. Eiser (eds.), Social Aspects, Attitudes, Communication, Care and Training, Academic Press, London

Williamson, J. (1981) "Screening, Surveillance, and Case Finding," In T. Arie (ed.), Health Care of the Elderly, Croom Helm, London

Williamson, J., Stokoe, I.H., Gray, S. et al. (1964) "Old People at Home: Their Unreported Needs," Lancet, 23 May

Williams, R. (forthcoming) "Concepts of Health: An Analysis of Lay Logic," Sociology,

Williams, T.F. (1981) "Barriers to Doctor-Elderly Patient Relationships: The Physician Viewpoint," In M.R. Haug (ed.), Elderly Patients and Their Doctors, Springer Pub. Co., New York

Zola, I.K. (1966) "Culture and Symptoms: An Analysis of Patients' Presenting Complains," American Sociological Review, 31

Zola, I.K. (1973) "Pathways to the Doctor - From Person to Patient," Social Science and Medicine, 7

Chapter 7

THE USE OF MEDICINES BY OLDER PEOPLE

Robert Anderson and Ann Cartwright

BACKGROUND

A comparative study of 12 areas in seven countries
(Kohn and White 1976) concluded that the large
volume of medicine consumption in all study areas
suggested two policy considerations:

> First, because of the enormous costs of these
> medicines ... it would be desirable to ensure
> that all medicines were in fact efficacious and
> that they were more likely to be useful and
> beneficial than to be useless or harmful for
> the purposes for which they were prescribed or
> advocated. Secondly, it would be important to
> consider the substantial potential both for
> adverse inter drug reactions and for general
> adverse drug reactions associated with excess-
> ive use.

The first suggestion may be too ambitious. In a
review of historical trends and international
comparisons in the use of medicines, Rabin and Bush
(1974) maintained, "No society has arrived at a
stage where all or even most medicine use is
rationally correlated with measurable outcomes." But
the second suggestion or warning about the potential
for adverse drug reactions is particularly relevant
for elderly people.
Bliss (1981), reviewing prescribing for the
elderly, identified seven reasons why the elderly
are "... the main victims of modern drugs and the
system by which they are administered." These were:
1. multiple pathology of the elderly; 2. poly
pharmacy; 3. increased sensitivity of the elderly to
drugs and side effects; 4. doctors' lack of training
in geriatric prescribing; 5. unsuitable drug packaging and instructions; 6. poor supervision of elderly

patients; and 7. dual prescribing systems in hospitals and primary care which prevent doctors from being fully responsible for their own prescribing. In addition, poor sight, inability to handle containers, loss of memory, and confusion may make it more difficult for elderly people to cope with "... a complex pattern of tablet taking which even a young alert person would find it difficult to maintain accurately ..." (Atkinson & al. 1977).

These are the problems. The issues addressed in this paper are: recent trends in drug taking; the types of medicines prescribed for and taken by elderly people; over-the-counter medicines; patterns of medicine taking; some characteristics of older people who use medicines; the role of older people in the taking -- or not taking -- prescribed medicines; and the role of general practitioners and hospitals.

INTERNATIONAL COMPARISONS AND RECENT TRENDS

Since most of the data quoted here relate to England or the U.K., it is appropriate to consider the few international comparisons that can be made. Rabin and Bush (1974) showed that the British Isles had the lowest expenditure on pharmaceuticals* per head of the population in the seven countries for which the data, relating to 1971, were available. (The other six countries were Sweden, Spain, Federal Republic of Germany, United States, Japan, and France.) Comparisons of the number of prescriptions dispensed per capita during the period 1962-1971 showed England and Wales had slightly higher rates than Sweden and, at the start of the period, Australia. England and Wales had somewhat lower rates than New Zealand and, at the end of the period, Australia, but considerably lower rates than the United States, Austria, and the Netherlands. Kohn and White (1976) included one English area around Liverpool in their study. They found that the patterns of rates for overall use of medicines and for use of prescribed medicines were roughly comparable, with relatively high rates for persons using medicines in the six North American study areas; intermediate rates in Helsinki, Liverpool, and Buenos Aires; and low rates in Lodz (Poland), Banat (Serbia, Yugoslavia), and Rijeka (Croatia,

* This includes prescribed and non-prescribed medicines

Yugoslavia). Among elderly people, similar area differences were found except that for them the rates in Helsinki were higher rather than intermediate.

So the data that are available are sparse and not very recent, but they suggest that England was not a comparatively high user of medicines.

TRENDS IN PRESCRIPTIONS DISPENSED

Turning to recent trends within England, the average number of prescription items dispensed per person per year on a general practitioner's list rose from 4.97 in 1959 to 5.51 in 1969 and 6.51 in 1981 (DHSS 1982). Data giving a breakdown for elderly people (men aged 65 or more and women of 60 and over) are available from 1977 and are presented in Table 7.1. These show that, whereas the average number of items prescribed per head of the population has remained relatively steady over the period 1977-1981, the average for elderly people has increased by 13 percent. In 1981, these elderly people made up 18 percent of the population, received 37 percent of the prescriptions and accounted for 39 percent of prescription costs.

While little or no variation has been seen in total prescribing rates, significant changes have appeared in the nature of these prescribed medicines. This is shown in Table 7.2, which is based on national data relating to a one in 200 sample of prescriptions dispensed, classified by therapeutic class (DHSS 1978 and 1982). This shows that over that four-year period when the total number of prescriptions increased by only 2.6 percent, the total population by 0.3 percent, and the population of the elderly (aged 65 or over) by 3.9 percent, prescriptions for cardiovascular drugs and diuretics rose by 21.3 percent, and those prescribed for rheumatism by 16.5 percent. Preparations acting on the nervous system fell by 5.5 percent, the decline in this group being greatest for sedatives and tranquillisers, least for minor analgesics.

The next section shows that the drugs which are being prescribed more frequently - those for the cardiovascular system and rheumatism - are used overwhelmingly by older people. This is consistent with the general finding that prescribing for elderly people has continued to rise, while that for younger sections of the population has stopped rising.

Table 7.1: Recent Trends in Prescribing Rates for the Total Population in England and for the Elderly (Men Aged 65+ Women 60+)

	1977	1978	1979	1980	1981
Prescription forms					
Average total population	3.9	4.0	4.0	4.0	3.9
Average elderly	6.1	6.3	6.4	6.8	6.7
Average non-elderly	3.4	3.5	3.5	3.3	3.2
Prescription items					
Average total population	6.4	6.6	6.6	6.5	6.4
Average elderly	11.6	12.1	12.4	13.2	13.1
Average non-elderly	5.3	5.5	5.3	5.1	4.9
Proportion of elderly in population	17.4%	17.5%	17.5%	17.7%	18.1%
Proportion of prescription forms dispensed to elderly	27%	27%	28%	31%	31%
Proportion of prescription items dispensed to elderly	32%	32%	33%	36%	37%

Source: Department of Health and Social Security (personal communication)

Table 7.2: Trends in Prescribing by Therapeutic Class

Therapeutic class	1977	1980	Proportional change
Preparations acting on the nervous system	74,649	70,527	- 5.5%
Sedatives and tran- quillisers	20,836	18,920	- 9.2%
Hypnotics	14,015	13,626	- 2.8%
Analgesics minor	17,578	17,409	- 1.0%
Anti-depressants	6,715	6,263	- 6.7%
Preparations acting on the cardio-vascular system and diuretics	39,711	48,159	+21.3%
Preparations acting on the heart	12,763	16,922	+32.6%
Diuretics	15,549	19,538	+25.7%
Anti-hypertensives	5,603	6,081	+ 8.5%
Preparations prescribed for rheumatism	13,595	15,839	+16.5%
All other prescriptions	167,701	168,811	+ 0.7%
All groups	295,656	303,334	+ 2.6%

Department of Health and Social Security. 1978 & 1982

AGE AND USE OF PRESCRIBED MEDICINES

Skegg, Doll, and Perry (1977), in their study of prescriptions issued by 19 general practitioners over a one-year period, related the prescriptions to the individuals receiving them. They showed that the proportion prescribed "antipsychotic tranquillisers" increased with age for men, while for women, although the general trend also increased with age, a slightly higher proportion of those aged 45-59 than of those aged 60-74 received such a prescription. The same variation with age emerged for those receiving any psychotropic drug, but when they considered the proportions receiving five or more prescriptions for psychotropic drugs there were clear increases with age for both men and women. Their data for three age groups, 45-59, 60-74, and 75 and over are summarised in Table 7.3.

Skegg and colleagues also found a pronounced increase with age in the proportion prescribed drugs acting on the cardiovascular system. Among those aged 75 or more, 33.3 percent of the men and 34.7 percent of the women received one or more of these drugs. Over a third of the prescriptions in this group were for diuretics. And the proportion receiving preparations other than psychotropic drugs acting on the nervous system (mainly analgesics) also increased with age. Among adult males, the proportion prescribed antimicrobial drugs (mainly penicillins) increased with age.

The most recent data about the types of prescribed medicines consumed by a nationally representative sample of elderly people come from a survey carried out in 1977 (Cartwright and Anderson 1981). The proportions of elderly (aged 65 or more) people who reported that they had taken different types of medicines in the previous two weeks are compared with the proportions for younger people in Table 7.4.

Higher proportions of elderly people were taking psychotropic drugs, preparations acting on the cardiovascular system and diuretics, endocrinological drugs and preparations prescribed for rheumatism.

Table 7.3: Drugs Prescribed for Older Patients in a Year by
19 General Practitioners

	Men			Women		
	45-59	60-74	75+	45-59	60-74	75+
Proportion prescribed						
Any drug	55.5%	63.1%	75.7%	69.4%	69.8%	78.2%
Five or more prescriptions	23.2%	37.2%	55.4%	37.7%	46.5%	61.2%
Twenty or more prescriptions	4.8%	10.4%	20.2%	8.6%	15.7%	24.3%
Any psychotropic drug	15.3%	18.2%	27.2%	33.0%	31.5%	37.7%
Five or more prescriptions for psychotropics	4.7%	6.6%	13.3%	12.9%	14.7%	20.2%
Sedatives or hypnotics	11.6%	14.3%	21.4%	24.9%	24.7%	29.9%
Antipsychotic tranquillisers	3.1%	4.4%	8.0%	7.5%	6.9%	12.6%
Anti-depressants	4.4%	4.4%	7.2%	11.2%	8.7%	8.9%
Any antimicrobial drug	18.7%	22.4%	30.6%	25.1%	25.5%	27.1%
Five or more prescriptions for anti-microbial drugs	1.2%	2.4%	4.3%	1.4%	1.9%	1.7%
Population (=100%)	2,984	1,992	415	3,118	2,108	945

Source: Skegg, Doll, and Perry 1977

Table 7.4: Proportions of Elderly People and others Taking Different Types of Prescribed Medicines in a Two Week Period in 1977

Therapeutic class	People aged 18-64 %	People aged 65+ %
Psychotropic *	10	20
Other nervous system	8	9
Gastrointestinal	4	4
Cardiovascular or diuretic	5	28
Respiratory or allergic	5	9
Rheumatism	3	11
Anti-microbial	4	4
Endocrinological **	2	8
Nutrition or blood	3	4
Skin, eyes or mucous membrane	5	6
Other	-	1
Number of people (=100%)	650	161

Source: Cartwright and Anderson 1977 study

* Sedatives, hypnotics, tranquillisers, anti-depressants, stimulants, and appetite suppressants

** Excluding oral contraceptives

AGE AND USE OF NON-PRESCRIBED MEDICINES

Only limited information is available about these. One source is a survey in 1969 of a random sample of adults in Great Britain (Dunnell and Cartwright 1972). This found that in a two week period two-thirds of the 281 elderly people (aged 65 or more) were using some over-the-counter medication, while somewhat fewer (56%) used prescribed drugs. The average number of the different types of medicines they used was 1.6 over-the-counter, 1.3 prescribed. Eighty-five percent were using medicines of one sort or the other, but no significant correlation, positive or negative, was found between the use of the two types. At that time, many of the names of prescribed drugs were not recorded on the containers so that 31 percent of those being taken by older people could not be identified. Table 7.5 shows the types of medicines the older people and other adults said they were using in a two-week period and the proportion of the different types that were prescribed. More older people than younger ones were taking health salts, indigestion remedies, and laxatives. Most of these types of medicines were purchased over-the-counter and not prescribed, although nearly a quarter of the laxatives and a fifth of the indigestion remedies taken by older people were obtained on a prescription. In addition more of the elderly people were taking sedatives, sleeping pills, or tranquillisers, nearly all of which were prescribed, and they were also more likely to use surgical clothing, trusses, bandages, or elastic stockings. Fewer older people had taken cold relievers, vitamin tablets, or aspirins or other pain killers during the two-week period, but they were more likely to get their pain-killers on a prescription.

Younger adults took aspirin for their minor self-limiting conditions; these were self-prescribed and taken comparatively irregularly and infrequently. Older people took analgesics for the relief of chronic conditions like rheumatism and arthritis. They were more likely to get these medicines from the doctor and to take them frequently. These various trends lead to a different age pattern in the taking of medicines in a 24-hour period. Over this time, rather more older than younger people had taken them: 17 percent of those aged 65 or more, 13 percent of those under 65.

Another source of some limited information on the types of prescribed and non-prescribed medicines

Table 7.5: Proportion of Elderly People (65+) and Other Adults (21-64) Using Different Types of Medicines in a Two Week Period and the Proportion of the Medicines that Were Prescribed

	Proportion taking medicines		Proportion of medicine used that were prescribed	
	Adults 21-64	Elderly 65+	Those taken by 21-64	Those taken by 65+
	%	%		
Gargles or mouthwashes	5	6	3% (58)	*
Health salts	7	15	0% (77)	2% (42)
Indigestion remedies	12	22	11% (151)	19% (69)
Laxatives	6	19	11% (73)	23% (56)
Suppositories	1	1	*	*
Throat or cough medicines or sweets	13	13	23% (167)	33% (40)
Cold or congestion relievers	5	2	36% (61)	*
Aspirin or other pain-killers	43	33	14% (528)	27% (99)
Sedatives, sleeping pills, tranquillisers	8	18	99% (101)	96% (55)
Anti-depressants, stimulants, pep pills	1	1	*	*
Skin ointments, antiseptics	15	13	32% (196)	26% (38)
Eye drops, lotions, ointments	4	5	24% (42)	*
Embrocation or ointment to rub in	6	9	19% (74)	19% (26)
Inhalants, drops, or things to sniff	4	5	39% (46)	*
Diarrhoea remedies	1	2	*	*
Corn pads, foot powders or ointment	6	9	1% (68)	19% (26)
Tonics, rejuvenators	4	6	51% (51)	38% (21)
Slimming aids	2	-	36% (22)	*
Vitamin tablets	7	2	22% (92)	*
Medicinal foods	3	7	2% (47)	0% (23)

Surgical clothing, elastic stockings	7	13	40% (78)	67% (39)
Alcohol for medicinal purposes	3	5	0% (40)	*
Hormones or contraceptive pills	5	–	100% (52)	*
Travel or other kind of sickness pills	1	–	*	*
Other	18	36	87% (292)	90% (176)
Number of people (=100%)/All medicines	1127	281	33%(2360)	45% (801)

The figures in brackets are the numbers on which the percentages are based (=100%)

Source: Dunnell and Cartwright 1969 study

* indicates a base of less than 20

consumed by elderly people and others is the General Household Survey 1972 and 1973 (OPCS 1975 and 1976). The main emphasis was on analgesics, and, like Dunnell and Cartwright, it showed that the proportion taking self-prescribed analgesics decreased with age while the proportion taking prescribed analgesics increased. Considering both types of analgesic, the proportion who had taken them in the last seven days was highest among adults aged 16-44. The differences between those aged 45-64 and 65 and over were less marked in the opposite direction in the two periods for which the data were collected. But what does emerge clearly, as is shown in Table 7.6, is that those aged 65 and over were taking analgesics containing aspirin more frequently during the seven day period.

This underlines the importance of considering the pattern of medicine taking since the numbers of prescriptions dispensed, the proportion of people taking a drug in a day, a week, a fortnight or a year are all quite different measures, each influenced in different ways by the amount and frequency with wich drugs are taken. The implications of using different medicines are also affected by the numbers and types of other medicines taken and by the duration of use.

POLYPHARMACY

Results from the national survey carried out in 1977 (Cartwright and Anderson 1981) indicate that, altogether, older people consume twice as many types of prescribed medicine per person as younger adults. The number of prescribed medicines (excluding oral contraceptives) taken in the previous two weeks is shown in Table 7.7.

As previously mentioned, Dunnell and Cartwright (1971) found that among people aged 65 and over rather more were using non-prescribed than prescribed medicines; the average number of medicines of both types taken or used during a two week period was 2.9. An American survey of people aged 65 and over living in the community reported 89 percent of people to be taking some medicine; these elderly people were using an average of 3.2 medications, almost half of which were non-prescription drugs (May & al. 1982).

In the United Kingdom, several general practitioners have looked at drug use among their patients. In one such study of patients aged 75 and

Table 7.6: Frequency with which Analgesics Containing Aspirin Taken during the Seven Days Ending "Yesterday" by Age and Sex

Number of times taken	Males			Females		
	16-44	45-64	65+	16-44	45-64	65+
	%	%	%	%	%	%
1	57	48	32	50	36	24
2	21	18	23	22	23	20
3	8	11	14	11	13	10
4-6	8	11	7	9	9	12
7 or more	6	11	23	8	19	34
Base (=100%)	999	521	166	1411	823	402

Source: General Household Survey Great Britain - 1973

Table 7.7: Proportions of Older (65+) and Younger Adults Taking Different Numbers of Prescribed Medicines in the previous Two Weeks

Number of medicines	People aged 18-64	People aged 65+
	%	%
0	66	43
1	17	20
2	10	16
3	4	9
4 or more	3	12
Average	0.6	1.3
Number of people (=100%)	665	162

Source: Cartwright and Anderson 1977 study

over, Law and Chalmers (1976) found that 87 percent of these patients were taking some medicine regularly. The number of drugs taken "regularly" averaged two to three per patient, but "... a third of our patients took three or four drugs a day ..." Nearly three-quarters of the drugs identified in this study were prescribed medicines. In another study, based in an inner city general practice, Kiernan and Isaacs (1981) interviewed 50 patients aged 65 or over. All but four patients said they were using medicine: 66 percent were taking a prescribed medicine "regularly" and 36 percent reported taking three or more prescribed medicines "regularly;" only six percent said they took any non-prescribed medicine "regularly."

Some evidence indicate that elderly people in hospital or other institutional care are more likely than those in the community to be using several medicines together. A one-day cross-sectional survey of elderly patients in Dundee Hospitals (Christopher & al. 1978) reported that patients aged 65 and over were taking an average of 3.3 prescribed medicines (compared with 1.4 and 1.3 respectively in the general population surveys of Cartwright and Anderson 1981, and Dunnell and Cartwright 1972). On the geriatric wards in the Dundee hospitals, the average was 4.0 prescribed medicines per patient; altogether one elderly person in seven was receiving six or more prescribed drugs.

In Finland, Hemminki and Heikkila (1975) studied 217 people in homes for the aged. One third had taken four or more prescribed medicines in the previous week, and only 23 percent had taken no prescribed medicine in the previous week. When the pharmacological substances were counted separately, almost half the residents had taken at least four prescribed substances in the previous week. These authors also looked at the nature of the drugs and report that psychotropics figured largely among the drugs taken -- a result similar to that found in studies of inpatients on geriatric wards (Christopher & al. 1978; Scott & al. 1982). The frequent use of psychotropic drugs in combination with some other prescribed medicine was evident in our survey, too (Cartwright and Anderson 1981). Nearly 4/5 of the people aged 65 and over who were using a psychotropic drug were also taking some other prescribed medicine; specifically, 47 percent were also taking a diuretic or medicine acting on the cardiovascular system. Put another way, psychotropic drugs were being used by at least a fifth of those taking other prescribed medicines, and by a third or more of people taking prescribed medicines in the rheumatism and cardiovascular or diuretic therapeutic classes. The widespread use of psychotropic drugs among elderly people with chronic physical illnesses has been extensively documented by Cooperstock and Hill (1982).

In summary, these studies of use of medicines by older people in the community, general practice, and hospital indicate that over a two-week period, 3/4 or more of older people take at least one medicine and that the average number taken is about three. However, the studies are difficult to compare because they come from several countries, are based on sample populations which may vary in their demographic characteristics, and because they sometimes fail to specify the time period over which drug use was identified, or to define what is meant by "regularly." The findings about use of prescribed medicines are more consistent than those for use of over-the-counter drugs. This propably reflects differences in the definition of non-prescribed medicines and in the methods employed to collect the data (e.g. interviewer check-list versus general practitioner's record). Systematic community studies (Dunnell and Cartwright 1972; May & al. 1982) indicate that about 2/3 of elderly people were using non-prescribed medicines around the time of the interview. There are conflicting findings about the relationship between use of prescribed and over-the-counter medicines (Blum and Kreitman 1981) but this appears to vary with age -- the greater use of drugs by elderly people is almost entirely due to an increase in use of prescribed drugs; the proportion using over-the-counter medicines is fairly constant across age groups (Dunnell and Cartwright 1972; May & al. 1982).

REPEAT PRESCRIPTIONS

In the United Kingdom, about 3/4 of prescribed medicines issued to adults are repeat prescriptions (Dunnell and Cartwright 1972; Anderson 1980 a). This proportion appears to increase with age: in our 1977 survey (Cartwright and Anderson 1981) the proportion of medicines that had been prescribed at least once previously increased from less than a third of those reported by people aged 18-24 to more than 4/5 of prescribed medicines used by people aged 65 and over. Murdoch (1980) recorded prescribing in an urban general practice over a six-month period and classified drugs according to the length of time for which they were continued. No distinction was made between prescriptions issued at a consultation and those issued without the patient seeing the doctor. He reports that the number of repeat prescriptions per patient showed a "very highly significant rise with age," but that the increase with age did not seem to apply to one-off prescribing. Among patients aged 65 and over, nearly 60 percent of items were "long-term" repeats (items repeated for 90 days or more): "Indeed, approximately 30% of the total items prescribed in the practice were long-term repeats prescribed to those over 65 years." Tulloch (1981) in a study of his patients from an Oxford general practice, found that in a six month period, almost half of those aged 65 or over were receiving a repeat prescription, defined as one that had been issued at regular intervals for more than three months.

Most repeat prescriptions regimens are long-standing; in both 1969 (Dunnell and Cartwright 1972) and 1977 (Anderson 1980 a) 70 percent of repeat prescriptions had been initiated one year or more previously. The more recent survey (Cartwright and Anderson 1981) showed a trend with age from two percent of people aged 18 to 24, to 42 percent of people aged 65 or over, in the proportion taking any medicine on a long-term prescription (first received one year or more previously). Twenty-seven percent of people aged 65 and over reported two or more medicines first prescribed a year or more previously, and 13 percent reported three or more. Das (1977) found that among a random sample of old people in Salford, 2/3 said they had been taking some prescribed or non-prescribed medicine for more than one year. This higher proportion is not surprising since, in general, non-prescribed medicines have been taken for longer than prescribed drugs (Dunnell and Cartwright 1972).

Considering the types of prescribed medicines used for long periods, in the 1977 study (Cartwright and Anderson 1981) 24 percent of people aged 65 and over reported using a diuretic or medicine acting on the cardiovascular system which was first prescribed one year or more previously, and 14 percent were taking a psychotropic drug on a long-term prescription. In Murdoch's (1980) study of prescriptions to people aged 75 and over, more than 20 percent were receiving diuretics which had been repeated for 90 days or more; over 10 percent were receiving hypnotics, and over 10 percent tranquillisers which had been repeated for this period. Several other studies have shown that older people are more likely to use psychotropic drugs for long periods of time (Williams & al. 1982; Dennis 1979).

SOME CHARACTERISTICS OF OLDER PEOPLE WHO TAKE MEDICINES

Health

It would be surprising if people who were in poorer health did not take more medicines. The study by Dunnell and Cartwright (1972) shows that, for all age groups, those who reported more symptoms of ill-health were more likely to be using both prescribed and non-prescribed medicines. Among people aged 65 and over, data from the 1977 study (Cartwright and Anderson 1981) indicate that the individual's assessment of his or her health was related to use of prescribed medicines: 11 percent of medicine takers rated their health for their age as "poor," but only one percent of those not taking a prescribed medicine said this; however, 17 percent of medicine takers still rated their health for their age as "excellent," as did 38 percent of those not taking any prescribed medicine. Although variations in the frequency with which patients consult their doctor is not, in general, an adequate indicator of differences in the use of prescribed medicines (Anderson 1980 b), the people in our survey aged 65 and over who used prescribed medicines reported an average of 5.8 consultations with a general practitioner in the previous twelve months, compared with an average of only 1.3 among those not taking any prescribed medicine. Nevertheless 11 percent of older people taking prescribed medicines said they had not consulted their doctor at all in the previous twelve months.

Sex

Women report more symptoms of illness than men, and make greater use of health services (Nathanson 1977). These characteristics are thought to make some contribution to explaining the general finding that women consume more medicines than men, of both prescribed and non-prescribed types (Cooperstock 1978, Dunnell and Cartwright 1972). Data from studies of prescribing indicate, however, that these sex differences are significantly diminished among older people (Skegg & al. 1977, Murdoch 1980).

Two local studies in England (Wadsworth & al. 1971, Jefferys & al. 1960) reveal no marked differences in use of medicines by older men and women. However, in the national survey carried out by Dunnell and Cartwright (1972), women aged 65 and over were more likely to be taking some medicine and were consuming a higher number of them -- an average of 3.3 medicines in the previous two weeks, compared with an average of 2.2 medicines by older men. This difference was mainly attributable to greater use of non-prescribed medicines by women. Although a higher proportion of Women were taking prescribed medicines (because of a difference among people aged 65 to 74), no significant differences were seen by sex in the average number of prescribed medicines used by men and women aged 65 and over. The figures are in Table 7.8

In the 1977 survey (Cartwright and Anderson 1981) no differences were found in the proportions of men and women aged 65 and over using prescribed medicines, nor in the numbers of prescribed medicines taken. There were, however, two small differences in the nature of the medicines used by people aged 65 and over; 11 percent of men, but no women, reported using medicines acting against infections; and three percent of men, but 14 percent of women said they were taking some prescribed medicine for rheumatism. The difference in use of drugs against infections has been noted previously on the basis of prescribing data (Bytheway 1976, Skegg & al. 1977). It would also have been consistent with these prescribing data to find that older women were using psychotropic drugs more than men of the same age, but in our 1977 study, the difference was not statistically significant (16 percent of men and 22 percent of women aged 65 or over reported taking a psychotropic drug in the previous two weeks).

Age

In Dunnell and Cartwright's (1972) survey, the proportion of people taking prescribed medicines increased with age among the elderly (see Table 7.8), but the average number of prescribed medicines used was not significantly different in the two age groups, nor were there any differences in the use of non-prescribed medicines. Overall, however, more people aged 75 or over were using some medicine, and the average number used was significantly higher among people aged 75 and over compared to those aged

Table 7.8: Use of Prescribed and Non-prescribed Medicines by Age and Sex for those Aged 65 or more

	Men			Women			Men and Women		
	65-74	75+	65+	65-74	75+	65+	65-74	75+	65+
Prescribed medicines									
Proportion using any	40%	73%	49%	58%	70%	62%	49%	71%	56%
Average number	1.0	1.5	1.1	1.4	1.6	1.4	1.2	1.5	1.3
Non-prescribed medicines									
Proportion using any	57%	64%	59%	71%	76%	73%	65%	71%	67%
Average number	1.0	1.3	1.1	1.9	2.0	1.9	1.5	1.7	1.6
All medicines									
Proportion using any	74%	88%	78%	89%	94%	91%	82%	92%	85%
Average number	2.0	2.8	2.2	3.3	3.6	3.3	2.7	3.2	2.9
Number of people (=100%)	88	33	121	106	54	160	194	87	281

Source: Dunnell and Cartwright 1969 study

65-74. The figures are in Table 7.8.

Polypharmacy is probably more prevalent among the older elderly people. Moir and colleagues (1980) found that people aged 85 or over were more likely than those aged 65-74 to be taking four or more medicines, and in the 1977 survey (Cartwright and Anderson 1981) 19 percent of those aged 75 and over reported taking four or more prescribed medicines compared with only seven percent of people aged 65-74. This difference was not quite significant, but the older elderly were more likely to be taking several long-term prescribed medicines together: 13 percent of people aged 75 and over said they were using four or more medicines first prescribed one year or more previously, but only two percent of people aged 65-74 reported this. The greater use of regularly repeated prescribed medicines by the older elderly is suggested too in the research of Tulloch (1981) and Skegg and colleagues (1977). The 1977 study (Cartwright and Anderson 1981) showed no differences by age among older people in the nature of the medicines consumed either in general or as long-term prescriptions.

Social Class
No significant social class differences were found in data from the 1969 survey (Dunnell and Cartwright 1982) for use of either prescribed or non-prescribed medicines. In 1977 (Cartwright and Anderson 1981) there were, similarly, no differences by social class in the proportions using prescribed medicines or in the average number taken, nor were there any such differences in use of long-term prescribed medicines. This lack of differences may be because social class, derived from reports of previous occupation, is not a sensitive indicator of the life-style of older people. Furthermore, both these studies were done in the United Kingdom where older people are exempt from charges for prescribed medicines; thus, the ability to pay for prescriptions is not a factor; elsewhere the cost of prescribed medicines may influence use only among the "very poor" (Blum and Kreitman 1981).

There were two small differences in the types of prescribed medicines used by elderly women in 1977: first 18 percent of working-class women compared with six percent of middle-class women were taking some medicine prescribed for rheumatism. This is probably a reflection of the higher rate of chronic illness among working class people (OPCS

1979). Secondly, 15 percent of working class women but only three percent of middle-class women were taking a medicine other than a psychotropic acting on the central nervous system (nearly all were minor analgesics). This difference in the use of central nervous system drugs by older women may be associated with differences which lie in the consulting room. Both Whittington and colleagues (1981) and Cooperstock (1978) have pointed to the attitudes and behaviour of doctors as factors which may explain some of the sex difference in the use of prescribed medicines, particularly the use of central nervous system drugs. It may be important to look further at differences in the behaviour of doctors associated with the social and economic characteristics of patients. As Dunnell and Cartwright (1972) suggest, in the consultation "... middle class patients may communicate their demands and anxieties more effectively, or the doctor may respond to their symptoms differently ..."

THE ROLE OF OLDER PEOPLE

Herxheimer and Stimson (1981) have suggested that "... all medication is to some extent self-medication, even if it is not self-prescribed ...it is usually the case that medication can take place only at the initiative of or with the consent of the patient ..."

In the case of non-prescribed drugs the doctor may suggest that the patient buy these medicines or the decision may be influenced more directly by the patient's ideas. Dunnell and Cartwright (1972) found that older people were more likely to regard a daily bowel movement as important, so this may contribute to their higher consumption of laxatives. Older people are likely to have grown up in an age when a regular dose of laxatives was often considered appropriate (Reid 1956). Dunnell and Cartwright also suggested that older people may regard themselves as suffering from sleeplessness because they do not realise they need less sleep as they grow older. Certainly, on that study the proportion of people reporting sleeplessness increased with age. This may lead them to suggest that doctors prescribe sedatives.

However, older people may be, in general, less likely to contribute to the decision to prescribe. Further analyses from the 1977 study (Cartwright and Anderson 1981) show that only four percent of the elderly, compared with 12 percent of younger people, were critical of their doctor for being either too inclined or too reluctant to give prescriptions. (More of the younger patients thought their doctors were too inclined to give them prescriptions than thought that they were reluctant to do so). There were no age variations in the proportions who said they had expected or hoped for a prescription before a recent consultation. Evidence that patients do not want prescriptions as often as doctors think they do comes from a variety of sources. Sheldon, a general practitioner, reported that he started to ask patients for whom a drug might be marginally helpful: "Would you like me to give you something for this?" and was surprised how many said no. Stimson (1976) found that general practitioners estimated that a high proportion of patients expected a prescription: 4/5 of the doctors believed that prescriptions were expected at 80 percent or more of consultations, and he contrasts this with studies of patients showing that between 2/5 and a half of them expect a prescription at a consultation.

Patients who want a prescription probably find it easier to convey their wishes to the doctor than patients who do not want one. It appears gratuitous to say they do not want one before it is offered, and a rejection of the doctor's help to do so afterwards. So, although patients may be becoming increasingly reluctant to take drugs, they may have difficulty in communicating this to their doctors. Herxheimer (1976) has drawn up a list of questions which patients might be encouraged to ask about their treatment. This includes: "How important is it for me to take these tablets?" and "What is likely to happen if I do not take them?"

Results from our 1977 study (Cartwright and Anderson 1981) show that a third of older people who were taking prescribed drugs said they felt they did not know enough about the medicines they were taking -- what they were and how they were likely to help. This is similar to the proportion among younger people. But the expectations and level of knowledge of older people may be somewhat lower. Of the medicines being taken by people aged 65 and over only 39 percent were known by name without reference to the container, compared with 51 percent of those being taken by younger adults. Older people may also be reluctant to admit to or report problems: relatively few of them, one percent, said they had any problems taking the medicines in the prescribed amounts at the prescribed times; nine percent of younger medicine-takers reported such problems. In addition fewer of the elderly people thought their drugs were likely to have side effects, 11 percent compared with 26 percent. So, although elderly people are most prone to adverse reactions because of reduced excretion, slower metabolism, and also probably increased sensitivity (Williamson 1978), they seem to be less aware of the possibility of side effects.

The question arises then whether older people are more or less likely to take their medicines as prescribed. Atkinson, Gibson, and Andrews (1978) concluded an investigation into the ability of elderly people continuing to take prescribed drugs after discharge from hospital as follows: "It would appear essential that doctors treating elderly patients should face up to the fact that in practice their patients are very frequently not taking the drugs prescribed to them in the doses prescribed." This was based on a study of 50 elderly patients. However, Drury, Wade, and Woolf (1976), in a study in general practice based on a sample of prescriptions, found no difference in compliance with age. They found 86 percent complied with both dose and time, three percent with dose only, four percent with time only, and seven percent with neither. There was relatively poor compliance over antibiotics. Ettlinger and Freeman (1981) in their study of patients aged 16-84 who were given a prescription for a new antimicrobial drug also found no significant association between compliance and age, but compliance with the prescription was found to be strongly associated with whether the patient felt he or she knew the prescribing doctor well. The proportion of "full compliers" was 57 percent among "the identifiers" -- those who felt they knew the doctor well, 22 percent among the "non-identifiers," while the proportions of "non-compliers" were eight percent and 57 percent in the two groups. Most of the patients, (81%) were "identifiers." Drury, Wade, and Woolf also concluded that the "... biggest variable in securing compliance is the doctor."

Multiple sources of prescribed drugs can lead to complications. In a study which recognised the potential of the interface between hospital and community for producing deviations from prescribed therapy, Crooks and Parkin (1977) studied 134 patients (3/4 of whom were aged 60 or more) discharged home from four general medical wards with one or more drugs prescribed which had to be taken regularly for a period exceeding 14 days following discharge. Four patients (3%) relied entirely on others to give them their drugs. Crooks and Parkin regarded it important to distinguish between non-comprehension and non-compliance. They found 35 percent did not <u>understand</u> the prescribed regimen correctly, making some error in reporting doses or times. Among those who understood correctly, roughly 3/4 complied without taking additional drugs, so just under half were on the correct therapy. Neither non-comprehension nor non-compliance was associated with the age of patients. "Most of the patients making dosage errors were unsure of the correct dosage or took their medicines only when they felt they were necessary." There was a strong association between making these types of errors and having taken one or more of the drugs of the current regimen before hospital admission. In addition errors were associated with the number of drugs scheduled and the frequency of daily doses.

Wandless, Mucklow, Smith, and Prudham (1979), in a study of elderly (aged 65 and over) patients in a single practice, investigated the frequency of error in medicine taking, the types of error made and the extent to which patients making errors could be identified easily and reliably. They found the correct dosage regimen was known for 92 percent and the correct purpose for 72 percent of all medicines taken. One compliance index (number of tablets taken as a percentage of those recommended to be taken) was between 90 percent and 110 percent for slightly less than half the medicines (47%), and they concluded that poor comprehension could not be responsible for this. They contrasted this finding with that of Parkin, Crooks, and their colleagues (1976) and suggested that the length of time their patients had had to become familiar with their treatment might account for the difference. Another possibility is the confusion between instructions from the hospital and the general practitioner on the Crooks and Parkin study. Wandless and her colleagues (1979) note that their compliance rate was considerably lower than that of Drury and his collaborators (1976) and ascribe this to the less frequent contact with the doctor. Certainly, the role of the doctor and the relationship between hospitals, general practitioners, and patients seem crucial.

ROLE OF GENERAL PRACTITIONER AND THE HOSPITAL

General practitioners account for over 80 percent of the drug expenditure in our National Health Service (DHSS 1982). But it is sometimes argued that hospital doctors initiate a substantial proportion of prescribing regimens which are then continued by general practitioners. Cartwright and Anderson (additional unpublished data) found that 81 percent of the prescribed drugs currently taken by elderly people had been initially prescribed by general practitioners and 19 percent by the hospital.

The prescription of medicines often takes place without contact between patient and doctor. For general practice, Drury (1982) has estimated that "... between a quarter and a third of all prescriptions now written are issued without a consultation taking place at that time ..." In our 1977 survey (Cartwright and Anderson 1981), more than half of repeat prescriptions and, therefore, about 2/5 of all prescribed medicines were obtained without the patient seeing the doctor. Elsewhere, Cartwright (1983) has argued that the proportion of prescriptions obtained without a face-to-face consultation with the doctor increased between 1969 and 1977.

Further analyses from the 1977 survey (Cartwright and Anderson 1981) show that the medicines taken by older people are more likely to be prescribed outside the consultation; the proportion of repeats obtained without the patient seeing a doctor increased from 29 percent of medicines for people aged 18-34 to 64 percent of medicines for those aged 65 and over. This proportion was not significantly different for any specific therapeutic category of prescribed medicine. Altogether, 57 percent of medicine takers aged 65 and over had obtained the most recent prescription for at least one medicine without seeing the doctor, and this proportion fell to 18 percent of those under 25. In addition, and as might be expected, the more prescribed medicines a person was taking the greater the chance that at least one of the current prescriptions had been obtained without seeing a doctor: the proportion rose from 37 percent of those taking one medicine to 51 percent of those taking four or more. Among people aged 65 and over the probability of contact with the doctor for receipt of a prescription was not clearly related to the duration of treatment with that drug. Considering the extent of polypharmacy in this age group, it may be that doctors tend to prescribe all their medicines, of both long and short duration, to-gether.

Obviously, it is important when doctors are prescribing drugs for them to be aware of what other drugs the patient is or may be taking. Problems can arise when patients receive treatment from more than one source. For example, Price (1983) has shown that when patients receiving treatment for chronic simple glaucoma, a condition which increases dramatically with age, were admitted to hospital for non-opthalmic reasons, over a third (37%) received no eye medication. Arcand and Williamson (1981) in an evaluation of home visiting of patients by phys-icians in geriatric medicine found that 23 percent of patients were taking prescribed drugs not mentioned by the general practitioner, although the general practitioners were asked about the patients' medication at the time of referral. The implication of this finding is not only that geriatricians and other hospital consultants may not be aware of the drugs their patients are taking if they rely only on the information provided by general practitioners, but the general practitioners themselves may not always be aware of them. This is supported by findings from three other studies.

Bowling and Cartwright (1982) reported that 82 percent of a sample of elderly widowed patients said they were taking some prescribed medicine in the months following the death of their spouse, but their general practitioners recorded that only 63 percent of these same people were taking prescribed medicine during that time. Cross analysis showed that 22 percent of the widowed were taking pre-scribed drugs, of which their doctors were apparent-ly unaware.

In another study of consultations between elderly patients and their general practitioners it was found that when patients were taking prescribed medicines in addition to those prescribed at the study consultation, doctors were not aware of this in a third of the instances (Cartwright, Lucas, and O'Brien 1974).

Finally, Patrick, Peach, and Gregg (1982), in a series of studies of the disabled, designed an enquiry to assess general practitioners' knowledge of their disabled patients. In a personal communi-cation, Peach revealed some additional unpublished data.

> With the help of case notes, general prac-titioners were asked to complete a question-naire which enquired after the names of the

drugs the disabled patients were taking at the time of their being interviewed by the field-workers. ... They knew of only 39% of the drugs the patients told the interviewers they were taking. When the survey results were fed back to the general practitioners they admitted that although they had recorded prescribing more drugs in the case notes they were uncertain as to whether the patient was still taking the drugs.

All these findings relate only to prescribed drugs. Doctors' awareness of the non-prescribed drugs their patients are taking is likely to be more sketchy and unreliable.

How does it happen that general practitioners do not know about so many of the prescribed drugs taken by their patients? One explanation, suggested by Peach, was that the drugs had been taken over a long period and doctors were unaware that they were still being prescribed and taken. Bowling and Cartwright (1982) identified minor tranquillisers as the type of drug doctors were likely to have forgotten in this way and it seemed likely that a relatively high proportion of repeat prescriptions in that group had been obtained without seeing a doctor -- 67 percent compared with 45 percent of all repeat drugs, but the numbers were small and the difference might have occurred by chance.

SAFETY OF DRUG USE BY OLDER PEOPLE

Given that so many older patients obtain their repeat prescriptions without any regular review (Das 1977, Law and Chalmers 1976) or without even seeing the doctor, there are questions about whether their use of drugs can be safe and effective. Shaw and Opit (1976) suggest that reliance on self-referral by elderly infirm patients does not guarantee adequate supervision of their medical needs and, although their specific research has been challenged (Crombie & al. 1976), there is a well-documented problem of adverse drug reactions among elderly patients.

In a study of patients aged 65 or more Martys (1982) found 36 percent of elderly drug takers had a possible drug related symptom or sign. This assessment was made by "... the practice drug monitor, a State registered nurse ... trained ... in techniques of drug monitoring ..." She interviewed the patients and used a check-list of specific symptoms. Gibson and O'Hare (1968) assessed the safety of drug taking among elderly people at home. They visited 273 patients and found 86 percent were taking drugs. They estimated that out of all 273, 31 percent were "unsafe" in the sense that they were taking four or more drugs daily or had inadequate supervision or were not fit to supervise their own drug taking.

A study of adverse reactions to prescribed drugs in 1,998 elderly patients admitted to 42 units in geriatric medicine departments (Williamson and Chopin 1980) found that 81.3 percent were receiving prescribed drugs and of these 15.3 percent were suffering adverse reactions. In 209 instances, i.e. 13 percent of those taking drugs, the adverse reaction contributed to the admission. The risk of adverse reaction was greatest with hypotensive drugs, antiparkinsonian drugs, psychotropics and digitalis, but the largest number of adverse reactions were due to diuretics which were by far the most commonly prescribed drugs for these patients.

A study of potential adverse drug reactions among 353 elderly hospital in-patients was carried out by Scott, Stansfield, and Williams (1982). They identified 30 potentially harmful drug reactions in 23 (6.5%) of the patients and three actual inter-actions. Balme (1977) reviewed the drugs taken by 78 patients referred to a geriatric department. He found 83 percent were taking some drugs. After his review he stopped or reduced the drugs of half of those taking drugs (all of whom had drug induced symptoms), started a quarter on new drugs and left a quarter on the same drugs.

Clearly the frequency with which unwanted effects of drugs occur depends on the population studied and on how and by whom they are identified. What is clear is that for a wide variety of reasons the elderly are particularly exposed to and vulner-able to unwanted effects.

IN CONCLUSION

Much of the material presented in this paper has been based on new analyses, for people aged 65 and over, of data from two national surveys, carried out by the Institute for Social Studies in Medical Care in 1969 and 1977. This reflects the lack of other detailed reports on drug use among representative samples of people aged 65 and over. On the whole, analysis by demographic characteristics was not very successful in distinguishing elderly people who use medicines. There were some differences by age and sex, indicating that women and the older elderly took more medicines, but these differences were generally small and were not maintained across several studies. On their own, "... age and sex are not good predictors of the number of drugs taken by an individual ..." (May & al. 1982). Many other factors, from problems with housing or money (Green 1982) to the patient's knowledge of medicines and attitudes to illness, may influence use, and these important factors may not be linked in any clear way to simple demographic characteristics (Blum and Kreitman 1981).

There is, therefore, wide scope for research in this field, documenting first who uses what medicines when, and including the use of non-prescribed medicines, and secondly considering the role of some factors, other than the demographic, as influences upon the use of medicines, particularly, perhaps, the meaning and significance of medicine use from the patient's perspective. There is a need to establish the frequency of drug problems in the elderly and to identify the medicines with which these problems are associated: from study of side effects and difficulties in using medicines, to identification of medicines which are not used when they could be helpful, and of other medicines which continue to be used when they are no longer helpful and may be hazardous.

Balme (1977) clearly feels that an overhaul is needed in general practitioner prescribing methods. He states that "... drug toxicity is frequently due to excessive dosage ..." and that "... the main reason for excessive drug doses in old age is that doctors lack the knowledge of the extent to which dosage in old age should be reduced compared to the conventional adult dose which is tailored to the needs of the middle aged or young patient." It is not only the prescribed doses that may be questioned, but the numbers of different types of medicines that are prescribed.

The need for caution and vigilance when prescribing for older people is frequently advised:

> ... on pharmacological grounds alone, there are good reasons for special care in prescribing for old people, but the situation is made much worse because two, three and sometimes five or

more drugs are often prescribed simultaneously. Adverse reactions are common and increase with the number of drugs given ... The greatest risk was with drugs affecting the cardiovascular system (diuretics, antihypertensives, and digitalis) and central nervous system (hypnotics, psychotropic agents and rigidity controllers) ... (Lancet 1977).

In the 1977 study (Cartwright and Anderson 1981), these categories of drugs constituted 2/3 of the medicines taken on a long-term prescription by people aged 65 and over.

Results from several research studies indicate little value in treating older people for extended periods with either diuretics (Burr & al. 1977, Myers & al. 1982) or psychotropic drugs (Tyrer 1978). The potential for reducing the prescription of repeat items to elderly patients had been assessed by Tulloch (1981) in his own practice. Ten percent of these prescriptions were thought to be no longer necessary, and for 28 percent the need was described as "equivocal" ("... when one drug could be stopped experimentally subject to the patient being well briefed, co-operative and under close surveillance ..."). The largest group of "unnecessary" prescriptions (1/3) was for psychotropic drugs; while 1/3 of the medicines described as "equivocal" were diuretics or drugs acting on the cardiovascular system.

The problems of dosage, polypharmacy and inappropriate prescribing are compounded by the use of non-prescription drugs, and, as we have shown, by the general practitioners' lack of knowledge of even the prescribed drugs that elderly patients may be currently taking. So if one implication is a need for continuing education in the complications and differences in prescribing for the elderly, another need is for an improved information or record-keeping system which ensures that all drugs being taken are reviewed at least whenever a new one is prescribed and preferably at every consultation so that doctors are alert to possible side effects and interactions. Although many doctors themselves urge more regular review and audit of their prescribing, they also note that regular monitoring of drug use could greatly increase the general practitioner's workload (Manasse 1974, Murdoch 1980). Perhaps pharmacists in general practice and the community could contribute to regular monitoring (Kiernan and Isaacs 1981, Frolund 1978), particularly as they are often the source of the patient's non-prescribed medicines.

How can older people be helped to use medicines more safely and effectively? Many studies have looked at "compliance" with instructions and how it can be improved (Sackett 1978). MacDonald, Mac-Donald, and Phoenix (1977) attempted to find ways to improve the drug compliance of elderly people after discharge from hospital. In their study of 165 consecutive discharges from a department of geriatric medicine, they found that counselling was effective, patients who were counselled making less than a third of the number of errors made by the uncounselled. A tear-off calendar improved results modestly but a "pill wheel" increased errors, and a tablet identification card was unhelpful. However, a study in Finland of elderly people's compliance with prescriptions and the quality of medication (Hemminki and Heikkila 1975) suggested that "... non-compliance with prescription instructions is not necessarily to be condemned as such. If drugs are prescribed in unreasonably large quantities, "under use" is a way for the patient to avoid ingesting excessive amounts of drugs..." This study also indicated that if a drug was considered important, it was taken more carefully.

A leader in the Journal of the Royal College of General Practitioners (1979) maintained: "It is no longer enough to ensure that the patient gets the right prescription: the doctor today must think ahead and consider if the patient understands the treatment, agrees with it and is likely to take it." Another leader in the British Medical Journal (1979) stressed a different problem: "Paradoxically, just as doctors have become concerned about the failure of some of their patients to take their medicines so have medical attitudes changed: increasing self awareness, helped sometimes by peer review, is persuading these same doctors that they can be wrong and that, on some occasions, their instructions are best ignored." That leader went on to pose the question: "What is the real problem: compliance or unnecessary prescribing?" Further, it referred to Sackett's (1978) hard-nosed questions: "Do we know that low compliance interferes with the achievement of the clinical goals of treatment?" And "Has it been established that treatment does more good than harm to those who do comply?"

The most important message that emerges from the various studies is that the prescribing and use of medicines must be regarded as a collaborative exercise between patients and doctors. As Banks (1979) has put it:

Too often the doctor is asking the patient to comply with directions which are either illogical or not based on scientific rationale ... The tendency is to blame the patient ... The answer ... is to question everything we do as practising clinicians, to stop and listen to what patients say, because often they will tell us the answers but we do not hear what they say.

If doctors should listen more, patients should probably be encouraged to ask more pertinent questions, of both their doctors and their pharmacists.

The high level of use of prescribed medicines by the elderly may be due, at least in part, to the limitations of a medical response to their common problems. Murdoch (1980) concluded his review of prescribing in a general practice in this way: "The evidence here is that general practitioners respond to the problems of ageing by the repeated prescribing of drugs." Older people and their doctors need to consider more regularly whether the use of medicines, often over many years, is a safe and effective answer to their problems.

REFERENCES

Anderson, R. (1980 a) "The Use of Repeatedly Prescribed Medicines," Journal of the Royal College of General Practitioners, 30, 609-613

Anderson, R. (1980 b) "Prescribed Medicines: Who Takes What?" Journal of Epidemiology and Community Health, 34, 4, 299-304

Arcand, Marcel, and Williamson, J. (1981) "An Evaluation of Home Visiting of Patients by Physicians in Geriatric Medicine," British Medical Journal, 283, 718-720

Atkinson, Leigh, Gibson, Iris I.J.M., and Andrews, James (1977) "The Difficulties of Old People Taking Drugs," Age & Ageing, 6, 144-150

Atkinson, Leigh, Gibson, Iris I.J.M., and Andrews, James (1978) "An Investigation into the Ability of Elderly Patients Continuing to Take Prescribed Drugs after Discharge from Hospital and Recommendations Concerning Improving the Situation," Gerontology, 24, 225-234

Balme, R.H. (1977) "Overhaul is Clearly Needed in GP Prescribing Methods," Modern Geriatics, 7, 6-8

Banks, D.C. (1979) (Letter) "Non-compliance: Does it Matter?" British Medical Journal, 2, 1585-1586

Bliss, M.R. (1981) "Prescribing for the Elderly," British Medical Journal, 283, 203-206

Blum, R., with Kreitman, K. (1981) "Factors Affecting Individual Use of Medicines," In Blum, R., Herxheimer, A., Stenzland, C. and Woodcock, J. (Eds.) Pharmaceuticals and Health Policy: International Perspectives on Provision and Control of Medicines, Croom Helm, London, 122-185

Bowling, Ann and Cartwright, Ann (1982) Life after a Death: a Study of the Elderly Widowed, Tavistock, London

British Medical Journal (1979) "Non-compliance: Does It Matter?" British Medical Journal, 2, 1168

Burr, M.L., King, S., Davies, H.E.F., and Pathy, M.S. (1977) "The Effects of Discontinuing Long-term Diuretic Therapy in the Elderly," Age & Ageing, 6, 38-45

Bytheway, B. (1976) "Prescribing and the Pensioner," In: Prescribing in General Practice. Journal of the Royal College of General Practitioners, Vol. 26, Supp. 1, 40-44

Cartwright, Ann (1983) "Prescribing and the Doctor-patient Relationship," In: Doctor-patient communication, David Pendleton and John Hasler (Eds.), Academic Press, London 177-191

Cartwright, Ann, Lucas, Susan, and O'Brien, Maureen (1974) "Exploring Communication in General Practice, A Pilot Study," Institute for Social Studies in Medical Care, Cyclostyled

Cartwright, Ann, and Anderson, Robert (1981) General Practice Revisited, Tavistock, London

Christopher, L.J., Ballinger, B.R., Shepherd, A.M.M., Ramsay, A., and Crooks, G. (1978) "Drug Prescribing Patterns in the Elderly: A Cross-Sectional Study of In-patients," Age & Ageing, 7, 74-82

Cooperstock, R., (1978) "Sex Differences in Psychotropic Drug Use," Social Science and Medicine, 12B, 179-186

Cooperstock, R., and Hill, J. (1982) The Effects of Tranquillisation: Benzodiazepine Use in Canada, Health & Welfare, Canada

Crombie, D.L., Green, C.M., Pearce, A.J., Benn, A., and Dewsbury, A. (1976) "Supervision of Repeat Prescribing," British Medical Journal, 1, 713

Crooks, J. and Parkin, D.M. (1977) "The Problem of Compliance in Drug Therapy," In: Topics in Therapeutics, 3, R.G. Shanks (Ed.) Pitman Medical

Das, B.C. (1977) "Drug Taking Is a Hazardous Business for the Old," Modern Geriatrics, 7, (1), 22-23

Dennis, P.J. (1979) "Monitoring of Psychotropic Drug Prescribing in General Practice," British Medical Journal, 2, 1115-1116

Department of Health and Social Security (1978) Health and Personal Social Services Statistics for England 1978 London: HMSO

Department of Health and Social Security (1982) Health and Personal Social Services Statistics for England 1982 London: HMSO

Drury, V.W.M., Wade, O.L. and Woolf, E. (1976) "Following Advice in General Practice," Journal of the Royal College of General Practitioners, 26, 712-718

Drury, V.W.M. (1982) "Repeat Prescribing - A Review," Journal of the Royal College of General Practitioners, 32, 42-45

Dunnell, K. and Cartwright, A. (1972) Medicine Takers, Prescribers and Hoarders, Routledge & Kegan Paul, London

Etlinger, P.R.A. and Freeman, G.K. (1981) "General Practice Compliance Study: Is It Worth Being a Personal Doctor?" British Medical Journal, 282, 1192-1194

Frolund, F. (1978) "Better Prescribing," British Medical Journal, 2, 741

Gibson, Iris I.J.M., and O'Hare, Margaret M. (1968) "Prescription of Drugs for Old People at Home," Gerontologia Clinica, 10, 271-280

Green, B. (1982) "Structural Antecedents of Psychoactive Drug Use Among the Elderly," Ageing and Society, 2, 77-94

Hemminki, E. and Heikkila, J. (1975) Elderly People's Compliance with Prescriptions, and Quality of Medication," Scandinavian Journal of Social Medicine, 3, 87-92

Herxheimer, A. (1976) (Letter) "Sharing the Responsibility for Treatment, How Can the Doctor Help the Patient?" Lancet, 2, 1294

Herxheimer, A., and Stimson, G.V. (1981) "The Use of Medicines for Illness," In: Blum, R., Herxheimer, A., Stenzland, C. and Woodcock, J. (Eds.) Pharmaceuticals and Health Policy: International Perspectives on Provision and Control of Medicines, Croom Helm, London, 36-60

Jefferys, M., Brotherston, J.H.F., and Cartwright, A. (1960) "Consumption of Medicines on a Working Class Housing Estate," British Journal of Preventive and Social Medicine, 14, 64-76

Journal of the Royal College of General Practitioners (1979) "Compliance," *Journal of the Royal College of General Practitioners*, 29, 387-389

Kiernan, P.J. and Isaacs, J.B. (1981) "Use of Drugs by the Elderly," *Journal of the Royal Society of Medicine*, 74, (3), 196-200

Kohn, R., and White, K.L. (Eds.) (1976) *Health Care: an International Study*, Oxford University Press, London

Lancet (1977) Editorial: "Drugs and the Elderly," *Lancet*, 2, 693-694

Law, R., and Chalmers, C. (1976) "Medicines and Elderly People: A General Practice Survey," *British Medical Journal*, 1, 565-568

MacDonald, Elspeth T., MacDonald, J.B., and Phoenix, Margaret (1977) "Improving Drug Compliance after Hospital Discharge," *British Medical Journal*, 2, 618-621

Manasse, A.P. (1974) "Repeat Prescriptions in General Practice," *Journal of the Royal College of General Practitioners*, 24, 203-207

Martys, C.R. (1982) "Drug Treatment in Elderly Patients: GP Audit," *British Medical Journal*, 285, 1623-1625

May, F.E., Stewart, R.B., Hale, W.E., and Marks, R.G. (1982) "Prescribed and Non-prescribed Drug Use in an Ambulatory Elderly Population," *Southern Medical Journal*, 75, 522-528

Moir, D.C., and Dingwall-Fordyce, I. (1980) Letter. "Drug Taking in the Elderly at Home," *Journal of Clinical and Experimental Gerontology*, 2, 329-332

Murdoch, J.C. (1980) "The Epidemiology of Prescribing in an Urban General Practice," *Journal of the Royal College of General Practitioners*, 30, 593-602

Myers, M.G., Weingert, M.E., Fisher, R.H., Gryfe, C.I., and Shulman, H.S. (1982) "Unnecessary Diuretic Therapy in the Elderly," *Age & Ageing*, 11, 213-221

Nathanson, C.A. (1977) "Sex, Illness and Medical Care: A Review of Data, Theory and Method," *Social Science and Medicine*, 11, 13-25

Office of Population Censuses and Surveys, Social Survey Division (1975) *The General Household Survey 1972*, HMSO, London

Office of Population Censuses and Surveys, Social Survey Division (1976) *The General Household Survey 1973*, HMSO, London

Office of Population Censuses and Surveys (1979) *General Household Survey 1977*, HMSO, London

Parkin, D.M., Henney, C.R., Quirk, J., and Crooks, J. (1976) "Deviation from Prescribed Treatment after Discharge from Hospital," British Medical Journal, 2, 686-688

Patrick, D.L., Peach, H., and Gregg, I. (1982) "Disablement and Care: A Comparison of Patient Views and General Practitioner Knowledge," Journal of the Royal College of General Practitioners, 32, 429-434

Peach, H. (Personal communication)

Price, N.C. (1983) "Importance of Asking about Glaucoma," British Medical Journal, 286, 349

Rabin, D.L., and Bush, B.J. (1974) "The Use of Medicines: Historical Trends and International Comparisons," International Journal of Health Services, 4, 61-87

Reid, J.J.A. (1956) "Regular Use of Laxatives by School Children," British Medical Journal, 2, 25-27

Sackett, D.L. (1978) "Compliance Trials and the Clinician," Archives of Internal Medicine, 138, 23-25

Scott, P.J.W., Stansfield, J., and Williams, B.O. (1982) "Prescribing Habits and Potential Adverse Drug Interactions in Geriatric Medical Service," Health Bulletin, 40, 5-9

Shaw, S.M., and Opit, L.J. (1976) "Need for Supervision in the Elderly Receiving Long-term Prescribed Medication," British Medical Journal, 1, 505-507

Sheldon, M.G. (Personal Communication)

Skegg, D.C.G., Doll, R., and Perry, J. (1977) "Use of Medicines in General Practice," British Medical Journal, 1, 1561-1563

Stimson, G.V. (1976) "Doctor-patient Interaction and Some Problems for Prescribing," In: Prescribing in General Practice, Journal of the Royal College of General Practitioners, 26, Supplement No. 1, 88-96

Tulloch, A.J. (1981) "Repeat Prescribing for Elderly Patients," British Medical Journal, 282, 1672-1675

Tyrer, P. (1978) "Drug Treatment of Psychiatric Patients in General Practice," British Medical Journal, 2, 1008-1010

Wandless, Irene, Mucklow, J.C., Smith, Andrew, and Prudham, D. (1979) "Compliance with Prescribed Medicines: a Study of Elderly Patients in the Community," Journal of the Royal of General Practitioners, 29, 391-396

Wadsworth, M.E.J., Butterfield, W.J.H., and Blaney, R. (1971) Health and Sickness: The Choice of Treatment, Tavistock, London

Whittington, F.J., Petersen, D.M., Dale, B. and Dressel, P.L. (1981) "Sex Differences in Prescription Drug Use of Older Adults," Journal of Psychoactive Drugs, 13, 175-183

Williams, P., Murray, J. and Clare, A. (1982) "A longitudinal Study of Psychotropic Drug Prescription," Psychological Medicine, 12, 201-206

Williamson, J. (1978) "Prescribing Problems in the Elderly," Practitioner, 220, 749-755

Williamson, J., and Chopin, Jean M. (1980) "Adverse Reactions to Prescribed Drugs in the Elderly: A Multicentre Investigation," Age & Ageing, 9, 73-80

Chapter 8

SELF-MEDICATION AMONG OLDER ADULTS IN THE UNITED
STATES

Susan Brown Eve

INTRODUCTION

Self-medication by older people involves two major
components: 1. self-administration of medicines, and
2. self-treatment with medicines. Self-administration refers to the taking of prescribed medications as a part of a total plan of treatment for
some condition, while self-treatment refers to
"using medications that were not obtained by a visit
to a physician" (50). Older adults may treat
themselves using prescription medicines, non-prescription medicines or social drugs. Prescription
medicines may be used for self-treatment when older
adults use left-over medicines that were prescribed
for a previous illness to treat a current illness or
when they obtain prescription medicines from informal, non-medical sources such as relatives or
friends. Non-prescription medicines are most commonly used for self-treatment, although physicians may
on occasion suggest or prescribe the use of these
medicines as part of a treatment plan. Older people
may also self-medicate with substances not usually
considered to be medicines, including socially
accepted drugs such as alcohol, nicotine, and
caffeine. Self-medication with social drugs among
older adults will be reviewed in the context of
possible interaction with prescription and non-prescription medicines.

Whenever possible, this review of the research
literature on the use of prescription and non-
prescription drugs among older adults in the United
States will distinguish between drugs used for
self-administration and self-treatment, although
many of the studies reviewed did not make this
distinction. Researchers have generally assumed that
prescription medicines are self-administered and

that non-prescription medicines and social drugs are used for self-treatment. The review will focus on identifying recent trends in the quantity and frequency of use of the two major medicine categories, the types of the medicines used, the characteristics of the users and the non-users and the appropriateness of the use. The findings will be organised in the context of the Andersen and Newman health care services utilisation framework of predisposing, enabling and need variables (2). Finally, the two major problems with drug use among the elderly in the United States -- 1. non-compliance with instructions for use of medicines in self-medication, and 2. drug reactions and interactions due to polypharmacy, i.e., the use of multiple drugs for self-medication -- will be discussed.

PRESCRIPTION MEDICINES

The growing interest concerning drug use among the elderly in the United States, especially use of prescription drugs, is reflected in the amount of empirical research on the topic during the last decade. These studies reveal that older adults consume a disproportionately large share of prescription medicines in general and psychoactive prescription medicines in particular.

Prescription Medicines in General

Prevalence of Use. Older adults who comprise approximately 10 percent of the population of the United States, consume more than 25 percent of the prescription medicines. Research in the past two decades has consistently shown that the use of medicines increases with age (3, 26, 34, 39, 42, 46, 47). Furthermore, the data indicate that the proportion of older adults who use prescription medicines is increasing. In 1963 just over half of older adults reported that they had used prescription medicines in the past year, compared to 3/4 reporting such use in 1977 (3,47). The average number of prescription medicines taken also increases with age and the sharpest increase occurs between middle-age and old age with older adults taking an average of 11 to 13 different prescription medicines in a given year compared to seven to eight among the middle-aged and two to four among young adults (39, 42, 46, 47).

Types of General Prescription Medicines Used. The major types of general prescription medicines used change with age, reflecting the age-related shift in major health problems from acute diseases among the young to chronic diseases among the old. Medicines for cardio-vascular diseases, including heart disease, high blood pressure and other conditions of the circulatory system, are the most commonly prescribed drugs for older adults, accounting for 30 to 40 percent of all prescription drugs used by the non-institutionalised older population and for 20 percent of all drugs provided or prescribed in office visits to a physician. Other major chronic conditions leading to use of prescribed medicines include arthritis and disorders of the bones and joints, accounting for eight to ten percent of all prescribed medicines; mental and nervous conditions, six to seven percent; and conditions of the digestive system and diabetes, about five percent each (40, 42, 46).

Determinants of Prescription Medicine Use. Older women are more likely to use prescription medicines and to use a greater number than are older men (18, 26, 34, 39, 42, 49). A slight tendency has been found for less educated older adults to use more prescription medicines than the more educated (39, 42). Research since the 1960s has shown that whites use more prescription medicines than their non-white counterparts (8, 39, 42).

Three studies of older adults have found belief variables to be important in predicting the use of prescription medicines. Back and Sullivan found that middle-aged and older women who use prescription medicines tend to be insecure, to adopt the sick role more readily and, ironically, to be afraid of medicine. They speculate that this fear and readiness to accept the sick role may encourage women to visit a doctor sooner than men would when they become ill, making them more likely to take medicines (4). Guttmann found that older adults who take prescription medicines are less likely to be satisfied with life, are less likely to perceive older adults as capable, and have better knowledge of health resources than older adults who are not using such medicines (18). Sharpe and Smith found that use of prescription medicines among older adults is positively related to anxiety (37).

The effects of income and insurance on the use of prescription medicines has changed in the United States with the introduction of the Medicare programme for retired workers and their families and the Medicaid programme for qualified indigents. Research on the use of prescription medicines conducted prior to the passage of the Medicare and Medicaid legislation in 1965 generally found income and private health insurance had a positive effect on the use of prescription medicines, while more recent research has found a negative relationship between income and prescription medicine use and no effect due to private insurance coverage (39, 42).

Prescription medicines are provided under Medicare only while older adults are being treated in a hospital. Medicaid, a programme for the medically indigent of all ages, is financed jointly by the federal and state governments with the states determining eligibility requirements. Because of the restrictiveness of these requirements, 39 percent of the elderly below the poverty line are not eligible for coverage by the programme (30). Prescription medicines are covered under the Medicaid programme but the number of prescriptions that can be filled per month is limited, usually to not more than three prescriptions. Research conducted since the passage of the Medicare and Medicaid programmes indicates that 3/4 of the expenses for prescription medicines among older adults were paid for out-of-pocket (42, 47).

Because they are less likely to have private health insurance, older adults pay a slightly higher proportion of the cost of their prescription medicine expenses out-of-pocket than do younger adults. Choi found that among older adults, the proportion of out-of-pocket expenses differed little by category; the very poorest paid 67 percent of these expenses as compared to 80 percent paid by the highest income group (42). The extent to which limitations in coverage of prescription medicines create hardships for the elderly poor does not appear to have been explicitly investigated, but Sharpe and Smith found that among the 35 percent of older adults who were eligible for Medicaid in their Mississippi sample, 81 percent knew that Medicaid covered prescription medicines but only 20 percent knew of the monthly limit on the number of prescriptions. A pharmacist had refused to fill a prescription for seven percent because of the monthly limit, which suggests that the needs of a significant number of poor, older persons are not being met (37).

Relationships between the rise of prescription medicines and urban/rural residence have been found. Studies by Choi and Wilder showed that older adults living in the South, which is the least affluent of the four regions of the United States and has the fewest health care services per capita, used more prescription medicines than residents of other regions. The same studies also indicated that older adults in rural areas used more prescription medicines than those in urban areas (39, 42). Perceived accessibility of medical care has been found to be positively related to use of prescription medicines (8).

As might be expected, the most consistent determinant of use of prescription medicines by older adults is poor health. Usage has been shown to increase as self-evaluation of health decreases, as the number of symptoms and the number of chronic conditions increases, as number of bed days and/or restricted activity days increases, and as the degree of limitation or disability increases (8, 18, 26, 37, 39, 41, 42, 52).

Psychoactive Prescription Medicine Use

Psychoactive drugs account for approximately seven to eight percent of all drugs taken by older adults (40, 42, 46). Furthermore, older adults receive a disproportionate share of psychoactive medicines prescribed by physicians. Prentice reported that in 1975, people 65 and older, who represented ten percent of the population, received 1/5 of all orders for psychoactive drugs, excluding stimulants for which older adults received less than five percent of the prescriptions (33).

Prevalence and Frequency of Use. Based upon the studies reviewed, four generalisations can be made concerning prevalence and frequency of use of psychoactive medicines among older adults. Firstly, although the data were collected at various times in the past two decades, a consistent finding has been that approximately 1/5 to 1/4 of the older population was currently using some type of prescription psychoactive medicine (18, 27, 45, 49); that approximately 1/3 had used a prescription psychoactive medicine in the past year (28, 29, 31, 45);

and that approximately 1/2 had ever used psycho-active medicines (44). Secondly, the percent of the total population using a prescription psychoactive medicine tends to increase with age, with the sharpest increases occurring between youth and middle-age and smaller increases occurring between middle and old age (28, 31, 45, 48). Thirdly, minor tranquillisers and sedatives are the most commonly used psychoactive medicines in all age groups (1, 18, 28, 29, 31). Furthermore, the percentage of the population using minor tranquillisers and sedatives, hypnotics, and antidepressants tends to increase with age while the percentage using stimulants tends to peak among young adults and decline with age. Use of major tranquillisers and antipsychotic medicines among the non-institutionalised populations is fairly constant across age groups because most adults needing these types of medication are likely to be institutionalised (28, 31). Finally, women of all ages are generally more likely than men to take psychoactive medicines (28, 29, 31, 48).

Data on frequency of use indicate that psycho-active medicines, especially the minor tranquil-lisers and sedatives, the most commonly used psychotropic medicines, are used less than daily. A nationwide survey by Parry & al. found that older adults were less likely than mature and middle-aged adults to be using prescription psychoactive medi-cines daily (31). Guttmann and Stephens & al. found bimodal patterns of frequency of use for minor tranquillisers, sedatives, and hypnotics, with most respondents reporting use of the drug either daily or infrequently, while antidepressants and anti-psychotics were most likely to be used every day (43). These patterns are very similar to patterns reported by Mellinger and Balter for the total adult population (28).

Determinants of Use. Among the predisposing vari-ables, use of psychoactive medicines has been found to increase with age and to be greater among women than men (1, 28, 29, 30, 42, 48, 51). Older adults who do not live alone, who are satisfied with their family relationships, who are married, who are working, and who report higher life satisfaction are less likely to be taking these medicines than others (18, 51). Among the enabling variables, income has been found to be negatively related to current use of psychoactive medicines but positively related to ever having taken psychoactive medicines (45, 51).

Illness-morbidity variables are the most strongly related to current use of psychoactive medicines in all studies. Watson & al. (1980) found that the total number of chronic conditions and hospitalisations in the past year both correlated positively with use of psychoactive medicines. Respondents in Guttmann's study who used psychoactive medicines reported that they were in poorer health, were more disabled, and needed more help with services such as house cleaning and legal matters than non-users. Stephens & al. also found that poor self-assessed health was associated with increased use of prescribed psychoactive medicines (18, 45, 51). Using secondary data that did not distinguish between prescription and non-prescription medicines, Eve and Friedsam focused on developing predictive models of use of psychoactive substances among older adults. They found that the best model that explained use of sleeping pills and tranquillisers among older Texans was the social stress model that has been widely used in social epidemiological studies of mental health. The two major types of variables that have been found to affect mental health are social stressors and social integration. Using this model, Eve and Friedsam found that the major stressors among older adults were loss of a spouse, low income, transportation problems, health problems, and housing problems. Both objective measures of these problems (e.g., monthly income) and subjective measures (e.g., how well income satisfies needs) were used. Interestingly, the subjective assessments of the social stress variables were more predictive than the objective measures. Similarly, subjective dissatisfaction with the frequency of interaction with family, friends, neighbours, clubs and organisations, and reported frequency of feelings of loneliness were more predictive of taking tranquillisers than were objective measures of actual frequency of visits with family, friends, neighbours and clubs and organisations (13).

NON-PRESCRIPTION MEDICINES

Use of non-prescription medicines has not been studies as extensively as use of prescription medicines. patterns of use of non-prescription medicines differ from those for the use of prescription medicines while the determinants of use of the over-the-counter medicines are interesting for their similarities and dissimilarities to the determinants of prescription medicine use.

Non-prescription Medicines in General

Prevalence and Frequency of Non-prescription Medicine Use. In contrast to the use of prescription medicines, use of non-prescription medicines in general decreases with age, although nearly all older people use at least one non-prescription medicine in a year. Recent studies of older adults in widely diverse settings have found that 50 to 70 percent of older adults report current use of non-prescription medicines. Older adults take fewer non-prescription medicines than prescription medicines, with all studies reviewed reporting averages of one to two different non-prescription medicines currently being used (18, 26, 37, 44, 52, 54).

Types of Non-prescription Medicines Used. The most commonly used types of non-prescribed drugs are pain relievers. Approximately half of the respondents in most of the studies reviewed reported recent use of such drugs with up to 75 percent reporting use within the past year (18, 26, 37, 54). In a national survey, Bonham and Leaverton found that regular use of aspirin increased with age for women from 17 percent at ages 20 to 25 to 35 percent at ages of 75 or more, and among men from 10 percent to 25 percent (44). In his study in Washington, D.C., Guttmann found that 35 percent of his sample took aspirin when necessary but only 13 percent took the medicine daily. Other common non-prescription medicines used include vitamins, cold and cough medicines, laxatives, antacids and skin ointments. Over-the-counter sleeping pills and tranquillisers are among the least used non-prescription drugs (18, 26, 37, 54).

Determinants of Non-prescription Medicine Use. Among predisposing variables, a consistent finding is that women use more over-the-counter medicines than men (8, 9, 39, 44, 53). Among social structure variables, a positive relationship between education and use of non-prescribed medicines has been shown (8, 26). Whites have been found to use non-prescription medicines more than non-whites (8). As with psychoactive medicines, Guttmann found that older adult users tended to have lower life satisfaction than did non-users; and that they also had poorer perceptions of their own and others' abilities (18). Back and Sullivan found that users of medicinal drugs were more likely than non-users to be insecure (4).

Among enabling variables, income, accessibility to health care, and morbidity have been examined in several studies. While data which predates Medicare and Medicaid found income had a curvilinear effect with the lowest and highest income groups spending the most for non-prescription medicines, more recent studies have found that income has no effect on use of over-the-counter medicines (8, 26, 39). Accessibility of medical care has been found to be negatively related to use of non-prescription medicines (8).

Among the illness variables, morbidity has been found to be related to the use of non-prescription medicines among the general adult population, especially in a sample of respondents having one or more chronic illnesses (8, 26). Among a population of older adults, the majority of whom had at least one chronic illness, self-rated health was negatively related to use of non-prescription medicines while visits to a physician and use of prescription medicines have been found to be negatively related to the use of non-prescription medicines, which suggests that non-prescription medicines are an alternative to use of the formal health care system (8, 18, 26). Sharpe and Smith found a moderately positive relationship between use of prescription and non-prescription medicines, suggesting that the two may complement each other rather than being alternatives (37).

Two recent studies of the use of medicines among older adults suggest that the determinants of the use of specific non-prescription medicines differ considerably. Whittington, Welchel and Petersen found that the major predictor of use of pain-killers was being female; the major predictors of use of laxatives were poor health, a recent physician visit, and low income; and the major predictor of the use of cough and cold medicines was age, which was negatively related to use (54). In research designed to distinguish between medicines used for different purposes, Eve and Friedsam also found that determinants of use differed for specific types of medicines. Using vitamins as an example of a medicine frequently taken for preventive purposes and laxatives as an example of a medicine often taken for a curative purpose, they found that taking vitamins was positively related to socioeconomic status and beliefs in the value of preventive health while use of laxatives was negatively related to health, self-reported assessment of income, and accessibility of physicians (14).

Non-prescription Psychoactive Drug Use

Studies of the prevalence of non-prescription psychoactive drug use indicate that usage of such medicines is less prevalent than the use of prescription psychoactive drugs. Mellinger & al. and Parry & al. found that less than 10 percent of older adults in their samples reported any use of over-the-counter stimulants, sleeping pills or tranquillisers in the past year, and Mellinger and Balter found that only four percent of older men and older women had used over-the-counter sleeping pills or tranquillisers in the past year.

Patterns of use vary by type of psychoactive non-prescription medicine. Data from the two national samples indicate that non-prescription psychotropic drug use peaks in young adulthood, especially for use of stimulants, but that a second smaller peak occurs in the oldest age group for use of sleeping pills. These studies also show that males of all ages are more likely than females to use stimulants and that females are more likely to take tranquillisers and sleeping pills but that use of non-prescription medicines tends to be short term and sporadic (28, 29, 31).

COMPARISON OF THE USE OF PRESCRIPTION AND NON-PRESCRIPTION MEDICINES

Comparison of use and determinants of both general and psychoactive prescription and non-prescription medicines discussed above reveals some interesting similarities and differences in the self-medication behaviours of older adults. The major similarities and differences are discussed below.

There are three variables which have consistently been found to be related to the use of all four categories of medicines reviewed. Firstly, poor health is the best predictor of use in all cases. Secondly, women are more likely than men to be using medicines in all categories. Thirdly, variables which measure quality of life such as the measures of life satisfaction consistently indicate that drug use increases as the perception of the quality of the older person's life decreases.

There are also differences in the determinants of use of prescription and non-prescription medicines. The most consistent difference is related to age. Use of prescription medicines has been found to increase with age while use of non-prescription medicines decreases. Secondly, most of the studies that have examined accessibility of health care services have found that accessibility is positively related to the use of prescription, but negatively related to the use of non-prescription medicines. The issue of accessibility is directly related to the unresolved issue of the relationship between the use of prescription and non-prescription medicines. Two studies conducted in the urban Northeast region, one using a general adult population and the second using an older adult population found a slight inverse relationship between use of the two types of medicines suggesting that use of prescription and non-prescription medicines are alternative avenues of treatment. A third study conducted in a more rural county of the South found a moderate positive relationship suggesting that the use of the two types of medicines are complementary (8, 18, 37).

DRUG MISUSE

Because of the high proportion of the elderly who take drugs and because older adults frequently take several drugs simultaneously, they are the age group at the greatest risk of misusing drugs (5). The most frequently discussed problems of misuse include overuse, underuse, contraindicated use, drug inter-actions, and drug related disorders and death. Misuse may result from errors in self-administration of prescribed medicines or self-medication of health problem using medications, usually non-prescription, obtained without a visit to a physician. Responsibility for errors may be due to or shared by the patient, the physician, and the pharmacist.

Overuse and Underuse of Prescription and Non-prescription Medicines
Studies of self-administration behaviour by patients generally report that 1/3 to 1/2 of patients do not comply with the instructions for using prescription medicines and that age is not consistently related to compliance (20). In a recent follow-up survey of 545 patients released from Johns Hopkins University over a nine-month period, Klein & al. found, one month after discharge, that among patients both under and over 65 years of age, more than half were

taking their medicines as frequently as they should and approximately were taking as much medicine as they should. In fact, older adults are more likely to underuse than overuse medicines (23). Green reported that only 16 percent of her community sample of older adults overused prescription medicines while 36 percent underused them (17). Stephens & al. found that only 6.9 percent of older adults misused prescription medicines and that of these non-compliers, 86.8 percent took less, while only 13.2 percent took more than was prescribed (37). Schwartz & al. reported that underuse was the most common form of non-compliance in a survey of 178 chronically ill patients seen in a New York hospital, and Raffoul & al. noted that 72 percent of the non-compliers in a local Kentucky sample underused their medicines (36). Similarly, Doyle and Hamm reported that 2/5 of a Florida community sample of 405 adults 60 years of age and older discontinued taking medicines they disliked (11).

Reasons for patient misuse of medicines that have been investigated include patient demographic characteristics, patient attitudes, and communication gaps between health care professionals and patients. Studies of compliance have not found consistent relationships with demographic characteristics including age, sex, race and ethnicity, but a relationship between non-compliance and several factors that are correlated with age has been shown, including lack of education, living alone, being unmarried, low income, and a belief that medicines were too expensive (7, 20, 37, 38). Poor health, including patient incompetence, psychological illness and chronic illness, have also been found to be related to non-compliance (20, 36). The most common reasons given by patients for misusing medicines involve voluntary choice. Older adults have reported that they feel better when they stop taking their medicines, they take their medicine only when they feel they need it, they do not like the medicine or the dosage, they get better results using the medicines their way, and they do not like the side effects (38).

Human error also contributes to drug misuse. Stephens & al. found that 23 percent of the older adults in their study admitted that they had trouble remembering to take their medicines and another eight percent had trouble taking their medicines at the right time (38). Professional errors that affect patient compliance include incomplete instructions for taking medicines and inadequate monitoring of patients (25, 26). Pharmaceutic packaging may also affect compliance. Thirty-seven percent of older adults in one study reported difficulty in opening medicine containers, nine percent reported problems with reading the label, and six percent reported difficulties in preparation of their medicines (37).

Schwartz & al., Lundin and Green have suggested that compliance would improve if patients were more knowledgeable about the medicines they are taking, but other research indicates that this may not be true (17, 25, 36). As much as 80 to 90 percent of prescription medicines in general and as much as 100 percent of psychoactive prescription medicines have been correctly identified by older adults. The two most frequently incorrectly identified prescription medicines were cardiovascular drugs and nutrient supplements (18, 25, 37). In the study of recently released hospital patients, however, adults under 65 correctly identified the purpose of 81 percent of their medicines while adults 65 years and older correctly identified only 74 percent; 72 percent of the younger adults but only 50 percent of the older adults correctly identified the purpose of all their prescription medicines. Both differences remained even when the number of medicines prescribed was controlled, but knowledge of purpose was not related to compliance in either age group. Of the patients who correctly identified the purpose of their medicines, 75 percent were in compliance for the frequency and 85 percent were in compliance for the quantity of the medicines being taken; the corresponding percentages of those incorrectly identifying the purpose of the medicines were 70 percent for frequency and 81 percent for quantity. Thus, the relationship between knowledge and compliance is weaker than is generally thought (23).

Although studies that have examined compliance by older adults with directions for using non-prescription medicines for self-treatment were not found, a study of 242 older adults in Washington D.C., in which prescription and non-prescription drugs were not distinguished, found than 15 percent of all medicines were used for reasons other than those given in the Physician's Desk Reference. Among drugs which are commonly available without a prescription, the findings were that aspirin was misused 15 percent of the time; laxatives, 2.7 percent of the time; vitamins, 9.9 percent; antacids, 6.3 percent; cough and cold medicines, 6.1 percent; and antihistamines, 33.3 percent (10).

Almost 3/4 of Guttmann's sample thought they knew the purpose of the non-prescription medicines they were taking, and 95 percent of Sharpe and Smith's sample correctly identified the purpose of their over-the-counter medicines. Analgesics and anti-infectives were incorrectly identified most frequently (36). Thus, older adults appear to use non-prescription medicines as appropriately as they do prescription medicines and appear to be as knowledgeable about non-prescription medicines as prescription medicines. Other community studies have found much lower percentages of potentially harmful interactions. Only six percent of older adults in the study by Stephens & al. reported currently using psychoactive drugs and alcohol, while Raffoul & al. found that 11 percent of the instances of drug abuse in their sample of older adults involved drug/drug or drug"alcohol interactions (35).

In summary, the research on prescription medicine use suggests that 1/3 to 1/2 of adults do not comply with prescription medicine instructions, but that age does not affect compliance. Older adults who are non-compliers are much more likely to underuse than to overuse their medicines. Non-compliance among older adults has been found to be negatively related to education and income and positively related to poor health, patient incompetence, psychological illness, and chronic illness. The major reasons given for underuse by older adults included voluntary choice (they felt better, did not like the medicine, etc.), economic necessity, and incomplete instructions and/or monitoring from the physicians.

Polypharmacy
Increasing age is associated with physiological changes which increase the risk of hazardous drug reactions and interactions among older adults. After reviewing research on these changes, Bender concluded that the pharmokinetic functions of absorption, distribution, metabolism and excretion of medicines decreases with age and that pharmacodynamic changes at the receptor sites changes the action of medicines in older people, e.g., reducing the action of stimulants and enhancing the action of depressants. In a review of the literature on polypharmacy among adults, Krupka and Veneer concluded that the risk of reactions and interactions increases with the number of medicines taken (6, 24). In a study by James, only 19 percent of

patients taking one to five drugs as compared to 81 percent taking six to ten had an adverse reaction (22). In a nine-week study of 120 ambulatory geriatric patients in a health clinic, Eberhardt and Robinson documented 43 drug interactions and 25 percent of the patients reported some unpleasant side effects (12). Sharpe and Smith reported that 216 of their 300 respondents were taking multiple drugs and identified 140 potentially interactive drug pairs involving 23 percent of the respondents. Of the 140 drug interactions identified, 43 percent were classified as minor in terms of their potential to harm the patient, 53 percent as moderate and four percent as major (37).

Prescription medicines may also interact with non-prescription and social drugs. Although no studies have systematically explored the prevalence of potential interactions among older adults, some data exists on the extent of combined use of these three types of drugs. In the Guttmann study, 17.4 percent of the older adults reported concurrent use of prescription medicine, non-prescription medicine and alcohol; 25.3 percent use prescription and non-prescription medicines; 8.4 percent use prescription medicines and alcohol; and 12.3 percent use non-prescription medicines and alcohol. Thirty-five percent of the older adults who used psycho-tropic medicines also reported that they used alcohol, a combination known to be dangerous (18).

Several studies have used existing records to measure the extensiveness of harmful drug reactions and interactions. The National Institute of Drug Abuse routinely monitors drug related incidents in hospitals, emergency rooms and medical examiners' offices as part of its Drug Abuse Warning Network. DAWN data for 1974-75 indicate that adults 50 years and older were involved in only six percent of the drug incidents in hospitals and emergency rooms that involved barbiturates, sedatives, tranquillisers, or alcohol/drug interaction, the lowest incidence for any age group. Only five percent of the incidents with adults 50 years of age and older involved alcohol/drug interactions (19). These data are consistent with those based on emergency room records in Dade County, Florida, where Petersen and Thomas found that only 5.4 percent of 1,128 admissions related to psychoactive drug-abuse-involved adults 50 years of age or older. Most incidents involving older adults, 80.9 percent, were reactions to psychoactive drugs and only 8.3 percent involved alcohol/drug combinations (32). A follow-up study that examined Dade County hospital emergency room records from January 1972 to June 1976 revealed that only 2.6 percent of the drug-related incidents involved adults 60 years of age or older. Although data indicate a low incidence of serious drug reactions, they obviously do not reflect the occurrence of drug incidents in which the person experiencing the reaction does not reach the emergency room or hospital (21). It is sobering to note that the DAWN data indicate that 62 percent of all references to death from psychoactive or psychoactive/alcohol combinations among adults 50 years of age and older were attributed to suicide, a rate that is more than twice as high as that for any other age group (19).

Even when not fatal, the use of non-prescription and social drugs simultaneously may have negative effects on the older person's health. Krupka and Veneer report anecdotal evidence on a 79-year-old male who lived in his own residence, had seven chronic illnesses and consumed 13 different drugs on a daily basis. When the respondent's total drug intake was examined, potential reactive and interactive hazards became evident, including twice as high an intake of caffeine as is recommended for a person with severe heart disease, and a potential aspirin/alcohol/vitamin C interaction that could exacerbate his ulcers and cause aspirin toxicity and kidney damage (24). The authors emphasise the need for health professionals to consider the total drug exposure of older adults including both pre-scription, over-the-counter and social drugs.

The potential for hazardous results from polypharmacy is increased by negligent or unsafe practices by health professionals as well as by older adults. In the study by Raffoul & al. the major correlates of drug misuse were the number of prescribing physicians and the number of dispensing pharmacies (35). Stephens & al. indicate that only a small percentage of older adults were asked by their physicians if they were seeing other physicians, ranging from 7.9 percent among those currently taking no medications to 21.5 percent among those taking four or more. Only 24.3 percent of those taking no medicines and 42.9 percent of those taking four or more were asked by the physicians if they were taking any other medicines (48).

Patients also have a responsibility to be careful about their prescriptions. Doyle and Hamm found that 71.6 percent of older adults did not discuss the prescriptions of one doctor with another doctor; 74.8 percent asked no questions about content, side effects, or cost when receiving a prescription; and only 13 percent of patients went to visit a physician when they needed a prescription. Thirty percent called the doctor to get their prescription and another 30 percent had the pharmacist call the physician (11). Guttmann, however, found that 75.8 percent of tne older adults who were taking prescription medicines reported that they consulted with a physician before taking other drugs in combination and 62.4 percent of those taking other prescription medicines did so. Sharpe and Smith found that 41.3 percent of the prescriptions taken by the older adults in their sample were refills, 39.3 percent were written by a physician, and 14.5 percent were ordered over the phone without a doctor's visit (37).

Other studies have reported that older adults may also engage in self-treatment with prescription medicines. Doyle and Hamm found that 12.8 percent of their sample keep old medicines because they think they might need them, 13.3 percent believe that sharing medicines is not dangerous and 12.6 percent had shared or would consider sharing medicines (11). Lundin also found that 10 percent of older adults took medicines from others (25).

Older adults usually treat themselves when using non-prescription drugs. For example, 2/3 of the older adults in Guttmann's study reported relying on their own judgement in choosing non-prescription medicines, with the remainder almost evenly divided between having asked a physician's advice or having sought advice from friends, relatives, and other health professionals. Similarly, only 1/4 of Sharpe and Smith's respondents had asked for a physicians' advice about over-the-counter medications and only one percent asked advice from a pharmacist. Furthermore, only 40 percent of over-the-counter medicines were purchased in a pharmacy, the bulk being purchased in grocery, discount and convenience stores, thus minimising the availability of professional advice (37).

In summary, polypharmacy increases the risks of drug reactions and drug interactions. The greater the number of prescribing physicians and of dispensing pharmacies involved, the greater the likelihood of drug reactions and interactions. The limited data on drug reactions and interactions suggest that as many as 1/4 of older adults take drug combinations that are potentially interactive and that approximately half of these interactions have the potential for producing moderate to major effects in the older adult. Most of the single drug reactions among older adults are in reaction to psychoactive prescription medicines. While concurrent use of alcohol and psychoactive medicines is rare, concurrent use of alcohol with other prescription and non-prescription medicines is not and represents a potential hazard for older adults. Most older adults do not discuss the prescription of one doctor with another.

CONCLUSIONS

Use of drugs among teenagers and young adults received increased research attention in the United States in the 1960s when use and abuse of illicit drugs began to capture public interest, but use among older adults is an area that has only recently begun to receive similar attention. The expansion of public awareness of the broader problem of drugs in American society in the past two decades has been reflected in the growth of related research literature, both in terms of the scope of the population affected by the problem and by the types of drug use that have come to be recognised as parts of the problem. The public and scientific community have come to realise that middle-aged and older adults are also a part of the drug problem, and concern with types of drugs now includes prescription drugs and licit non-prescription and social drugs. This review of the self-medication behaviour of older adults has focused on the prevalence and frequency of use of prescription and non-prescription medicines and the determinants of the use of these medicines and the extent of their misuse. Six major gaps in knowledge of self-medication among older adults in the United States have been identified including 1. lack of theoretical models, 2. neglect of multi-disciplinary perspectives, 3. absence of studies of relationships among the use of prescription, non-prescription and social drugs, 4. failure to refine the concept of self-medication, 5. neglect of subgroups of medicines, and 6. absence of empirical research in drug reactions and interactions.

Most of the research on self-medication is descriptive and atheoretical. Researchers have tended to focus on prevalence of use of prescription and non-prescription medicines and on social and demographic correlates of use, but have not focused on the reasons for the relationships. The relationships among the predictor variables and drug use that have been discovered should be explored in more detail. As one example, the finding that women are more likely to use medicines than men is consistent in the literature but no studies have demonstrated why gender should make a difference. Another example of an area in which research is lacking is in studies focusing on how problematic the obtaining of medicines is for older adults, especially poorer older adults despite the fact that lack of, or inadequacies in, coverage of prescription medicines in public insurance programmes and private medigap insurance means that even the poor must pay for most of their medicines out-of-pocket and that a major reason given by older adults for underuse of prescribed medicines is lack of money to pay for them. The extent to which income creates a barrier to prescribed medicine use is not known and should be investigated since not using medicines may contribute to deterioration of existing conditions that may be both more difficult and more expensive to treat later.

Another shortcoming in the existing literature is the limited amount of research based upon a multi-disciplinary approach. Reasons for taking prescripton medicines and non-prescription medicines are influenced by physical signs and symptoms, mental signs and symptoms, personality character- istics, social characteristics, attitudes and be- liefs related to health and illness and economic status. Multi-disciplinary multi-variate predictive models that include all relevant factors are necessary to achieve a full understanding of self-medication behaviour. Depending upon the scope of a study, a research team may require a physician, pharmacist, nurse, psychiatrist, psychologist, soci- ologist, social worker, and economist among others.

The relationships between self-medication and the use of prescription, non-prescription and social drugs also needs further examination. Previous research on these interrelationships is inconsistent with the finding by some studies that the use of these three different types of drugs are alterna- tives, while others find that they are complemen- tary. Folk medicines may also play an important role among some population subgroups. In the United States, for example, older Mexican-Americans, Indians, Blacks, and Applachian whites have been found to cling to folk beliefs about disease and treatment of disease, even though the younger generations have relinquished these beliefs and practices as they become more educated and affluent.

The concept of self-medication itself needs to be refined. Glantz has recently suggested that inappropriate drug use can be further subdivided into drug misuse and drug abuse. The major distinction that he makes between the two is that drug misuse is inadvertant, while drug abuse occurs when a person knowingly uses a drug in a non-sanctioned or non-therapeutic way. Drugs can be misused or abused both by underutilisation as well as over-utilisation, and this can apply to use of prescription, non-prescription and social drugs (15, 16). Just as self-administration must be distinguished from self-treatment, a measure of the appropriateness or inappropriateness of use must be developed. A model can be found in research on health care services' utilisation which has recently begun developing measures of appropriateness of use of physicians' services that involve using a panel of experts, usually physicians, to judge whether a visit to a physician was appropriate or inappropriate based on the respondent's reported signs and symptoms.

Researchers need to examine the determinants of medicine use more closely by type of medicine used. For example, researchers have found that the determinants of the use of psychoactive medicines, whether prescription or non-prescription, differ from those predicting the use of prescription medicines in general. Other research has found that the determinants of use differ with the purpose for which the drug is taken -- i.e., preventive, curative, or maintenance. The determinants of use of social drugs such as alcohol and caffeine may also vary. Although analysis of the broad categories of prescription, non-prescription and social drugs may yield generalisations about the determinants of most of the use of drugs in a category, the use of the broad categories may obscure some important differences as well.

Finally, much anecdotal evidence suggests that drug reactions and interactions are not uncommon among older adults, but little systematic scientific evidence is available assessing the prevalence of reactions and interactions among older adults living in the community and the reasons for the reactions. Given the potentially serious consequences of the reaction and interactions, further study of this area is essential.

In conclusion, the research reviewed in this chapter has identified the basic dimensions of the problem of self-medication among older adults and has raised many issues that need to be addressed in future research. Future research can build on the previous research by developing multi-disciplinary theoretical models that are explanatory and predictive and by focusing on research issues that have been identified, but not thoroughly researched in the previous studies.

The author would like to thank Hiram J. Friedsam, Ph.D., Professor, Center for Studies in Ageing, North Texas State University and editor of The Gerontologist (1982-1984) and Kathryn Dean, Ph.D., co-editor of this volume, for their very helpful comments and suggestions of the various drafts of this manuscript.

NOTES

(1) Abelson, H.I. and Atkinson, R.B. (1975) Public Experience with Psychoactive Substances. Cited in the Aging Process and Psychoactive Drug Use, National Institute of Alcohol, Drug Abuse and Mental Health Administration, U.S. Public Health Service Publication No. 79-813, U.S. Government Printing Office, Washington, D.C., 1979, pp. 22-24.

(2) Andersen, Ronald and Newman, John F. (1973) "Societal and Individual Determinants of Medical Care Utilization in the United States," Milbank Memorial Fund, 51, pp. 95-124.

(3) Andersen, Ronald, Smedley, Bjorn, and Anderson, Odin W. (1970) Medical Care Use in Sweden and the United States: A Comparative Analysis of Systems and Behavior, Center for Health Administration Studies Series No. 27, Center for Health Administration, Chicago, IL.

(4) Back, Kurt W. and Sullivan, Deborah A. (1978) "Self-image, Medicine, and Drug Use," Addictive Diseases: An International Journal, 3, pp. 373-382.

(5) Basen, M.M. (1977) "The Elderly and Drugs: Problem Overview and Problem Strategy," Public Health Reports, 92, pp. 43-48.

(6) Bender, A.D. (1975) "Pharmacodynamic Principles of Drug Therapy in the Aged," Journal of the American Geriatrics Society, 7, pp. 296-303.

(7) Brand, F.N., Smith, R.Y., and Brand, P.A. (1977) "Effect of Economic Barriers to Medical Care and Patient Non-compliance," Public Health Reports, 92, pp. 72-78.

(8) Bush, P.J. and Osterweiss, M. (1978) "Pathways to Medicine Use," Journal of Health and Social Behavior, 19, pp. 179-189

(9) Bush, P.J. and Rabin, D.L. (1976) "Who's Using Nonprescribed Medicines?" Medical Care, 14, pp. 1014-1023.

(10) Chien, C., Townsend, E.J., and Ross-Townsend, A. (1978) "Substance Use and Abuse among the Community Elderly: the Medical Aspect," Addictive Diseases: An International Journal, 3, pp. 357-372.

(11) Doyle, J.P. and Hamm, B.M. (1976) Medication Use and Misuse Study among Older Adults, The Cathedral Foundation of Jacksonville, Inc., Jacksonville, Florida. Cited in U.S. Department of Health and Human Services, Public Health Services, Alcohol, Drug Abuse and Mental Health Administration, Drugs and the Elderly, edited by Meyer D. Glantz, David M. Petersen, and Frank J. Whittington, Research Issues 32. U.S. Government Printing Office, Washington, D.C.

(12) Eberhardt, R.C. and Robinson, L.A. (1978) "Medical Problems of the Elderly in Non-metropolitan Illinois," Journal of Gerontology, 33, pp. 681-689.

(13) Eve, Susan Brown and Friedsam, Hiram J. (1981) "Use of Tranquilizers and Sleeping Pills among Older Texans," Journal of Psychoactive Drugs, 13, pp. 165-173.

(14) Eve, Susan Brown and Friedsam, Hiram J. (1981) "Factors Influencing Older Persons' Use of Nonprescription Medicines for Prevention and Cure," a paper presented to the XII International Congress of Gerontology, Hamburg, Germany, July 12-17, 1981

(15) Glantz, Meyer D. "Drugs and the Elderly." In U.S. Department of Health and Human Services, Public Health Service, Alcohol, Drug Abuse and Mental Health Administration, Drugs and the Elderly, edited by Meyer D. Glantz, David M. Petersen, and Frank J. Whittington, Research Issues 32. U.S. Government Printing Office, Washington, D.C., pp. 1-3.

(16) Glantz, Meyer D. (1981) "Predictions of Elderly Drug Abuse," Journal of Psychoactive Drugs, 13, pp. 7-16.

(17) Green, C.E. (1977) "A Study of Drug Use and Misuse by the Elderly in Osceola County, Florida, The Door of Central Florida's Training Program for Service Providers to the Elderly, Osceola County, Florida." Cited in Richard C. Stephens, C. Allen Haney, and Suzanne Underwood, Drug Taking among the Elderly, Treatment Research Report. U.S. Government Printing Office, Washington, D.C.

(18) Guttmann, David (1977) A Survey of Drug Taking Behavior of the Elderly, Catholic University of America, Washington, D.C.

(19) Heller, F.J. and Wynne, R. (1975) "Drug Misuse by the Elderly: Indications and Treatment Suggestions." In E. Senay, V. Shorty, and H. Alkene (eds.) Developments in the Field of Drug Abuse, Schenkman Publishers, Cambridge, Massachusetts.

(20) Hussar, D.A. (1975) "Patient non-compliance," Journal of the American Pharmaceutical Association, 15, pp. 183-190.

(21) Incaiardi, J.A., McBride, D., Russe, B.R., and Wells, K. (1978) "Acute Drug Reactions among the Aged: A Research Note," Addictive Diseases: An International Journal, 3, pp. 383-388.

(22) James, I. (1976) "Prescribing for the Elderly: Check the Interaction and Cut down your Calls," Modern Geriatrics, 6, pp. 7-14.

(23) Klein, L.E., German, P.S., McPee, S.J., Smith, C.R., and Levine, D.M. (1982) "Aging and its Relationship to Health Knowledge and Medication Compliance," The Gerontologist, 22, pp. 384-387.

(24) Krupka, Lawrence R. and Veneer, Arthur M. (1979) "Hazards of Drug Use among the Elderly," The Gerontologist, 19, pp. 90-95.

(25) Lundin, D.V. (1978) "Medication Taking Behavior of the Elderly: a Pilot Study," Drug Intelligence and Clinical Pharmacy, 12, pp. 518-522.

(26) Macukanovic, P., Rabin, D.L., Mabry, J.H., and Simc, D. (1976) "Use of Medicines." In R. Kohn and K.L. White (eds.) Health Care: An International Study, Oxford University Press, London, pp. 223-277.

(27) Manheimer, Dean, Mellinger, Glen D., and Balter, Mitchell B. (1968) "Psychotherapeutic Drug Use among Adults in California," California Medicine, 109, p. 447.

(28) Mellinger, Glen D. and Balter, Mitchell B. (1981) "Prevalence and Patterns of Use of Psychotherapeutic Drugs: Results from a 1979 National Survey of American Adults." In G. Tognoni, C. Bellantuono, and M. Lader (eds.) Epidemiological Impact of Psychotropic Drugs, North-Holland Biomedical Press, London, pp. 117-135.

(29) Mellinger, Glen D., Balter, Mitchell B., and Manheimer, Dean I. (1971) "Patterns of Psychotherapeutic Drug Use among Older Adults in San Francisco," Archives of General Psychiatry, 25, pp. 385-394.

(30) National Impact (1980) "The Health Care Crisis in the USA: Analysis and Recommendations for Public Policy," National Impact, August, 1980.

(31) Parry, H.J., Balter, Mitchell B., Mellinger, Glen D., Cisin, I.H., and Manheimer, Dean I. (1973) "National Patterns of Psychotherapeutic Drug Use," *Archives of General Psychiatry*, 28, pp. 769-783.

(32) Petersen, David M. and Thomas, Charles W. (1979) "Acute Drug Reactions among the Elderly." In D.M. Petersen, F.J. Whittington and B.P. Payne (eds.) *Drugs and the Elderly: Social and Pharmacological Issues*, Charles C. Thomas, Springfield, Illinois.

(33) Prentice, R. (1979) "Patterns of Psychoactive Drug Use among the Elderly." In *The Aging Process and Psychoactive Drug Use*, National Institute of Alcohol, Drug Abuse and Mental Health Administration, U.S. Public Health Service Publication No. 79-813, U.S. Government Printing Office, Washington, D.C.

(34) Rabin, D.L. and Bush, P.J. (1975) "Who's Using Medicines?" *Journal of Community Health*, 1, pp. 106-117.

(35) Raffoul, Paul R., Cooper, James K. and Love, David W. (1981) "Drug Misuse in Older People," *The Gerontologist*, 21, pp. 146-150.

(36) Schwartz, Doris, Wang, Mamie, Zeitz, Leonard, and Goss, Mary E.W. (1962) "Medication Errors Made by Elderly Chronically Ill Patients," *American Journal of Public Health*, 52, pp. 2018-2029.

(37) Sharpe, T.R. and Smith, M.C. (1983) "Final Report: Barriers to and Determinants of Medication Use among the Elderly: July 1, 1982-June, 1983, "AARP Andrus Foundation, Washington, D.C., 1983.

(38) Stephens, R.C., Haney, C.A., and Underwood, S. (1981) "Psychoactive Drug Use and Potential Misuse among Persons Aged 55 Years and Older," *Journal of Psychoactive Drugs*, 13, pp. 75-83.

(39) U.S. (1966) Department of Health, Education and Welfare, Public Health Service, *Cost and Acquisition of Prescribed and Nonprescribed Medicines*, by Charles S. Wilder. Vital and Health Statistics Series 10, No. 33, U.S. Public Health Service, U.S. Government Printing Office, Washington, D.C.

(40) U.S. (1968) Department of Health, Education and Welfare, Task Force on Prescription Drugs (1968) *The Drug Users*, Office of the Secretary, U.S. Department of Health, Education and Welfare, U.S. Government Printing Office, Washington, D.C.

227

(41) U.S. (1969) Department of Health, Education and Welfare, Public Health Service, Inter-national Comparisons of Medical Care Utilization: A Feasibility Study by Kerr L. White and Jane H. Murnaghan. Vital and Health Statistics Series 2, No. 33, U.S. Government Printing Office, Washington, D.C.

(42) U.S. (1977) Department of Health, Education and Welfare, Public Health Service, Out-of-Pocket Cost and Acquisition of Prescribed Medicines by Jai W. Choi. Vital and Health Statistics Series 10, No. 108, U.S. Government Printing Office, Washington, D.C.

(43) U.S. (1979) Department of Health and Human Services, Public Health Service, A Study of Legal Drug Use by Older Americans by David Guttmann, Services Research Report. U.S. Government Printing Office, Washington, D.C.

(44) U.S. (1978) Department of Health, Education and Welfare, Public Health Service, National Center for Health Statistics, Use Habits among Adults of Cigarettes, Coffee, Aspirin and Sleeping Pills by Gordon Scott Bonham and Paul E. Leaverton. Vital and Health Statistics Series 10, No. 131. U.S. Government Printing Office, Washington, D.C.

(45) U.S. (1982) Department of Health and Human Services, Public Health Service, Alcohol, Drug Abuse and Mental Health Administration, Drug Taking among the Elderly by Richard C. Stephens, C. Allen Haney and Suzanne Underwood, Treatment Research Report. U.S. Government Printing Office, Washington, D.C.

(46) U.S. (1982) Department of Health and Human Services, Public Health Service, Drug Utilization in Office Practice by Age and Sex of Patient: National Ambulatory Medical Survey, United States, 1980 by Hugh H. Koch. Advance Data from Vital and Health Statistics No. 81, Public Health Service, Hyattsville, Maryland.

(47) U.S. (1982) Department of Health and Human Services, Public Health Service, Prescribed Medicines: Use, Expenditures and Source of Payment by Judith A. Kaspar, Data Preview 9. U.S. Government Printing Office, Washington, D.C.

(48) U.S. (1983) Department of Health and Human Services, Public Health Service, National Center for Health Services Research, Psychotropic Drugs: Use, Expenditures and Sources of Payment by Gail A. Cafferata and Judith A. Kaspar, Data Preview 14. National Center for Health Services Research, Hyattsville, Maryland.

(49) Warheit, G.J., Arey, S.A., and Swanson, E. (1976) "Patterns of Drug Use: An Epidemiological Review," Journal of Drug Issues, 6, pp. 223-237.

(50) Warren, F. (1979) "Self-medication Problems among the Elderly." In B.P. Payne, D.M. Petersen, and F. Whittington (eds). Drugs and the Elderly, Charles C. Thomas, Springfield, Illinois, pp. 105-125.

(51) Watson, Jack Borden, Eve, Susan Brown, and Reiss, Edith McBride (1980) "Use of Psychotropic Prescription Medicines among Older Adults," paper presented at the Gerontological Society of America meetings, San Diego, California, November, 21-25, 1980.

(52) White, Kerr L., Andjelkovic, Dragana, Pearson, R.J.C., Mabry, John H., Ross, A., and Sagen, O.K. (1967) "International Comparisons of Medical Care Utilization," The New England Journal of Medicine, 277, pp. 516-522.

(53) Whittington, Frank J., Petersen, David M., Dale, Barbara, and Dressel, Paula L. (1981) "Sex Differences in Prescription Drug Use of Older Adults," Journal of Psychoactive Drugs, 13, pp. 65-73.

(54) Whittington, Frank J., Welchel, Lucy B., and Petersen, David M. (1981) "Correlates of the Over-the-counter Drug Use by Older Persons," paper presented at the XII World Congress of Gerontology, Hamburg Germany, July 12-17, 1981.

Chapter 9

DOCTOR-PATIENT RELATIONSHIPS AND THEIR IMPACT
ON ELDERLY SELF-CARE

Marie R. Haug

INTRODUCTION

On the dust cover of a recent book on geriatric
care there is a photograph of a little old lady
and a middle-aged man, presumably a doctor. The
little old lady is caressing the man's hand, in
a posture of adoration and gratitude. Practitioners familiar with the health care of the
elderly recognize that this is as much an
erroneous stereotype as another possible picture, of a little old lady angrily whacking a
doctor over the head with her cane.

This opening paragraph in a collection of
papers on elderly patients and their doctors (Haug
1981) epitomises two contrasting views on the
doctor-patient relationship involving old people:
utterly dependent versus fiercely independent
patients. Neither stereotype is accurate, of course,
but their implications for self-care would appear to
be evident. Conventional wisdom would hold that the
physician-dependent eschew self-care, while the
independent prefer not to rely on doctors, but
manage their own problems. However, the issues
involved are much more complex than simple personal
attitudes toward doctors.
This paper will attempt to show that anti-
professional beliefs need to be considered. Indeed,
it has been argued that anti-professionalism is a
prime factor in self-care decisions of the in-
dependent-minded. By positing a link between issues
in doctor-patient relationships and self-care, this
paper's underlying theme is that negative experiences in that relationship can predispose those with
symptoms at least to postpone visiting a physician,
if not foregoing a visit altogether, unless the

symptoms grow much worse. This does not imply that general anti-professionalism is the major motivator. There are other issues as well, including a range of sources of strain between providers and aged recipients of care in the doctor-patient relationship that may influence a person's decision to engage in self-care. These sources of strain can arise from personal characteristics, from situational contexts, and from specific prior experiences.

Many studies of doctor-patient interactions have been conducted, but most of these focus on problems of compliance, revolving around physician communication skills and presumed patient inability to understand, with virtually nothing related to the meaning of advanced patient age. Conceptual models, both those in medicine and in sociology, place the physician in the dominant role in a therapeutic relationship. This is particularly the case in medicine, where it has been so taken for granted the physician should be in charge that dominance is a given rather than a concept to be stated and justified theoretically and empirically. The theoretical, but not the empirical, underpinning for physician control was offered by sociology (Parsons 1951). His sick role concept is based on the notion that sickness is a form of deviance upsetting to the social order. The ill are excused from normal role obligations, provided they seek professional help and cooperate in getting well. The physician is the agent of social control, and the "competency gap" between practitioner and patient legitimates the norm of medical authority and patient obedience (Parsons 1975).

Modifications of these approaches relative to doctor-patient relationships have been developing in recent years from various quarters. Dr. George Engel (1980, 1981) has put forward the biopsychosocial model, which extends the physician's scientific expertise to the social and behavioural aspects of the ill person's condition, including family, community and cultural aspects relevant to an illness. Even with the most benign intentions, this broadens the potential scope of a physician's dominance and suggests that the competence gap encompasses not only medical but also psychosocial knowledge.

A constriction of that range of dominance is proposed by those who argue for a negotiated model of the relationship in which practitioners and patients are viewed as equals who work out a mutually agreeable course of action in the process of their interaction (Lazare, Eisenthal & Stoeckle 1978). Such a model is consonant with a consumerist perspective, where seller (provider) and buyer (patient) come to terms on the sale of a product (medical care) (Reeder 1972; Haug & Lavin 1983). Moreover, this reformulation of an appropriate "active" sick role is congruent with current demands for physician accountability with respect both to treatment decisions and costs. The effects of differing physician and patient interaction styles on a person's selection of self-care in the face of symptoms and the variables that impinge on these styles and their realisation are one possible explanation for self-care behaviour. These effects have never been studied, although their relevance is implied by those who place self-care activities in the context of an anti-professional movement.

Cross-cutting prior and anticipated doctor-patient relationships as factors in self-care are the sets of variables found in models of health behaviour and physician utilisation. The work of Rosenstock and Kirscht (1979) and Becker (1974) focused on psychosocial factors in preventive health care, while Andersen (1968) originally analysed families' use of health services in more structural terms. Their sets of predictors, designed to forecast physician use, should also be applicable to physician non-use, which in the face of identified symptoms would be likely to include some specific self-care actions along with ignoring the complaints.

The Rosenstock and Becker models include assessment of the seriousness of a health problem, the likelihood that care will produce positive results, cues to action from significant others and the media, as well as the standard demographic variables. Andersen postulated three sets of variables, predisposing, enabling, and need: Predisposing variables include demographic factors such as age, gender, race, and education; enabling variables cover accessibility and availability of care, both geographic and economic; while need involves the health problem generating the seeking of a physician's advice. None of these models were particularly successful in predicting actual utilisation behaviour, although they have been frequently used for a multi-aged sample (e.g., Andersen & Aday 1980) and occasionally with the elderly (e.g., Coulton & Frost 1982; Wolinsky & al. 1983).

Moreover none of the studies included attitudes

concerning relationships with physicians as an explanatory factor, a shortcoming partially corrected in a national project using the Andersen model (Haug & Lavin 1983), in which consumerist relations with physicians were entered in a path analysis. Again, however, the amount of variance explained was low, although the consumerism measure did enter the equation. In another analysis of these utilisation data, two measures of challenge of physician authority affected age-differential use of services for some common complaints (Haug & Lavin 1980).

Although self-care can be viewed as the other side of the coin of physician care, utilisation studies are no substitute for an examination of the phenomenon itself. Here the researcher runs into problems of defining just what self-care is. There have been several attempts to create conceptual models for self-care study, most of which suffer from definitional diffuseness. One model views it as an emerging social movement, related in part to the rise of interest in holistic health and public skepticism of medicine (Levin, Katz & Holst 1976). Another model focuses on self-help groups as a form of self-care (DeFriese & Woomert 1983), while Butler and colleagues (1979) include everything from everyday activities like good diet and adequate exercise to self-treatment such as taking throat cultures in their rubric. Similarly a nine-category scheme of personal actions by experienced illness (Giachello, Fleming & Anderson 1982) make self-care so all-inclusive as to limit its utility for research purposes.

These diverse concepts illustrate the importance of carefully defining the scope of self-care at the individual behaviour level. Illsley (1981) makes this point, describing symptom recognition, diagnosis, and treatment as the most significant aspects of self-care. This definition, however, should not be assumed necessarily to eliminate the seeking of professional help. One person experiencing symptoms may ignore them or take care of them on his or her own, without ever seeing a physician or other therapist; another may try self-treatment for a while and, if it does not solve the problem, then turn to a physician for help. Both these individuals have engaged in the self-care process described by Illsley (1981), except that the latter ultimately combined self-care with professional care. Only the individual who consults a physician at the first signs of symptoms without engaging in any personal remedial action can be excluded from the self-care category.

These criteria have been employed in two large-scale empirical investigations, one in Denmark (Dean 1980) and the other a secondary analysis of a United States survey (Giachello, Fleming & Anderson 1982). Neither of these studies focused on the elderly or took into account the respondents' feelings about and experiences in doctor-patient relationships as factors in self-care behaviour. Secondary analysis of a subset of 330 older respondents from a 1975 interview study (Haug & Lavin 1977) also failed to take the effect of doctor-patient relationships into account, but did succeed in expanding on earlier work by developing categories of different types of treatment used in self-care by older persons. Self-care was defined as intentional behaviour in response to one's own health problems or symptoms, exclusive of current professional health care. Self-care included diag- nosing or naming the problem or symptom, deciding on a course or courses of action, and tending to oneself with the intention of alleviating or palliating the symptom or problem.

Respondents had been asked open-ended questions on how they would handle each of five common symptoms -- depression, difficulty sleeping, stomach gas, heavy cold, and infected cut. Responses were evaluated from three age cohorts, those 46 to 59, 60 to 74 and 75 and over. Older persons were generally more likely than younger to avoid professional care. Biserial correlations demonstrated that self-care was the increasingly favoured response to symptoms as age increased, except for the cold symptoms, where there was no relationship between age and care type. The analysis uncovered seven substantive and distinct self-care practices: 1. use of ingested over-the-counter medicines; 2. use of ingested home remedies; 3. use of non-ingested over-the-counter remedies; 4. use of non-ingested home remedies; 5. change of activity; 6. "fighting it off;" and 7. doing nothing/waiting.

The type of home remedy projected by this elderly sample for possible use varied by ailment. For example, 45 percent claimed they would use an activity change for depression, while 25 percent suggested an over-the-counter remedy for difficulty sleeping; almost 40 percent proposed a combination of treatments for a cold, while about 60 percent would treat stomach gas by a drug-store remedy. Clearly, self-care can involve a range of possible activities that might be influenced by attitudes toward physicians as evolved in prior relationships. For example, high rates of self-care for difficulty sleeping and stomach gas, if these symptoms are conceived as concomitants of aging, might be related to doctor-patient encounters in which patients were advised to accept the symptoms of growing old without complaining to the doctor.

If, indeed, concerns about physician response militate against professional utilisation and encourage self-care, variables that might produce such concerns among the elderly are worthy of analysis. Sources of strain in the relationship between physicians and their aged patients are one such set of variables. Such sources include physician characteristics, patient characteristics, and the circumstances in which the therapeutic encounter occurs. The balance of this paper raises theoretical issues in each of these domains and relates them to potentials for self-care. Some preliminary, ancillary data are involved in support of these speculations, although the current lack of research that deals specifically with the impact of negative doctor-patient relationships and presumed anti-professional attitudes severely limits the availability of empirical information.

PHYSICIAN CHARACTERISTICS

Stereotyping of the elderly is the physician characteristic that former NIA Director, Dr. Robert Butler (1977), has dubbed "ageism." Among the younger public, this stereotype involved lumping all those aged 65 and over into one category, whose members are considered to be in declining or ill health, suffering from loneliness, and generally economically deprived, unhappy, sexless, and doomed to ultimate senility. Conscious and unconscious discriminatory practices with respect to work and educational opportunities are bolstered by similar negative images in the media, particularly television and the movies.

But the ageism of physicians is more subtle. Doctors are unlikely to compress all elderly into one level of health and activity; they are aware of the differences between the vigorous and the frail elderly. What they may fail to realise is the extent of their lack of knowledge about the special diagnostic and treatment problems involved in elderly care, and the extent to which their own latent fears and boredom with repetitive complaints of the chronically ill impair their therapeutic attitudes and behaviour.

One physician characteristic perhaps most conducive to alienating the elderly from professional care is perceived lack of competence, as evidenced by a claimed history of medical errors made in diagnosis or treatment. Such errors are not inconceivable in light of the limitations of expert knowledge about the special characteristics of the aged's response to drugs and other treatments. More generally, physicians are not immune to mistakes, regardless of the patient's age, as evidenced in more than one study (e.g., Bosk 1979).

Whether or not an error actually occurred is irrelevant in this context, since the old person's belief in the event could generate the rejecting behaviour. The elderly are likely to have long memories in this regard. In a random sample of Ohio residents in 1975, a third of those over 60 reported an episode of medical error, ranging from insufficient information to mistakes that actually caused patient harm, although some dated back many years.

For example, one aged respondent complained that, 28 years before, a physician had misdiagnosed her husband's stomach cancer as sinus, and he died in great pain. Another reported, "Twenty years ago my brother felt run down and our doctor told him it was his teeth so he had them all out -- but he still felt run down, so he went to another doctor and they found he had TB." Even less life-threatening claimed errors were not forgotten. One respondent recalled that 42 years earlier an itch from clothing was incorrectly diagnosed, while another reported that 12 years before a doctor burned her husband's arm applying a heat lamp for bursitis. More recent errors were reported as well, including over-prescription of diuretics that depleted potassium levels and caused eye sight difficulties, failure to diagnose cracked ribs after a fall, and misdiagnosis of a gall bladder problem.

Although the nature of this particular research did not permit relating experience of medical error to self-care behaviour, it is theoretically conceivable that doubts and uncertainties from past episodes could encourage an individual to rely initially on his or her own resources on the grounds that visiting a physician might result in more harm than good. However, also worthy of note is that in most of the claimed instances of physician error, the individuals reported that the error was finally discovered by a second doctor. Past experiences could thus be as likely to encourage doctor shopping and second opinions as to explain rejection of all physician contact and the substitution of self-care.

One aspect of perceived physicians' incompetence relates to their ageist attitudes, which can produce misdiagnosis and errors in treatment plans. Expectations that "senility" is the normal accompaniment of aging are likely to mean not only overlooking treatable conditions such as depression, but even more mundane explanations of unusual behaviour. Weiss (1981) reported on a patient whose falls were attributed to increasing dementia, when in fact they were caused by improper footwear and an inadequate cane. In this instance, the effect of the error would have little to do with self-care decisions of the older person, but might affect decisions of the care-giver.

One consequence of provider ageism is that it causes the elderly patient to feel rejected because his ailments are intransigent and boring. Not wanting to bother a physician who has failed to emphasise or accept that his or her role and responsibility is to be "bothered" when a patient has health concerns is likely to be the most common rationale for self-care, a hypothesis that has not yet been tested empirically. The source of such patient feelings may arise not only from experience with the attitudes of a particular practitioner, but from a generalised image of the physician as very busy with really seriously ill patients, as well as of his high status and social importance. Thus, visiting the doctor for possibly minor and unworthy ailments is an imposition. Although these beliefs are properties of the elderly patient, they are a product of presumed physician characteristics as well, whether or not reinforced by the pattern of actual experience.

Marshall (1981) has analysed doctor-patient relationships with the aged patient in terms of physician characteristics from three perspectives: the authority relationship, the affective relationship, and the issue of the practitioner's therapeutic activism. He focuses on the issue of physician willingness to afford the patient respect. Given acceptance of the physician's authority in purely medical matters, "Patients -- and seemingly older patients especially -- want to be treated with respect. Respect is a term relevant in a model of the doctor-patient relationship...in which both doctor and patient are viewed as persons, and in which what goes on between them is viewed as interaction instead of the action of one on something the other has." (Marshall, 1981:100)

Compliance, in this view, is contingent on the patient's satisfaction that he is being treated with respect. Non-compliance can be conceptualised as one indicator of self-care; a person who changes a prescribed regimen, by addition or subtraction of medications or procedures, is in a sense taking charge, substituting his or her own criteria for those of the practitioner. This can be a reaction to lack of respect or, as Marshall insightfully suggests, "the patient's attempt to protect a little integrity in a kind of class conflict with the physician. Non-compliance is perhaps in some respects akin to industrial sabotage...failure to fully adhere to clinical regimens (is)...a kind of role-distancing behaviour in which the patient asserts individuality...making a claim to some personal control over aspects of the doctor-patient relationship." (Marshall, 1981:103)

The affective coloration of the relationship is related to the respect issue. Elderly patients, particularly those with chronic illnesses, may not really be liked by physicians; indeed, they may be actively disliked by persons whose work satisfaction comes from achieving successes -- i.e., cures. For such physicians, the therapeutic activists, who may well constitute a majority, dealing with the elderly is stressing and painful to their egos, which thrive on positive achievement. For them, successful management may not be enough, particularly because in the end they must face the death of their patients and the burden of bringing the sad news to a distraught family.

To protect their own feelings, physicians may experience difficulty in maintaining a therapeutic viewpoint, they may give up on the patient and pass on to other members of the health care team or to the family responsibility for dealing with the patient's problems (Breslau 1980, 1981). Although Breslau does not mention the possibility, when a provider gives up on the elderly patient, the family might be spurred to try various home remedies or other self-care activities. On the other hand, he suggests that the physician's own feelings of helplessness could be transmitted to the family, where strained relationships may recur in a downward spiral of care, with repeated attempts at more desperate self-care measures. A family's search for cure by way of bizarre diets, unproved medications, and other last-resort treatmets are examples of the results of physicians' inability to face their own feelings about their difficult elderly patients.

PATIENT CHARACTERISTICS

Ageism is not limited to physician attitudes. Older patients can accept the stereotype as well. The attribution of symptoms to aging can abort a doctor-patient relationship. The elderly sufferer will consider it pointless to seek professional help for a condition believed endemic to the aging process and may rely on home remedies to alleviate pain and discomfort instead of seeking expert advice and getting to the root of the problem. The ageism of the elder and the ageism of the physician may indeed reinforce each other. Since for many elderly a doctor is a respected, even feared, authority figure, his or her stereotyping of the old will be taken as normal and right. Concurrently the old person's acceptance of the idea that age is responsible for their aches, pains, and other bodily ills will validate the practitioner's easy assumption that this is actually the scientific fact.

Such habits of attribution do not necessarily mean that the aged are indifferent to their health, or generally are dubious about the utility of medical care. A recent national survey (Haug & Lavin 1977) of 1,509 subjects demonstrated quite the contrary, replicating findings from other studies. For example, nearly three quarters of the respondents aged 70 and over (N = 161) gave the highest salience to good health, compared to less than 40 percent of those under 45 (N = 822). The oldest group was demonstrably sicker: Nearly half reported one or more chronic conditions that interfered with normal routines, as against less than 10 percent of the younger group with a similar level of disability. In congruent findings, fewer than 10 percent of the oldest considered their health excellent, in stark contrast to over 38 percent of the younger with this vigorous view. And in the face of experiencing one or more common, not life-threatening, complaints like cold, backache, or minor infection, more than 40 percent of the oldest group sought a doctor's care, while fewer than a third of the younger reported a similar action.

On the other hand, these attitudes and practices characterising the elderly may be less meaningful in structuring the doctor-patient relationship and its impact on self-care than four

239

basic demographic characteristics: the person's age cohort, gender, race, and social class.

Cohort differences in interaction with phys- icians and in self-care behaviour offer a rich field for speculation and virtually no data. One can hypothetically compare two cohorts of elderly -- those born in 1905 or before, who would be 75 and over by 1980, and those born between 1915 and 1925, who would be between 55 and 65 at the same point in time. Members of the senior cohort were born before the explosion of scientific discoveries changed medicine dramatically. If they were part of the wave of Eastern European peasant immigrants just after the turn of the century or if they were Black, they probably never saw a doctor in their childhood and survived entirely on home remedies administered by the mother of the family. They experienced two major depressions: hard times when money was scarce, unemployment compensation unknown, and visits to a doctor a luxury to be used only in the face of a dire, life-threatening emergency. Reaching retire- ment age in the 1960s or 1970s, they became eligible for Medicare. Thus, cost became less of an impedi- ment to a doctor visit, but a lifetime of reliance on self-care, possible language barriers, and lack of experience in dealing with the upper class, usually white practitioner might well discourage professional utilisation.

Members of the cohort born 10 to 20 years later had quite different experiences. Since they were infants or not yet born during World War I, that conflict and its hardships had little lasting effect, but the medical discoveries that began to develop at the time could contribute to their greater longevity and a more vigorous old age. They were likely to have enjoyed more education than the earlier cohort and to have been native born and, thus, might be more comfortable in dealing with physicians. They experienced the depression of the 1930s while still children or adolescents and entered working life during and after the World War II boom. For them various insurance plans like Blue Cross and Blue Shield buffered the cost of care, and made physician use a customary response to symptoms. Self-care might be in the form of over-the-counter medications, but such behaviour would be less a long-standing habit of non-physician use than a response to negative evaluations of the health care system, from personal experience or media reports.

Variations in exposure to historical events, in educational level, and in doctor-patient relationships distinguish different cohorts and can, in turn, produce variation in the use of self-care. The extent of these effects, however, is currently unknown and ripe for empirical investigation. Some hints are available from one national sample survey which showed that 56 percent of persons aged 50 to 59 in 1975 (N = 203) believed that physicians should have the main say in health matters, compared to 77 percent aged 70 to 79 (N = 116) (Haug & Lavin 1975). This cohort difference has implications for self-care. Persons who doubt that physicians should dominate health care decisions are candidates for self-care, and these persons are more common in the younger than in the older cohort.

The effect of gender on doctor-patient relationships and self-care is another understudied area, although it is well established that women suffer more morbidity and make more physician visits than men (Verbrugge 1983). This utilisation edge persists into old age (Haug 1981), but virtually disappears when both genders reach age 75. The higher use rate for "young-old" women could argue that they depend less on self-care because they see physicians more. However, studies have shown that frequent physician use is not necessarily a substitute for self-care (Dean 1981; Fleming N.D.). It might even be argued that women, more sensitive than men to bodily cues and more committed to maintenance of good health, would be likely both to employ more self-treatment and to consult a physician more often.

Two additional factors must be taken into account. Women are the "care-givers of first resort" in the family. As wives and mothers, they will be consulted by spouses or children uncertain about their symptoms in the first step of the lay referral system defined by Freidson (1961). Women may, therefore, determine whether or not a physician should be consulted and which self-care remedies, if any, are to be employed. Secondly, it is noteworthy that no significant differences emerged by gender in the extent of attitudinal or behavioural challenge to physician authority in one study of older adults (Haug 1979). This runs counter to a popular notion that women are more compliant than men, but is consistent with the findings of role reversals with aging, in which women take on more aggressive, supposedly male traits as they grow old (Guttman, forthcoming 1985). Again, however, we are faced with the fact that knowledge is scarce, in this instance both about women's behaviour in a doctor-patient relation and the prevalence and types of their self-care practices.

If the data on these issues with respect to gender are scanty, those on race are even scantier. The quality of doctor-patient relationships when the patient is an elderly Black can be presumed to be problematic because of probable differences in social class, response styles, and cultural beliefs about illness. However, evidence on the interaction itself is not available. Haug (1979) found no racial effect on challenges to physician authority among those 60 and over, either in attitude or behaviour. On the other hand, Santos, Hubbard, and McIntosh (1982) in a seminal paper on problems of elderly Blacks in relation to mental health therapists have pointed out sources of difficulty that could readily apply in any therapeutic encounter. For example, Blacks tend to be hesitant concerning self-disclosure, particularly in situations where they lack trust, as may well be the case when the provider is white, middle class, and young. Holding back may manifest itself in "sullen reserve or even misleading friendliness, smiling and talkativeness..." (Santos, Hubbard & McIntosh 1982:56). It should be recalled that the relatively small numbers of Black practitioners make it likely that most Blacks will be forced to seek care from whites, and if the locale of care is a hospital out-patient clinic, the provider could easily be young -- a resident -- as well.

The effect of these possible blocks to satisfactory relationships as generators of self-care practices can only be surmised. Fearing the effect of ageist and racist stereotypes, elderly Blacks could conceivably prefer to rely on home remedies and treatments remembered from their rural childhood rather than to deal with a physician. According to Jackson (1980), physician visits by non-white elderly poor do not differ materially from visit rates for white elderly poor. Data from general surveys provide apparently contradictory evidence. The National Medical Care Expenditure Survey revealed that in 1977 over a third of the Black pupulation had not used ambulatory doctor services, compared to 22 percent of whites without contact (NCHSR 1983). But information on persons aged 60 or over in the 1978 Health Survey indicates that being Black significantly predicted physician utilisation (Wolinsky & Coe 1984). Of course, use or non-use of medical providers offers only a slender clue to actual self-care. Indeed, no significant racial

differences in health practices were found by
Andersen and colleagues (1981) in their study of
self-care in five U.S. cities, although in a
secondary analysis of national data, rural blacks
were found least likely to use non-prescribed home
treatments (Giachello, Fleming & Anderson 1982). In
short, the effect of race on doctor-patient relationships or as a precursor of self-care behaviour
remains uncertain at best.

Social class differences in doctor-patient
relationships among the elderly is yet another topic
that has been insufficiently studied. In the past,
higher social class patients have been thought to
interact with their physicians more comfortably
because of similarities in educational level and
social status. On the other hand, studies have shown
that persons of higher education, one indicator of
higher social class, are more likely to be willing
to challenge a physician's authority, which for some
practitioners is a stance difficult to accept (Haug
& Lavin 1979) and might well lead to strained
relationships. When health knowledge was substituted
for educational level in an analysis specifically
concerning those over 60, the same associations
emerged (Haug 1979). Education is not, however, a
perfect indicator of social class, and that variable, taken by itself, did not predict issues in
doctor-patient interactions in these studies.

Assessing the link between social class and
self-care must rely more on indirect than direct
evidence. For example, Wolinsky and Coe (1984) found
that both higher education and higher income
contributed to physician utilisation among the
elderly in the 1978 Health Interview Survey. Higher
educational level, occupational rank, and income
were all related to elderly use of physician visits
in a Virginia study (Wan & Arling 1983). National
data, not differentiated by age (NCHSR 1983), show
that those with incomes of $20,000 or more in
1977-78, and those with a college education or
better were more likely than those less well-off or
educated to have had at least one ambulatory
service.

Yet Giachello, Fleming, and Anderson (1982)
report no relationship between higher education and
use of non-prescribed home treatments in an all-age
national sample; in fact, it was those with a high
school education who were the more likely to engage
in that form of self-care. Considering that these
researchers found those who used home treatments
less likely to visit physicians, logic suggests that

the lower class status of the elderly -- as indicated by education and perhaps income and occupation as well -- is most apt to predict self-care.

THE CONTEXT OF CARE

The locale and circumstances for the meeting between doctor and elderly patient are additional factors that influence the character of the relationship. As Goss (1981) has perceptively noted, when persons are seen in a hospital or nursing home the physician comes to the patient, who has little control over whether or not to accept the provider's visit. Persons who see physicians in their medical offices go to the provider and can consequently control whether or not an interaction takes place at all. This element of choice, however slim it might be in some situations, can put a different cast on the relationship. The patient does retain the option to break it off, and this may elicit more respect for the patient's dignity and personal concerns on the provider's part.

On the rare occasion of a home visit, a new factor is relevant. Now the patient is in his or her home territory, surrounded by familiar objects and family, and although undoubtedly sicker, nevertheless not subject to being intimidated by the trappings of the physician's turf (Zola 1981). The physician, on the other hand, in the presence of one or more witnesses, may feel constrained to show extra regard for the patient's feelings.

Family involvement can also occur at the doctor's office, however, and this is a circumstance that may lead to trouble. When an elder is accompanied to a consultant by a family member -- often a daughter, the encounter involves a triad. And triads can easily devolve into two against one. Rosow (1981) has reviewed the possible forms of these coalitions. Taking into account the fact that many of the old-old are from immigrant cohorts, with limited education, Rosow suspects that the most likely coalition is doctor plus adult child versus parent. Such a line-up is understandable in the face of an elder's incompetence. But as Rosow suggests, even when motives are benign, "The parent may seldom be accorded the courtesy of significant choices that are well within his or her competence. With the doctor's cooperation, all of this occurs in the name of the child's acceptance of responsibility. Because it is also a very efficient alliance, time pressures on the doctor are also conducive to it." (Rosow 1981:144)

The relevance of this aspect of doctor-patient relationships to self-care comes down to the issue of respect for the patient. To the extent that the circumstances surrounding a therapeutic encounter militate against a show of respect on the doctor's part, the consequence can be a reinforcement of anti-professional proclivities on the part of the elder. And if, indeed, one of the motivators of self-care is dislike and distrust of doctors, the net effect can be the encouragement of self-care behaviour.

SOME CONCLUSIONS

Although physician competence, ageism or burn-out, patient social and demographic characteristics, and the ambience of an encounter's setting may all be doctor-patient relationship issues that are implicated in accounting for self-care, the nature of the elder's health problem remains a critical explanatory variable. Chronic illness is by definition incurable, and in these terms nearly all elders eventually suffer from conditions that modern medicine cannot cure (Verbrugge, forthcoming, 1985). Some conditions can be managed and discomfort alleviated, but not eliminated.

Old people may live many years with their disease, and by way of experience become very knowledgeable about the condition, including the medications and procedures that work best for them in enhancing mobility and comfort. Indeed, the old person may come to believe, whether accurately or not, that he or she knows more about the disease than the doctor, whose only knowledge is academic (Haug & Lavin 1981). For the more highly educated who are able to keep up with the literature on their condition, this may not be too far off the mark, while for those whose only information is experimental, their beliefs may not jibe with the current state of knowledge.

Both groups can reasonably be expected to seek methods of their own such as home remedies handed down in the family or ideas gathered from the media or friends. Many of these may be physiologically useless, but psychologically therapeutic, providing placebo effects. A few may be dangerous, but that is a risk in any regimen: introgenic illness can follow

245

from a physician's prescription, oraflex for example, or from a bit of folk medicine, like kerosene for a cold. Perhaps a key ingredient is the satisfaction an old person can derive from the sense of achieving independence, not having to lean on a physician, particularly one who dismisses complaints as due to old age, which "you will have to live with." Not a few elderly are fiercely independent, even stubborn in their insistence on doing things for themselves, making decisions about their own health usages, and not wishing to appear weak.

The real dangers in self-treatment arise from failure to use expert advice as an important source of information. The blind rejection of physician services because of anti-professional ideology, just as the failure to seek care because of fears about a possible diagnosis, is an irrational response to disturbing symptoms. A past history of negatively perceived encounters with physicians, if in fact it generates anti-professional attitudes, can produce greater reliance on self-care. But no great harm will generally be done if the old person does not delay too long when symptoms persist or grow worse.

Physicians who deal with elderly patients can help to avoid dangerous outcomes by recognising the appeal of self-care as a source of feelings of independence and self-esteem. Most important, they can grasp the old persons' need for understanding and accord them the dignity of being listened to with patience and respect.

POSTSCRIPT

Does anti-professionalism encourage self-care among the elderly? Does antagonism against physicians make old people try home and drug store remedies before seeking professional help? As this paper has demonstrated, although the ideas have intuitive appeal, no empirical evidence currently supports them. The interplay of physician and patient characteristics, along with likely settings of care, may well play a role in self-care decisions, but conclusions remain speculative. Of particular note in this context are the ageist stereotypes that still pervade both medical and public belief systems and may account for one form of "self-care," waiting and neglect. However, while the negative aspects of doctor-patient relationships may be a necessary explanation for elderly self-treatment, they are certainly not sufficient. One might hypothesise, for example, that a practical issue such as cost should be added to the equation, along with psychological characteristics such as elderly depression or confusion. As with so many other concerns involving health and the elderly, there is plenty of room for research. The traditional last-sentence plea for more studies seems particularly apt in this context.

REFERENCES

Andersen, R. (1968) A Behavioral Model of Families' Use of Health Services. Chicago: Center for Health Administration Studies Research Series 25, University of Chicago

Andersen, R., & Aday, L. (1980) Health Care in the U.S.A.: Equitable for Whom? Beverly Hills: Sage

Andersen, R.M., Fleming, G.V., Giachello, A.L., Androde, P. & Spencer, B. (1981) Self Care Practices in the U.S.: Analysis of National Data. Chicago: Center for Health Administration Studies, University of Chicago

Becker, M.H. (Ed.) (1974) The Health Belief Model and Personal Health Behavior. Thorofare, N.J.: Charles B. Slack

Bosk, C.L. (1979) Forgive and Remember: Managing Medical Failure. Chicago: University of Chicago Press

Breslau, L. (1980) "The Faltering Therapeutic Attitude Toward the Institutionalized Aged." Journal of Geriatric Psychiatry, 13, 193-206

Breslau, L. (1981) "Problems of Maintaining a Therapeutic Viewpoint." In M. Haug (Ed.), Elderly Patients and Their Doctors. New York: Springer, pp. 119-127

Butler, R.N. (1977) "Questions on Health Care for the Aged." Papers on the National Health Guidelines: Conditions for Change in the Health Care System. U.S. DHEW, Pub. No. (HRA) 78-642, September

Butler, R.N., Gertman, G.S., Oberlander, D.L., & Shindler, L. (1979) "Self-care, Self-help and the Elderly." International Journal of Aging and Human Development, 10, 95-119

Coulton, C. & Frost, A.K. (1982) "Use of Social and Health Services by the Elderly." Journal of Health and Social Behavior, 23 (4), 330-338

Dean, K. (1980) Analysis of the Relationships Between Social and Demographic Factors and Self Care Patterns in the Danish Population. Unpublished doctoral dissertation. Minneapolis: University of Minnesota

Dean, K. (1981) "Self-care Responses to Illness: A Selected Review." Social Science and Medicine, 15A, 673-687

DeFriese, G.H., & Woomert, A. (1983) "Self-care among U.S. Elderly, Recent Developments." Research on Aging, 5 (1), 3-23

Engel, G. (1980) The Challenge of the Biopsychosocial Model. New York: Elsevier

Engel, G. (1981) "The Clinical Application of the Biopsychosocial Model." In M. Haug, (Ed.), Elderly Patients and their Doctors. New York: Springer, pp. 3-22

Fleming, G.V. Satisfaction with Medical Care. Unpublished manuscript. Chicago: Center for Health Administration Studies, University of Chicago, No date

Freidson, E. (1961) Patients' Views of Medical Practice. New York: Russell Sage Foundation

Giachello, A.L., Fleming, G.V., & Anderson, R.M. (1982) Self Care Practices in the United States: Final Report. Chicago: Center for Health Administration Studies, University of Chicago

Goss, M. (1981) "Situational Effects in Medical Care of the Elderly: Office, Hospital, Nursing Home." In M. Haug (Ed.), Elderly Patients and Their Doctors. New York: Springer, pp. 147-156

Guttman, D. (forthcoming 1985) "Developmental Perspectives on Diagnosis and Treatment of Psychiatric Illness in the Older Woman." In M.R. Haug, A.B. Ford & M. Sheafor (Eds.), The Physical and Mental Health of Aged Women. New York: Springer

Haug, M. (1979) "Doctor-patient Relationships and the Older Patient." Journal of Gerontology, 34, 852-860

Haug, M. (Ed.) (1981) Elderly Patients and Their Doctors. New York: Springer

Haug, M. & Lavin, B. (1977) Public Challenge of Physician Authority: final report, unpublished

Haug, M. & Lavin B. (1979) Public Challenge of Physician Authority, Medical Care, 17, 844-858

Haug, M. & Lavin, B. (July, 1980) "Final Progress Report: Challenging Physician Authority and Utilization Behavior." Grant ≠ HS02968, National Center for Health Service Research, DHHS

Haug, M. & Lavin, B. (1981) "Practitioner or Patient, Who's in Charge?" Journal of Health and Social Behavior, 22 (3), 212-229

Haug, M. & Lavin, B. (1983) Consumerism in Medicine. Beverly Hills: Sage

Illsley, R. (1981) "Self Care: What Is It and What Does It Mean for the Elderly and Health Care Providers?" Paper presented at Conference of Self Care of the Elderly, University of Michigan, (October)

Jackson, J. (1980) Minorities and Aging. Belmont, CA.: Wadsworth

Lazare, A., Eisenthal, S., Frank, A., & Stoeckle, J.D. (1978) "Studies of Negotiated Approach to Patienthood." In E.B. Gallagher (Ed.), The Doctor-patient Relationship in a Changing Health Scene. Washington, D.C.: U.S. DHEW, pp. 119-139

Levin, L.S., Katz, A.H., & Holst, E. (1976) Self-care: Lay Initiatives in Health. New York: Prodist

Marshal, V. (1981) "Physician Characteristics and Relationships with Older Patients." In M. Haug, (Ed.), Elderly Patients and their Doctors. New York: Springer, pp. 94-118

NCHSR (National Center for Health Services Research) (1983) Contacts with Physicians in Ambulatory Settings: Rates of Use, Expenditures and Sources of Payment. Data Preview 16, DHHS Publication No. (PHS) 83-3361

Parsons, T. (1951) The Social System. Glencoe: Free Press

Parsons, T. (1975) The Sick Role and Role of the Physician Reconsidered. Health and Society, 53, 257-277

Reeder, L.G. (1972) "The Patient-client as Consumer: Some Observations on the Changing Professional-client Relationship." Journal of Health and Social Behavior, 13, 402-416

Rosenstock, I. & Kirscht, J. (1979) "Why People Seek Health Care." In G. Stone, F. Cohen, & N. Adler (Eds.), Health Psychology. San Francisco: Jossey-Bass, pp. 161-188

Rosow, I. (1981) "Coalitions in Geriatric Medicine." In M. Haug (Ed.), Elderly Patients and their Doctors. New York: Springer, pp. 137-146

Santos, J.F., Hubbard, R.W., & McIntosh, J.L. (1982) "Mental Health and the Minority Elderly." In L. Breslau & M.R. Haug (Eds.), Depression and Aging: Causes, Care and Consequences. New York: Springer, pp. 51-70

Verbrugge, L.M. (1983) "Multiple Roles and Physical Health of Women and Men." Journal of Health and Social Behavior, 24 (1), 16-29

Verbrugge, L.M. (forthcoming 1985) "An Epidemiological Profile of Older Women." In M.R. Haug, A.B. Ford, & M. Sheafor (Eds.), The Physical and Mental Health of Aged Women. New York: Springer

Wan, T. & Arling, G. (1983) "Differential Use of Health Services Among Disabled Elders." Research on Aging, 5, 411-431

Weiss, H. (1981) "Problems in the Care of the Aged." In M. Haug (Ed.), Elderly Patients and Their Doctors. New York: Springer, pp. 79-90

Wolinsky, F.D., & Coe, R.M. (1984) "Physician and Hospital Utilization among Non-institutionalized Elderly Adults: An Analysis of the Health Interview Survey." Journal of Gerontology, 39 (3), 334-341

Wolinsky, F.D., Coe, R.M., Miller, D.K., Pendergast, J.M., Creel, M.S., & Noel, M.N. (1983) "Health Services Utilization among Non-institutionalized Elderly." Journal of Health and Social Behavior, 24 (4), 325-337

Zola, I.K. (1981) "Structural Constraints in the Doctor-patient Relationship: The Case of Noncompliance." In L. Eisenberg and A. Kleinman (Eds.), The Relevance of Social Science for Medicine. Boston, Mass.: D. Reidel Publishing Co.

Chapter 10

SELF-CARE AND HEALTH CARE: INSEPARABLE BUT EQUAL FOR
THE WELL-BEING OF THE OLD

Rosalie A. Kane and Robert L. Kane

PREMISES

We take as axiomatic that self-care activities have
potential for the elderly, not only for treatment of
disease, but perhaps even more for prevention and
treatment of disability and dysfunction. Further, we
contend that the self-care efforts of older people
should be mobilised in relationship to the formal
care-giving system.

This chapter considers self-care in relationship to health care. Some proponents of the
self-help movement object to any suggestion that
older people should learn to use to best advantage a
health care system that is ill-suited to their
needs. Consumer advocates bristle at the idea of
accommodating to the language, style, and practices
of the medical community. However, the elderly use
health care services and their self-care must
include efforts to get the most benefit and the
least harm from such care. Simultaneously, work can
take place on two other fronts: educating health
care providers to ways of fostering self-care and
self-help activities in their elderly clients; and
social action to try to reshape the health care
delivery system.

In tandem with efforts to educate health
professionals about the needs of older people, the
elderly can themselves become better equipped to
negotiate that system for their own best interest
and to use both their individual marketplace
decisions and collective action to bring about
improvements in the system. We argue for deliberate
strategies to activate health consumers and their
families into exercising "defensive health behaviour." At the same time, the difficulties of

251

achieving this goal are acknowledged and discussed.

Those who use the health-care system to greater advantage are in fact taking better care of themselves. Those who use the health-care system ineptly unwittingly put themselves at risk of increased dysfunction. Similarly, health-care providers who encourage self-care in their patients provide better health care. Indeed, because providers can influence the self-care activities of their clientele, health-care professionals should also be a target for educational approaches. The various structural arrangements governing relationships between health-care consumers and providers -- from reimbursement policies to conventions of care delivery -- should also be scrutinised for their effect on the older person's self-care abilities.

Why Emphasise Functioning?

When an elite, well-educated group of very old persons prepared essays on the experience of aging, over half the 52 subjects described health problems in detail; topping the list were functional disabilities such as deterioration in vision and hearing, loss of energy and diminution of manual dexterity (Hellebrand 1980). Conventional wisdom asserts that physical, emotional, social and even cognitive factors interact for better or worse to produce functional patterns in old age (Kane and Kane 1981). This statement holds for persons of all ages, but has particular import for self-care and health care among the frail elderly. Problems in functioning arise from one or a combination of physical, mental, and social (including financial and environmental) causes and can sometimes be ameliorated by changes on any one of these fronts. The goal of both self-care and health care is to enhance an individual's well-being. To this end, health-care providers must take a broad view in their diagnosis and treatment. Similarly, older persons must take a broad view in clarifying their preferences for how to live with their seniority.

Attention to functioning is as important as many diagnoses (Kane & al., USDHEW 1979 a). As they age, people acquire an assortment of diagnoses which fail to explain their functional abilities. Maintaining such functional abilities -- the capacity to handle intimate body functions, the capacity to manage one's home, money, and environment, the capacity to enjoy activities and friendships -- is a crucial goal for both self-care activities and health-care activities.

Lifelong habits often determine the risk of acquiring so-called life-style diseases in older age. The rhetoric of preventive health movements sometimes short-circuits careful consideration of the benefits expected from changing habits at various ages. For example, the effect on morbidity and mortality is unclear when dietary modification, exercise, or stress reduction is begun in old age. A rather small number of preventive health practices are on solid ground. It is useful to stop smoking at any age. It is generally useful to detect and treat hypertension at any age. But when functioning rather than disease becomes the guiding theme, the list of the preventable expands dramatically. In old age, actions instituted by the individual in conjunction with health-care providers can prevent or minimise (or make worse) sensory loss, immobility, sleep problem, memory problems, incontinence, depression, accidents, victimization, loneliness, and isolation. Eyeglasses, hearing aids, dentures, foot care, home modifications, convenience devices -- all these can increase functional capacity.

Why Relate Self-Care to Health Care?

Unless strategies to enhance self-care in the elderly are coordinated with strategies to improve health care and related services, the two efforts may end up at cross purposes. Consider that:

1. Chronic illness predominates among the old;
2. The multiple interacting problems of the old render medical diagnosis difficult;
3. Ambulatory care of older people is characterised by short encounters usually terminated by a prescription for medication;
4. Older people are likely to interact with health-care providers at times of crisis, and these providers can have far-reaching power over the older person's life;
5. Common preventable problems of older people are associated with too much, too little, or inappropriate health care;
6. For the age cohorts now elderly, health is salient and medical practitioners are well respected.

Age is associated with an increase in the prevalence of chronic diseases, which, by their very nature, accumulate over time. National data indicate that disability also rises with age, although the increase is not linear. The disability curve has a dramatic inflection beyond age 75. This change is associated with greater utilisation of health-care services, particularly hospitals and nursing homes; over 20 percent of those 85 and over are in nursing homes. Persons over age 65 account for 25 percent of prescriptions written, 33 percent of hospital beds occupied, and 30 percent of health-care bills paid (Dychtwald 1983).

Although the likelihood of dependency increases with age and the accumulation of chronic diagnoses, such dependency is by no means inevitable. In the United States, about 40 percent of noninstitutionalised persons over 85 claim to have no limitations on their usual activities. But the older person exists in a delicate equilibrium. Compensatory mechanisms permit functioning despite deficiencies in organ systems, social losses, psychological stress, and economic hardships. An additional stress may disrupt this homeostatic balance, resulting in a diffuse set of reactions. Because such a patient has an underlying substrate of chronic conditions, new problems appear not on a flat terrain but as a mild alteration in the overall jagged silhouette of a mountainous vista. This difficulty exacerbates the task of reaching an acute diagnosis. Older people need to use strategies that improve their physicians' chances of finding out what is wrong.

Many older people see doctors regularly. A large-scale Harris poll (1981) showed that 86 percent of elderly respondents received medical care from their own identified private physicians. Similarly, in a sample of clients of an Area Agency on Aging, all but six percent had a regular source of primary care, and only 12 percent needed any transportation help to get there (Kosidlak 1980).

Despite the increase of chronic disease and disability with age and the likelihood of having a doctor, older people are far from excessive users of physician ambulatory services. On the average, persons over 65 in the United States make only about one more doctor's visit per year than do younger adults, and that pattern persists with increasing age after 65. More striking, the actual contact time between physicians and their patients is less for older patients than younger ones (Keeler & al. 1982) despite the additional history and morbidity and sometimes slowed communication of the elderly. Moreover, few physicians in the U.S. have special

training or interest in geriatrics (Kane & al. 1981
b). In one small-scale study, a multidisciplinary
group of health professionals were unable to
separate physiological and functional conditions
accurately into those that are "normal aging" and
those that are "disease-related" (Dye & Sassenrath
1979).

Given the brevity and infrequency of encounters
between older people and physicians, patients must
time their visits well and use the time to best
advantage. Brody and Kleban (1981) suggest that
older people are unlikely to tell anybody about many
symptoms and are especially unlikely to consult
professionals. Haug (1981) found that, although the
elderly were more likely to receive regular checkups
and to seek medical attention for five specified
minor complaints, they were just as likely as their
younger counterparts to under-utilise medical care
for five complaints that physicians believe merit
attention. Kosidlak (1980) found that 90 percent of
her sample of seniors in a screening programme
needed to return to their doctors. Although suffering considerable discomfort, these patients were
uncertain what they should describe to their doctors
and what language to use. The current elderly
generation under-utilise dental care, and insurance
status does not predict dental use in old age
(Evashwick, Conrad, & Lee 1982).

Older people or their agents are likely to be
seen by health-care providers at times of crisis.
Such crises often rally the extended family, however
far-flung. Important decisions are made in an
atmosphere of chaos. Writing about adults of all
ages, Pratt (1978) suggests that the users of
medical care should be expert problem solvers, able
to choose among services and providers, plot the
implications of alternative choices for their own
well-being, and evaluate the results of care. Such a
stance is difficult under the best of circumstances
and, without considerable socialisation and social
sanction for the role, sick elderly persons are
unlikely to be able to carry it off. Yet at those
times of illness and crisis, far-reaching decisions
are made (including recommendations for care in
institutional settings). In the United States,
medical authorisation is needed for publicly funded
care in long-term care facilities or at home. A
physician's recommendation (or failure to recommend)
may be pivotal. Older people must develop knowledge
and skill to protect themselves against becoming
victims of professional snap decisions.

Although some older people suffer from lack of timely and accurate diagnostic and curative care, others suffer from iatrogenic problems. Some unavoidable iatrogenic complications arise because of the narrow window for therapeutic effect in the elderly. Health care interventions, most notably drugs and surgery, can be used efficaciously, but they can also produce toxic reactions. Drugs, for example, may accumulate because of age-related decreases in metabolism and excretion. Surgery represents an additional insult to the aging organism. Thus, the distance between a potentially helpful effect and a potentially harmful effect narrows as the individual gets older. The result may be inappropriate prescriptions, recommendations, and diagnostic lables. If the older person already has gathered prescription and nonprescription drugs from many sources, the prescriber may not even have a full information base before adding a new drug to the mix.

Bed rest and hospitalisations, if not carefully managed, can in themselves create irreversible functional impairment in the old. One study of hospital complications (Jahmogen & al. 1982) revealed a much higher overall rate in persons over age 65. In particular, the elderly accounted for almost all the drug reactions, physical trauma, infections, and "psychiatric deterioration."

Older persons are extremely concerned about their health and their health care. They are particularly worried about the high cost of physicians, drugs, and hospitals (Louis Harris and Associates 1981). The importance of health-care issues to older people is also evidenced in the popularity of health-related courses and programs at community colleges and senior centers. The cohorts who are now old also appear to hold the physician in great respect, viewing the appropriate patient role as deferential. Some may be self-effacing about their own abilities. Elderly persons facing surgery have been described as timid and fearful about asking questions lest they reveal ignorance, yet eager to describe their own symptoms and reactions adequately and retain the information they need (Nugent 1981). Because health is such a salient concern, many old people are susceptible to those who advocate (and sell!) a wide variety of nostrums and remedies. And because costs of care are a gnawing worry, elders are also vulnerable to persons selling insurance schemes, some of which offer benefits largely redundant with Medicare. Given that health is salient, yet misconceptions exist about health care, and given that deferential attitudes toward physicians are combined with vulnerability to health "pitches," self-care and health care should be linked.

DEFENSIVE HEALTH BEHAVIOUR

We define defensive health behaviour as strategies that maximise the benefits and decrease the costs (in morbidity, functioning and well-being, and dollars) that older persons incur as a result of interaction with the health-care system. Although this paper stresses medical care, the "health-care system" is construed here to encompass physicians, hospitals, nursing homes, pharmacies, dentists, and a wide array of therapists, including mental health providers.

First, defensive health behaviour requires new information or correction of faulty information in several categories, including general information about the aging process and accurate information about diseases and disabilities prevalent in old age -- heart disease, stroke, arthritis, cancer, osteoporosis, cataract. Some such information can help dispel fears -- for example, despite the favourable prognoses for many cancers of the elderly, that disease evokes stark fear in most elderly and is the subject of rampant misinformation (FallCreek & Mettler 1982). Older cancer patients tend to present with cancers in later stages, perhaps because of fatalism or perhaps because this group has not been instructed in early detection or in how to demand such screening from their physicians. Similarly, fear about possible loss of mental faculties is also strong enough to interfere with seeking help at the right time. Seniors also need to learn the characteristic way that physicians marshall information so they can observe and describe their own symptoms most usefully. For example, physicians speak of pain in terms of location, radiation, duration, associated symptoms, causative factors, and relief factors. Patients who organise their thoughts and observations along those lines are better prepared to provide meaningful input to the diagnostician.

A second general area of defensive health behaviour concerns medications, the cause as well as the cure of much geriatric disability. Some problems occur because older persons fail to comply with regimens, use prescription drugs incorrectly, or

257

self-medicate inappropriately with over-the-counter drugs. Other problems occur because the regimen itself is faulty -- e.g., too high a dosage, incompatible with other drugs being taken. Sometimes the individual neither asks nor is told specific important information about how and when to take the drug. Pharmacists specialising in geriatrics blame many parties for this misuse of medication, citing inadequate pharmacist knowledge and skills, poor patient compliance with physician's regimens, inadequate physician prescribing patterns, particularly overuse of psychoactive drugs; and communication problems with older clients (Pratt, Simonson & Lloyd 1982). A study of prescriptions written for medical/surgical hospital patients in a single day showed that a third of those over 60 received psychoactive drugs, with sleeping preparations heading the list. Antipsychotic drugs were used as analgesic or sedative agents for nonpsychotic patients (Salzman & van der Kolk 1980). Raffoul, Cooper, and Love (1981) found similar drug misuse in community-dwelling older persons. Considering all forms of misuse (e.g., overuse, underuse, using someone else's drug, improper storage or labelling, using drugs that interact negatively), more than 1/3 committed one or more drug errors. Interestingly, the number of prescribing physicians and the number of dispensing pharmacies was directly related to medication error. Thus, patients themselves need to develop the interest and skills to coordinate their medication use, asking the right questions, keeping the right records, and treating all medicine with respect tinged with skepticism.

Defensive health behaviour requires information about the health-care delivery system itself. Most patients use medical encounters poorly to find out things they later wish they knew: the alternative diagnoses the physician was considering, the purpose of tests, the treatment choices and their side effects, the aetiology of the disease, and the prognosis (Pratt 1978). Furthermore, users of medical care rarely understand the division of labour within the medical profession and among ancillary services such as laboratories. Yet the older persons may need to track down and refer themselves to health-related services rather than wait for a physician to propose or arrange it. For example, physicians tend to be conservative in their use of home health agencies (Trager 1980), and this might account in part for the lack of pressure on home health services to expand. Older people need to know the mechanics of seeking second opinions on matters like elective surgery, another source of iatrogenic disability.

Defensive health behaviour requires understanding and skilful use of health benefits. Despite the Health Care Financing Administration's efforts to prepare easily-understood brochures and manuals, Medicare's benefit structure and communications processes are Byzantine. Elders end up incurring unexpected costs while avoiding procedures that they mistakenly believe are not covered. An adequate income permits purchase of items and services that enhance independence. Therefore, a desirable health-related goal is to help older people weigh various claims on their own scanty resources in the name of health or protection.

Defensive health behaviour also means recognising and resisting the power of the pat diagnosis, particularly the label "senility." Fears about the spectre of losing one's mental faculties are rampant among older people (Hellebrand 1980). But studies have shown that senility is an overused term, substituting sometimes for diagnosis and treatment of remediable conditions (Garcia, Redding, & Blass 1981). Patients may also be labelled as incontinent without much attention to ways of reversing that functional problem. Geriatric assessment units, which look for treatable functional problems in addition to diseases, tend to find two or three remediable problems per admission (Rubenstein, Rhee, & Kane 1982). The patient or patient's agent must insist on better explanations than catch-all labels, which too often can become a self-fulfilling prophecy. Simply avoiding doctors entirely and resorting to an unencumbered self-help stance to prevent the possibility of diagnostic labelling would be a nihilistic solution. Modern health care can do too much good for people to voluntarily shun its benefits.

Confusion about the extent and prognosis of various conditions in the old can lead to inappropriate self-imposed restrictions or overzealous restrictions by care-givers. Anxiety can be reinforced by encounters with the care system. Older persons fearful of falling may dangerously narrow their activities and interests. If the first sign of forgetfulness on the part of an older person sends family members into panic, the results may be overprotection. The older person who is confident in his or her judgment, who has reviewed his or her priorities in the light of his or her own values, and who has explicitly discussed important issues with family members is in an advantageous position when a health crisis strikes and professional become involved. Yet few seniors discuss their wishes with responsible family members in advance of a crisis (Kulys & Tobin 1980), and many have a fatalistic pessimistic attitude to the merits of future planning for a time when they might be somewhat physically infirm (Kulys 1983).

Information must, therefore, be directed toward the relatives and friends of an older person who may inadvertently promote excess disability through risk aversion. Concerns about the potential dangers of leaving vulnerable elderly to function on their own may encourage a concerned family (or government) to become over-protective. Families need an opportunity to appreciate the ramifications of any decision to restrict freedom and to talk through thoroughly the pros and cons of such decisions. In the end, these decisions are heavily value-laden, but the underlying values are too often inadequately explored. Addressing the fears, articulating them, and acknowledging them may be sufficient to allow an individual to continue in a relatively independent mode, accepting a constant potential for adverse consequences.

In summary, defensive health behaviour calls for a posture that permits the older person to make more effective use of the health-care system, reaping its substantial benefits and avoiding its dangers. Such a stance can have a number of benefits. At times of critical decision-making, the values and preferences of the patient need to get adequate recognition lest others make decisions for him. Decisions about regular health-care need to be made in a more egalitarian way, with less dependence on the physician. This increase in self-sufficiency can result in savings for both the patient and the public purse. It should also result in better decisions leading to changes that are more comfortably accepted by the elderly patient. The activated elderly patient is more likely to make good decisions about when to see a physician and to provide useful information, both about the symptoms associated with the problem and reactions to prior therapy. Such input should facilitate physician decision-making and thus improve the quality of care.

The ultimate responsibility for coordination resides with the patient, who, after all, has the most to gain or lose. Although health care providers have a monopoly on some knowledge and competencies, the patient has unique areas of competence. Patients have a monopoly over: 1. experimential expertise (i.e., their own history and symptoms); 2. integrative expertise (i.e., total functioning apart from health or a subspecialty thereof); 3. the ability to initiate service; 4. the ability to give informed consent; and 5. their own behaviour (Howard 1978). These five factors could potentially be shaped into a powerful beneficial role.

STRATEGIES FOR PROMOTING DEFENSIVE HEALTH

Different Strategies for Different Subgroups

The requirements for information and skill differ among the age groups and according to the health status of the people concerned. Receptivity to and interest in specific information also varies. Although statistics may identify the start of aging at 65 or even 60, individuals in their late sixties and early seventies are likely to be in good health, and resemble 55-year-olds more than 80-year olds. Yet health education messages typically are not tailored for older Americans at all, let alone for well-targeted subgroups in that population.

Self-help behaviour among those with illnesses range from passive to active. For example, a passive but potentially salutary approach involves scrupulous adherence to medical advice and therapeutic regimens, including return for scheduled appointments and systematic observations of one's own symptoms and reactions to treatment. A more aggressive stance involves deliberate strategies to select physicians, to get second opinions, to question medical care providers closely about their choices, and even to apply checklists to be sure that health care providers are told and asked all that is necessary. For persons who are essentially well, the intensity of the self-care effort also varies. Some persons keep themselves informed by reading the lay literature on health matters, screen themselves for preventable problems, have regular check-ups, and take general steps to avoid accidents and diseases. Others embrace a vigorous effort to experience "positive health" through stress reduction and life-style changes.

Self-care efforts may be pursued individually or within the supportive atmosphere of a group. Groups of two types are becoming more common among

261

older people: 1. the disease specific group, which permits persons with the same ailment or disability to come together, share practical information, and encourage each other; and 2. the general group (either a purposely constituted or existing group), which provides a structured learning environment for curriculum on healthy life styles. Although the latter approach can include content about specific health problems and how to activate the health-care system, major themes are often general: i.e., nutrition, exercise, stress management. No research is available to suggest whether practical precepts about using drugs or dealing with physicians are best introduced as one plank of a "wellness" platform or whether the ideas become lost in that context.

Nursing home residents' self-care efforts are circumscribed by the rules and customs of the institution. They have no choice about whether they will take fewer or more medicines -- even the simple aspirin is professionally administered. They may have no choice over their life-style routines -- when and what to eat, sleeping patterns, and activities. Some nursing home residents with severe cognitive impairment or physical limitations may not be candidates for self-care in any realistic sense of the term. Others, however, could and would prefer to control many more aspects of their decision-making than is typically permitted. Without such opportunity for choice, "learned helplessness" is often seen (Seligman 1975). In the nursing-home context, lack of perceived control and choice is bad for the health of the elderly and may even hasten death (Langer & Rodin 1976, Schulz 1976, Mercer & Kane 1979, Ferrari 1962). But the strategy for empowering persons in institutions clearly differs from the approach to the community-dwelling persons. It requires simultaneous work on many fronts: nursing-home reform, education of care-givers, environmental changes, and eliminating structural barriers to the exercise of autonomy.

Habitually, a sharp dichotomy is drawn between those in and outside nursing homes. However, another large but unenumerated population group lives in sheltered residential settings outside the nursing-home system, e.g., board-and-care homes. Residents and staff in such homes are in a programmatic limbo. Board-and-care residents usually have more structural opportunity to exercise self-care than those in nursing homes, but they also tend to be an isolated group, cutt off from community contacts. Another

special population is the large group of seniors who
live in mobile homes and recreational vehicles. This
tends to be a rather low income and peripatetic
group that may be missed by outreach programs.

Sometimes self-care for the elderly could more
appropriately be dubbed family-care. Spouses, sib-
lings, and adult children of cognitively impaired
seniors are the logical persons who need to use the
defensive health behaviour and learn to negotiate
the system. Such care-givers need to understand the
condition of their relative, the drugs used, and the
service structure in the community. Care-givers
require special support and reassurance and constitute a separate target group for activation.

Compliance

Compliance with medical advice is an aspect of
recovery from disease and minimising dysfunction.
"Compliance" has unpleasant connotations, as if
following medical advice represents a loss of
autonomy. But when the advice is wise, the older
person benefits by following it without many
variations on the theme. Compliance is most often
discussed in terms of medication use, but has other
applications. People may comply or fail to comply
with suggestions for alleviating symptoms, returning
for appointments, or making life-style changes.

Improving patient compliance involves some
measure of self-care, albeit delimited by professional approaches. Research suggests that
patients are more compliant when they are satisfied
with the doctor-patient relationship, when the
regimen itself is less complex and of short
duration, when the patients have a stable family
situation, a previous record of compliance, and
nonpsychiatric status; when structural aids to
compliance (e.g., reminders) are used, and when the
conditions of the health belief model, discussed
elsewhere in this conference, are met (Sackett &
Haynes 1976, Kane & Glicken 1979). Assuming the
elderly are similar to other groups, they are at
risk of noncompliance. Many older people live alone
and lack stable family supports, are depressed or
cognitively impaired, have complex regimens, have
unsatisfying encounters with care-givers, have
health beliefs that reflect an earlier era of
medical knowledge and receive few explanations that
clarify reasons for various regimens.

Despite these factors, Klein & al. (1982) found
that older people were no less compliant than

younger subjects, though all age groups have room for improvement. Interestingly, however, the older clients had significantly less knowledge about their disease or the purpose of the medication, but these comparative deficits in information did not lead to comparatively poorer performance. Most of this sample were black, limiting the generalisability, but the results suggest that knowledge is not the whole answer.

Few deliberate efforts to improve drug com-pliance in the elderly have been reported. In a randomised trial of three methods of reducing medication errors in an ambulatory geriatric clinic (standardised instructions with accompanying video tapes and transcripts; colour-coded pill bottles; and colour-coded pill bottles matched to colour-coded weekly pill trays) only the last strategy was associated with improved compliance (Marten & Mead 1982). Such studies need repeating because they have important implications for practice. A growing minority of enlightened hospitals are now discharging patients with clear written statements about their drugs. Such strategies should be expanded if helpful; but if unreinforced instructional ap-proaches do not make a difference, we should un-deceive ourselves.

Patient-Activation Programmes

Support groups of all kinds are much in style in the United States today, and other chapters in this book deal with the phenomenon in more detail. Indeed, even when peer support and mental well-being rather than medical information and self-care are the programmatic goals, health-focused workshops are sometimes organised as a nonthreatening start. Health programmes have immediate, widespread appeal. Lectures on arthritis, nutrition, memory, heart conditions, and "how to winterise aching bones and joints" allow social groups to coalesce (Campbell & Chenoweth 1981). Giving and receiving help may be good for one's health. In a study of network patterns among elderly people in retirement hotels and apartments, those who neither gave nor received help functioned worse both physically and psycho-logically (Stein, Linn, & Stein 1982).

Below we describe programmes that deliberately attempted to change the patterns of interaction with health-care providers and improve the skills older people bring to the medical encounters. We ident-ified quite a few programmes that aspired to activate patients, although most had other agendas as well. These illustrative programmes vary in many aspects: sponsorship, content, intensity, teaching techniques, provision for follow-up, degree of professionalisation and costs. They also vary on the amount of attention given to "activated" patient behaviour compared to general health information.

Below are thumbnail sketches of seven sample programmes. (Descriptions date to May 1983 when this paper was originally presented.)

Senior's Health Programme, Augustana Hospital, Chicago. Begun as a one-year pilot under a drug abuse grant, this programme quickly became a small department in its host community hospital. Although the hospital now budgets for the program, perpetual fund-raising from service clubs, church groups, and private philanthropists, together with earnings from workshops for professionals and industries recovers most of the cost. The programme is staffed by two nurses and miscellaneous part-time staff and volunteers.

Initially the focus was community education on safe use of medications. The staff developed a presentation which it had offered to as many as possible of the 1,000 identified senior clubs in Chicago. A wallet-sized reminder card was developed with the key questions a person should have answered before swallowing any drug. Educational materials and cards are translated now into half a dozen languages. The second approach involved a series of topical presentations around six common conditions (e.g., arthritis, diabetes, hypertension). The presentations include a simple description of the condition, a statement of what a patient can do himself, and a discussion of how to interact with the medial system for that particular disease. Finally, the programme has moved cautiously into "wellness" instruction, which it has tried to anchor to scientifically defensible precepts. In ten weekly, one-hour sessions, participants are taught specially modified relaxation techniques, Ti Chi, and massage. The programme has produced a book, To Your Good Health (Skeist 1980).

Growing Younger, Boise, Idaho. Sponsored by the Boise Council on Aging and initially funded by a grant from the Center for Disease Control, this programme is a neighborhood-based effort to assist seniors in taking informed responsibility for their health. The method relies on identifying neighbourhoods with about 250-300 seniors and finding a community leader to host an initial gathering.

Similar to a "Tupperware party," project staff come to the first meeting, do a demonstration, and take sign-ups for a four-session programme conducted at Boise's Senior Center. Content covered includes how to talk to your doctor, how to prepare for an office visit, how to treat injuries, how to take one's pulse and find one's target heart rate, and how to use the Physician's Desk Reference (PDR) to look up side-effects of drugs. Demonstrations and materials are part of the plan. The handbook developed for the programme (Kemper, Deneen & Giuffre 1981) is a masterpiece of practical hints and techniques, including tools for keeping personal health records, all in a detachable loose-leaf form. Once the four sessions are over, a group may decide to continue on its own. From the 1,500 groups exposed to the content in three years, 60 (involving about 300 seniors) are continuing some type of regular structure. Leaders of these follow-up groups attend periodic meetings at the center, where their ideas are refreshed. Other spin-offs include a large walking group that dubs itself the Happy Hoofers.

The Growing Younger Programme has worked its way through Boise's neighbourhoods once and is starting again. The earliest recruits were the more vigorous, self-motivated seniors in the community, but with time frailer people have become involved. The programme has also reached unique neighbourhoods such as trailer parks. The evaluation has compared before-after blood pressure and similar physiological indicators and suggested improvements after the programme. Presently a programme called Growing Wiser is in the planning stages. Using a similar model, it will deal with ways to minimise the effects of memory loss and encourage mental health.

The Wisdom Club, Queens, New York. Funded by the Red Cross in collaboration with Long Island Jewish Medical Center, this programme provides health screening and direct care in senior centers in New York City's Queens area. A geriatric nurse practitioner staffs the health programme, and a health educator provides group instruction and individualised feedback on medications. Goals are to help people use the health care system effectively, recognise signs and symptoms, and become active decision-makers. Red Cross volunteers assist with transportation and accompany the participants if they need tests in the collaborating hospital (Lederman & al. 1983).

Self-Care for Senior Citizens, Dartmouth Medical School. This programme, sponsored by the

Institute for Better Health at Dartmouth, is dedicated to increasing medical self-care and independence. The 600 participants in the 13 two-hour sessions were taught to count their pulse, check their glands, evaluate sore throats, and measure blood pressure. Although details of the evaluation are skimpy, a quasi-experimental design is said to show that those in the programme had better self-care skills and were more likely to use a recommended book to help solve medical problems (Simmons, Roberts & Nelson 1983). The authors claim that 17 months later, 84 percent of the experimental group and only 41 percent of the controls had learned to communicate better with their doctor, and 71 percent compared to 18 percent of controls possessed a directory of local social service agencies.

Arthritis Self-Management Project, Stanford University Medical Center, California. This disease-specific programme has trained 60 arthritic persons (mostly seniors as lay volunteers. In turn, they have worked with 1,200 arthritics in groups. A randomised controlled trial, mentioned by Minkler (1981) but not located in the published literature, apparently showed that the experimental group had less pain and more knowledge of their disease. Groups seem to be self-sustaining, and when the leaders move to other communities, they start new groups there.

Wallingford Wellness Project, Seattle, Washington. A grant from the Administrtion on Aging to the Washington School of Social Work permitted the modelling of a preventive health approach in a senior center. A full programme was developed, organised on four "pillars": stress management, nutrition, physical fitness and personal and community self-help. Common health concerns, however, were a cross-cutting theme, with 15 selected areas for focus: accidents, alcohol abuse, arthritis, cancer, diabetes, foot care, heart disease, hypertension, insomnia, medications, normal changes of aging, oral health, sensory loss, smoking, and weight loss. For example, the medication segment taught participants to maintain drug records and monitor their symptoms. A list of questions was developed to apply to any prescription or over-the-counter drug before using: 1. What is the name of the drug? 2. What is it for? 3. How does it affect symptoms? 4. What are its side effects? 5. What do I do if I have a side effect? 6. When do I take it? 7. How long should I take it? 8. What instructions are there about how to take it -- e.g., on an empty stomach? 9. What substances should be avoided when taking this drug? 10. What does the drug cost? 11. Is there a generic substitute that is cheaper? 12. How should I store the drug? (FallCreek & Mettler 1982).

The September Club. (Aptekar 1983). Unlike the others, the final example involves a cost for participating seniors. Owned by a for-profit corporation of clinical social workers, the programme is a membership organisation that entitles paying members to a core package of services and the right to purchase optional services. The core package funds a case manager who reviews personalised regimens and plans and helps the member construct a package of services that includes: health education, opportunities to socialise, a mobile mini-market to allow people to make convenient purchases from their homes, volunteer and paid job placement, and arrangements for repairs and services from pre-screened, trustworthy tradesmen. Optional services include purchase of homemaking, counseling, and other services.

Other examples could have been chosen. The Healthy Life-style for Seniors programme (Warner-Reitz 1981) in Santa Monica, California, and in Arizona developed a formula that combined a geriatric nurse practitioner's monitoring with health education. The Senior Health and Peer Counseling Center in Santa Monica, California, developed a peer health advocacy programme wherein selected seniors receive relatively intensive training so that they can offer health-related counseling on a one-to-one basis with other older people. North Carolina has developed a state-wide fitness programme, Add Health to our Years (Jacobs & Abbots 1983). McMorran (1983) reports on the Health Advocacy Programme of the American Association for Retired Persons (AARP). This has several components: a personal health care planning effort that reaches a wide gamut of members with films and presentations; a consumer representation project in seven states wherein elders are positioned as members of community boards and committees and are trained for the roles; and an extensive programme by which volunteer health advocates in 15 states provide assistance to seniors in dealing with Medicare and Medigap insurance.

Several programmes have applied the concepts from Keith Sehnert's How to Be Your Own Doctor (Sometimes) (1975) to an older population. Using this model, Mountain States Health Corporation in

Idaho developed training materials and organised 12 of its ten-session, 20-hour activated patient courses for the elderly in rural communities of Idaho, Montana, Washington, and Oregon. Local sponsors for the programmes included health departments, community colleges, senior centers, and Councils on Aging. A key to success was the use of local seniors as programme coordinators (Gaarder & Cohen 1982). Earlier, Kosidlak (1980) used the same Sehnert material to forge a programme at the Peninsula Area Agency on Aging in Virginia.

The prototypic programmes just described represent a range. Some are reminiscent of the "school health model," wherein a travelling road show makes presentations at multiple sites. Other programmes are more analogous to the consciousness-raising in small groups that characterises the women's movement. Still others follow a community organiser's model of developing grass-roots organisations. The September Club, in contrast, is most analogous to the health spa. The service is limited to the wealthy, and the club in some ways is the antithesis of self-help. It offers yet another layer of purchased service that may require its own defensive strategies on the part of the consumer who wants to use it well. It is also a staging ground for vending a wide variety of "optional items." Although in theory a case manager's perspective dictates the recommendations, the incentives for a for-profit organisation to sell a product are present.

Commonalities do appear. Most programmes have multiple sponsorship, for two reasons: the advantage of delivering the programme in community locations, and having health professional involvement; and the ever-present need to piece together money to finance the effort. Programmes tend to be experimential and practical: the effort is to equip people with tools and checklists against which to consider their own health status and health care and to use in communication with providers. Evaluation of the programmes tends to be perfunctory, perhaps appropriately because such programmes defy scientific evaluation. A valid evaluation could cost much more than the programme itself and perhaps threaten its essence as well.

To at least some extent, each programme uses group process to consolidate commitment to both healthy life-styles and the desired defensive health behaviour. The group is also meant to be a supportive environment that will permit self-confidence to increase and at the same time allow for intrinsically pleasurable socialisation. Some models -- such as the Boise Growing Younger programme -- that are built around a neighbourhood have potential for a self-sustaining effort. Others emphasise individuation of each person's needs with tailor-made programmes for assertive health behaviour -- these typically use geriatric nurse practitioners and offer a component of health screening or treatment. In the Red Cross-sponsored programme in Queens, older people are literally provided the supportive presence of a volunteer to help them negotiate the clinics at Long Island Jewish Medical Center.

Evaluations tend to be expressed by counts of programmes conducted and persons reached, as well as the durability of self-care group structures. Physiological parameters such as blood pressure and weight are sometimes incorporated into an evaluation plan. Achievement of goals involving the relationship of the older person to the care-giving settings has not been systematically examined. At this time, therefore, no body of knowledge is available about the outcomes of efforts to encourage defensive health behaviour. What differences do such programmes make in the way people choose and use physicians? Seek second opinions? Request ancillary health services? Do patterns of drug use and surgery change for a group of activated patients? Would such a group be more likely to have and use appropriate visual, auditory, and dental appliances? And what kind of reinforcement -- e.g., of a peer group mechanism, a buddy system of volunteers, nurse practitioner -- instruction is most likely to bring about the desired results?

The National Institute on Aging (U.S. DHEW 1979 b) posits a hierarchy of self-care groups according to their function: i.e., self-care as self-knowledge, self-care as self-surveillance, and self-care as self-treatment. The relationship between professionals and a self-care group is often difficult to conceptualise, let alone implement. Authorities do agree that professionals should do no more than facilitate and serve as resource persons, with leadership coming from the group itself. The lines get murky, however, when a group has a clear-cut agenda that requires fund-raising, a national base, communication mechanisms, and political action. Paid staff then seems essential, but the organisation may be on its way to bureaucratization. Similarly, when a group's agenda includes activating elders to become skilful, self-protective consumers, some professional involvement is needed, if only to provide up-to-date technical information.

Media Activation and Interaction
The media offer an opportunity for supportive interaction for people who cannot easily get out. Although one frequently encounters radio programmes with two-way interaction capacity, few of these have been directed toward the health problems of elderly individuals. Because people presently old tend to enjoy radio, this idea has promise. Only a few television programmes exclusively address problems of elderly individuals and only occasionally do these deal with health topics. At a local level, cable television has been used on an experimental basis to enhance health-related communication, but the potential is only beginning to be tapped. Other technical solutions include the use of interactive communication mediated by various computerised systems. With the increasing prevalence of home computers, the feasibility for this kind of inter-action increases. However, some suggest that people now elderly are more likely to be averse to technology than are younger individuals.

Complementary Strategies for Health Providers
Health-care providers need to be educated and prepared to receive and encourage the activated elderly patient. With proper socialisation and incentives, the providers can enhance their patients' self-care abilities. First, they can adapt the conditions of care to correspond to the needs of the elderly. They can communicate clearly, taking into account visual, hearing, and perceptual dif-ficulties of their patient. The pace of the encounter can be geared to the needs of the individual. Written explanations can be provided. Compliance can be enhanced by specific reminders. Aids can be developed to help patients remember their medication schedules, record actual taking of medicines, and simultaneously note any side effects. If specific steps are useful for alleviation of recurring symptoms, they should be carefully taught. The potential for such self-care is poorly realised. Avery, March, and Brook (1980) found that adult asthmatics failed to perform various activities that could have relieved distress. Greater efforts may be needed to reach older persons with effective messages about how to alleviate their symptoms.

If the cost of physician attention is pro-
hibitively expensive, then substitutes must be
sought. Less expensive personnel may be more
effectively used. Certainly the substitution of
nurse practitioners for physicians is one effective
route. Similarly, pharmacists have an important role
in explaining drug regimens and anticipating side
effects, in taking drug histories, and in working
with patients to establish a monitoring mechanism
for the use of medications. Other kinds of individuals can be used as well. The growth of peer
counseling programmes offers great promise in
providing volunteer organisations, which can work
with elderly patients to assure that the individual
has understood the physician's instructions and has
a plan for incorporating them into daily activities.
For certain specialised information, particularly
developing practical strategies to alter the home
environment, the physician is not equipped to advise
but there is really no ready place in the delivery
system where this help can be sought.

Physicians need to consider their own entrench-
ed beliefs. A common tenet is that patients are
dissatisfied unless they leave the doctor's office
with a prescription (Comaroff 1976). A suggestive
study of a prepaid practice showed that persons who
did not receive prescriptions were more satisfied
with the communicative aspects of their visit than
those who did (Wartman & al. 1981). Controlling for
disease categories, patients were more satisfied
with the way their questions were answered, the
interest shown in them and the explanations they
received if they received no prescription -- and
their visits were longer besides. The only other
predictors of dissatisfaction were respiratory
disease and degree of anxiety at the time of the
visit, and physicians consistently underestimated
the patient's anxiety. This study bears replication
with an elderly sample.

If the fixed idea that patients want drugs can
be debunked, then physicians could also develop
practical substitute techniques. For example,
Fletcher (1982) has suggested some pragmatic ideas
to reduce prescription sleeping pills or over-the-
counter preparations for insomniacs, including
prescribing no more than ten pills in unrefillable
prescriptions, educating patients about sleep physiology and the way sleeping pills work and suggesting non-drug aids to sleep.

Physicians might also focus on geriatric
preventive health maintenance. Systematic regular

assessments are needed on a variety of factors that may cause disease and dysfunction. This argues for structured information gathering (Morrison 1981). Indeed, allied health practitioners such as nurses can collect data, and any primary care-giver should develop a health maintenance flow sheet as a reminder.

It behoves the provider to be aware of well-done books for the public in given areas, particularly those bearing the stamp of a well-respected programme. For example, The 36-Hour Day (Mace & Robins 1981) could be highly recommended as an explication of senile dementia for families of those affected and a gold-mine of practical suggestions. Similarly, Lorig and Fries' Arthritis Helpbook (1981) offers a wealth of practical suggestions. If care-givers become familiar with resources that are up-to-date and accurate as well as persuasive and reassuring, their recommendations can help consumers wend their way through the popular literature.

Although this discussion has emphasised physicians, all care-givers need to do their jobs in ways that make the consumer more informed and effective. This is equally true of social service organisations and long-term care providers. Frankfather, Smith, and Caro (1981) did a detailed study of a project that used family service social workers as case managers for the frail elderly. These case managers had funds to purchase additional goods and services to support the family as primary care-giver. The essence of this project was a negotiated care plan that was to be approved by the client. The evaluators noted, however, that the case managers tended to recommend the service they thought best. The consumers, for their part, tended to be unaware of the range of possibilities from which they selected the particular mix of services they received. In particular, the clients did not perceive the counseling and friendly visiting of the social workers as a service with a price tag that might prohibit other services. The researchers recommended displays of service menus, with detailed descriptions of each, including housekeeping, personal care, companion service, heavy-duty house-cleaning, home maintenance, counseling, friendly visiting, escort services, household modification, prosthetic equipment, transportation, financial aid, and assistance in getting specialty services (e.g., legal advice).

BARRIERS TO DEFENSIVE HEALTH BEHAVIOUR

At least four factors impede developing defensive health behaviour: The bewildering profusion of messages competing for the consumer's attention; the difficulty in developing agendas given the sheer volume of relevant technical information and the numerous gaps in knowledge; the anxiety attendant on the activated consumer role; and the absence of a policy or a mandate for any group to do the necessary work.

Competing Messages

The inquiring consumer contends with a maze of courses, workshops, popular books, manuals, and heavily advertised health programs. The popular demand for health information is seemingly high. Many newspaper columns feature health advice to seniors, and health topics are ubiquitous on television talk shows.

In this sea of information, it is all too easy for people to be uninformed or misinformed. The consumer-awareness initiatives in health represent both a social movement and big business. Neither phenomenon is easily controlled. The older person, bombarded with a variety of contrasting and often conflicting information, may be in a greater quandary than before. Unfortunately, the information presented with the greatest zeal and urgency may be that based on the least scientific evidence. Those with financial incentives may be eager to present their cures, nostrums, regimens, services, and devices in the best light. At the far end of the spectrum, blatant quackery abounds. Worthless devices are particularly reprehensible if they provide a false sense of security and eclipse the possibility of more effective help. Ducovny's (1969) accounts of frauds in the area of hearing aids and denture-repair kits are especially poignant. Consumers who buy improper hearing aids that fail to work often assume mistakenly that their own condition is not amenable to help, while others who truly are not candidates have wasted their money. Denture-makers who advocate "avoiding the middleman" cause damage and can do irreparable harm to the gums, as do many home-handyman denture-repairs techniques.

One potential solution to the problem of the quality of information is to develop creditable and even quasi-official sources, and familiarise people with their existence. Government reports, professional societies, disease societies such as the American Heart Association and the American Cancer Society and consumer groups such as the AARP can and do prepare information packets in a variety of forms for older people. The National Institute on Aging sponsored a series of informational flyers on specific topics -- Age Page -- distributed in conjunction with a drug-store chain in the Washington, DC, area.

However, commercial organisations are likely to have large sums of money to advertise and present attractively and effectively packaged information. Public health organisations will have difficulty competing. Commercial firms stand to gain enormous sums if they capture even small shares of certain markets. A cigarette company can gain millions if it influences but a minute percentage of smokers to adopt its brand. In contrast, a public health group cannot raise funds for a campaign unless large-scale results are anticipated (Wallack 1981).

Some propose that health messages be concentrated in official hands. In the United States today, a controversy surrounds whether prescribed medications should be marketed <u>directly</u> to the public. Should drug firms be allowed to advertise to the general public, who could then demand certain prescriptions from their physicians? Even if the worst scandals in the marketing of dentures, hearing aids, and other health paraphernalia are behind us, the potential exists for vigorous marketing in areas hardly exploited yet. For example, emergency buzzer systems, incontinence aids, and adult-parent-sitting services all could be sold. Nestle (1983) identifies only a few legitimate criteria for food supplements, yet vitamins and minerals are a booming business. Kahn and Kamerman (1982) depict a revealing trend in America's families toward purchasing a wide variety of services that provide advice and help with almost every aspect of life. A Florida-based firm sells families a service to check on their aging parents. As such programmes proliferate and become vigorously marketed, the potential for exploitation as well as benefit is there. Hospital chains and geriatric medical programmes may also increasingly indulge in advertising, and it will become very difficult for the consumer to identify sources of medical information that are disinterested but not uninterested.

Uncertainty about Knowledge
The Geriatric knowledge base has large areas of

275

uncertainty. One must decide whether to transfer the burden of uncertainty to health care users. In any event, the cautious messages of the balanced reporter stand a poor chance against the dramatic messages of convinced "salesmen." Business interests are only one source of confident messages. There are also "true believers" in vitamins, exercise, nutrition, and other similar strategies who bring the force of ideology to their arguments. In the United States, any efforts to control the dissemination of information tread on guaranteed constitutional freedoms.

Anxiety-Provoking Knowledge
Some professionals worry that knowledge about diagnosis, disease, dysfunction, medication, and complications will turn the trustful patient into an anxious one. If optimism and a belief in one's care-givers influence positive outcome, the activated patient is placed at a disadvantage.

Furthermore, one can legitimately question the effect of full knowledge about potential side-effects. When is a symptom a side-effect? Some years ago, Reidenberg and Lowenthal (1968) showed that 81 percent of persons without illness and taking no drugs showed a least one of 25 symptoms often associated with drug reactions.

Policy and Mandate
Public policy in the United States does not always support defensive health behaviour nor the effort to maximise functioning. Consumers who seek to maximise their mobility, vision, hearing, or dental health find these services are not excluded from Medicare. More positively, Medicare has lately underwritten the expense of a "second opinion" for those considering elective surgery.

Orthodox behaviour in hospitals, nursing homes, and medical settings encourages dependency, not responsibility. Medicines are typically administered, baths are supervised, and information is guarded. Even home health programmes may be organised to minimise the authority and decision-making of the consumer, with homemakers "taking their orders" from an agency rather than the homeowner.

Most important, no person or organisation has the authority to design and implement a scheme to help older persons develop knowledge and skills to act decisively in their own behalf. Whether those efforts are appropriate as public programs is unresolved. If answered affirmatively, should the effort stem from the health establishment or some other social authority in cooperation with health care professionals? Secondly, how much money should be invested, and should it be at the expense of direct care? In the United States, government officials have been attracted to self-care programmes as a way of possibly curbing high health-care costs. But this goal is probably illusory at best and manipulative at worst. More likely, self-help efforts can lead to more appropriate health-care costs.

CONCLUSIONS AND RECOMMENDATIONS

Our emphasis has been on the informed user of health, long-term care and related social services. We favour this approach because so much disability and dysfunction is the result of too little, too much, or inappropriate service. Simultaneous work is needed on many fronts, and the education and re-education of professionals is clearly important. Professional change, however, is influenced by many factors besides professional education. Medical providers are sensitive to the demands, requests, and preferences of their clientele, especially when these are clearly formulated and expressed. For example, some evidence indicates that changing practices in the surgical treatment of breast cancer were hastened by the changed expectations of a newly sophisticated group of consumers (Kane & al. 1981 a). In the same way, older people who continue to ask for information and to give feedback when they do not understand will recondition the care-givers.

Providers also respond to role models among their peers. The growing awareness of geriatrics gives legitimacy to increased attention to the old. The emergence of geriatric training programmes for the physician and the creation of models such as "the teaching nursing home" add the lustre of academe to the subject. And as for long-term care, the high costs and poor quality of many programmes has produced a climate ripe for reform. The time is auspicious to introduce new ideas to providers, including the idea of activating the consumer.

Both consumers and providers will be more effective if the efforts to modify their behaviour are planned in tandem. Our is frankly a middle-of-the-road stance, advocating neither self-care in isolation nor all-out efforts to promote patient compliance with the wise provider's recommendations. Improving the functional status of older people truly requires activation and change on the part of both users and suppliers of health care, and if the efforts are integrated, the changes should be mutually reinforcing. A check and balance system is needed to guard against professional domination on the one hand and misinformation or exploitation of the elderly on the other. A newly activated group of older people and health-care providers could work together toward producing the structural changes so necessary to maintain optimum functioning of older people. These include changes in reimbursement programs and in the delivery system.

Finally, a research agenda is needed. At the moment, at least in the United States, self-care for the elderly is on the crest of a social movement. A bewildering array of interventions are being proposed, developed, and sold. It would be impossible as well as inappropriate for health-care providers or planners to orchestrate events. But in the more limited sphere of developing and testing tools and techniques by which consumers can interact with and receive desirable results from the care system, the health providers and planners have an obligation to design and conduct the studies.

It would be ironic if self-help incentives became transmogrified into new authority and new orthodoxy. Consumers and providers working together to create the activated, defensive user of health-care services can guard against that eventuality.

REFERENCES

Aptekar, R.A. (1983) "The September Club: A Private Sector Wellness Program," Generations, 7:53-54ff

Avery, C., March, J., and Brook, R. (1980) "An Assessment of the Adequacy of Self-Care by Adult Asthmatics," Journal of Community Health, 5:167-180

Brody, E., and Kleban, M. (1981) "Physical and Mental Health Symptoms of Older People: Who do They Tell," Journal of the American Geriatrics Society, 10:442-449

Brody, E., and Kleban, M. (1983) "Day-to-Day Mental and Physical Health Symptoms of Older People: A Report on Health Logs," Gerontologist, 23:75-85

Campbell, R., and Chenoweth, B. (1981) "Health Education as a Basis for Social Support," Gerontologist, 21:619-627

Comaroff, J. (1976) "A Bitter Pill to Swallow: Placebo Therapy in General Practice," Sociological Review, 24:79-96

Ducovny, A. (1969) The Billion $ Swindle: Frauds Against the Elderly, New York: Fleet Press Corp

Dychtwald, K. (1983) "Overview: Health Promotion and Disease Prevention for Elders," Generations, 7:5-7

Dye, C., and Sassenrath, D. (1979) "Identification of Normal Aging and Disease-Related Process by Health Care Professionals," Journal of the American Geriatrics Society, 27:472-475

Evashwick, C., Conrad, D., and Lee, F. (1982) "Factors Related to Utilization of Dental Services by the Elderly," American Public Health Association, 72:1129-1135

FallCreek, S., and Mettler, M. (1982) A Healthy Old Age: A Sourcebook for Health Promotion with Older Adults, Washington, DC: Government Printing Office

Ferrari, N. (1962) "Institutionalization and Attitude Change in an Aged Population: A Field Study in Dissonance Theory," Doctoral Dissertation, Cleveland, OH, Case Western Reserve University

Fletcher, D. (1982) "Helping the Elderly to Sleep Without Drugs," Geriatric Consultant, 1:11-13

Frankfather, D.L., Smith, M.J., and Caro, F.G. (1981) Family Care of the Elderly, Lexington, M.A.: Lexington Books

Gaarder, L., and Cohen, S. (1982) Patient Activated Care for Rural Elderly, Boise, ID: Mountain States Health Corporation

Garcia, C.A., Redding, M.J., and Blass, F.P. (1981) "Overdiagnosis of Dementia," Journal of the American Geriatrics Society, 29:407-410

Gorrell, R. (1982) "Case History: Would You Have Overlooked This Test" Geriatric Consultant, 1:25

Haug, M. (1981) "Age and Medical Care Utilization Patterns," Journal of Gerontology, 36:103-111

Hellebrand, F. (1980) "Aging Among the Advantaged: A New Look at the Stereotype of the Elderly" The Gerontologist, 20:404-417

Howard, J. (1978) "Patient Centric Technologies: The Case for a Soft Science," In EB Gallagher (ed.) The Doctor-Patient Relationship in the Changing Health Scene (DHEW Publ. ≠ NIH 78-183) Washington, DC, John E. Fogarty International Center for Advanced Study in the Health Sciences

Jacobs, B., and Abbott, S. (1983) "Planning for Wellness: A Community-Based Approach," Generations, 7:57-59

Jahmogem, D., Hannon, C., Laxson, L., and LaForce, F.M. (1982) "Iatrogenic Disease in Hospitalized Elderly Veterans," Journal of the American Geriatrics Society, 30: 387-390

Kahn, A.J., and Kamerman, S.B. (1982) Helping America's Families, Philadelphia, Temple University Press

Kane, R.A., and Glicken, M. (1979) "Compliance and Consumerism: Complementary Goals of Social Work in Health Settings," In J. Hanks (ed.) Toward Human Dignity: Social Work in Practice, Washington, DC, National Association of Social Workers

Kane, R.A., and Kane, R.L. (1981) Assessing the Elderly: A Practical Guide to Measurement, Lexington, MA, D.C. Heath

Kane, R.A., Kane, R.L., Williams, C.E., Hopwood, M.D., Lincoln, T.L., Rettig, R.A., and Williams, A.P. (1981 a) The Breast Cancer Networks: Organizing to Improve Management of a Disease (R-2789-NCI), Santa Monica, CA, The Rand Corporation

Kane, R.L., Solomon, D.H., Beck, J.C., Keeler, E., and Kane, R.A. (1981 b) Geriatrics in the United States: Manpower Projections and Training Considerations, Lexington, MA, D.C. Heath

Kane,R.L., Ouslander, J., Abrass, I (1984) "Essentials of Clinical Geriatrics," New York, McGraw-Hill

Keeler, E.H., Solomon, D.H., Beck, J.C., Mendenhall, R.C., and Kane, R.L. (1982) "Effect of Patient Age on Duration of Medical Encounters with Physicians," Medical Care, 20:1101-1108

Kemper, D.W., Deneen, E.J., and Giuffre, J.V. (1981) Growing Younger Handbook, Boise, ID, Healthwise, Inc.

Klein, L., German, P., McPhee, S., Smith, C., and Levine, D. (1982) "Aging and Its Relationship to Health Knowledge and Medication Compliance," The Gerontologist, 22:384-387

Kosidlak, J.G. (1980) "Self-Help for Senior Citizens," Journal of Gerontological Nursing, 6:663-668

Kulys, R., and Tobin, S.S. (1980) "Older People and Their 'Responsible' Others," Social Work, 25:138-145

Kulys, R. (1983) "Future Crises and Very Old: Implications for Discharge Planning," Health and Social Work, 8:182-195

Langer, E., and Rodin, J. (1976) "Effects of Choice and Enhanced Personal Responsibility for the Aged," Journal of Personality and Social Psychology, 34:191-198

Lederman, E.O., Rothschild, M.F., and Spilka, L. (1983) "The Wisdom Project: A Community-Based Education Program," Generations, 7:48-49

Lorig, K., and Fries, J. (1981) The Arthritis Helpbook, Reading, MA, Addison Wesley Publishing Company

Louis Harris and Associates (1981) Aging in the Eighties: America in Transition, Washington, DC, National Council on Aging

Mace, N.L., and Rabins, P.V. (1981) The 36-Hour Day, Baltimore, Johns Hopkins

Martin, D., and Mead, K. (1982) "Reducing Medication Errors in a Geriatric Population," Journal of the American Geriatrics Society, 30:258-260

Mercer, S., and Kane, R.A. (1979) "Helplessness and Hopelessness in the Institutionalized Elderly," Health and Social Work, 4:90-116

Minkler, M. (1981) "Applications of Social Support Theory to Health Education: Implications for Work with the Elderly," Health Education Quarterly, 8:147-165

McMorran, W. (1983) "Older Participation, Advocacy Needed for Health Planning," Generations, 7:55-56

Morrison, J. (1980) "Geriatric Preventive Health Maintenance," Journal of the American Geriatrics Society, 28:133-135

Nestle, M. (1983) "Dietary Recommendations for Older Americans," Generations 7:20-22

Nugent, M. (1981) "Social and Emotional Needs of Geriatric Surgery Patients," Social Work in Health Care, 6:69-76

Pratt, C.C., Simonson, W., and Lloyd, S. (1982) "Pharmacists' Perceptions of Major Difficulties in Geriatric Pharmacy Practice," Gerontologist, 22:288-292

Pratt, L. (1978) "Reshaping the Consumer's Posture in Health Care," In E. Gallagher (ed.) The Doctor-Patient Relationship in the Changing Health Scene (DHEW Publ # NIH 78-183) Washington, DC, John E. Fogarty International Center for Advanced Study in the Health Sciences

Raffoul, P., Cooper, J., and Love, D. (1981) "Drug Misuse in Older People," Gerontologist, 21:146-150

Reidenberg, M.M., and Lowenthal, D.T. (1968) "Adverse Nondrug Reactions," New England Journal of Medicine, 279:678-679

Rubenstein, L.Z., Rhee, L., and Kane, R.L. (1982) "The Role of Geriatric Assessment Units in Caring for the Elderly: An Analytic Review," Journal of Gerontology, 37:513-521

Sackett, D., and Haynes, R.B. (1976) (eds.) Compliance with Therapeutic Regimens, Baltimore, Johns Hopkins

Salzman, C., and Van der Kolk, B. (1980) "Psychotropic Drug Prescriptions for Elderly Patients in a General Hospital," Journal of the American Geriatrics Society, 28:18-22

Schulz, R. (1976) "Effects of Control and Predictability on the Physical and Psychological Well-Being of the Institutionalized Aged," Journal of Personality and Social Psychology, 33:563-573

Sehnert, K. (1975) How to be Your Own Doctor (Sometimes), New York, Grosset and Dunlap

Seligman, M. (1975) Helplessness: On Depression, Development, and Death, San Francisco, CA, W.H. Freeman and Co.

Simmons, J.J., Roberts, E., and Nelson, E.C. (1983) "Self-Care: Tools, Strategies and Methods" Generations, 7:46-47

Skeist, R.J. (1980) To Your Good Health, Chicago, Chicago Review Press

Stein, S., Linn, M., and Stein, E. (1982) "The Relationship of Self-Help Networks to Physical and Psychosocial Functioning," Journal of the American Geriatrics Society, 30:764-768

Trager, B. (1980) Home Health Care and National Health Policy (Special issue of Home Health Care Services Quarterly), New York, Haworth Press

U.S. DHEW (1979 a) Healthy People: The Surgeon General's Report on Health Promotion and Disease Prevention (PHS No. 79-55071), Washington, DC, Government Printing Office

U.S. DHEW (1979 b) A Guide to Medical Self-Care and Self-Help Groups for the Elderly (NIH Publ # 80-1687) Washington, DC, Government Printing Office

U.S. DHHS, PHS, NIH (1980) Perspectives on Geriatric Medicine (81-1924) Washington, DC, Government Printing Office

Warner-Reitz, A. (1981) Healthy Lifestyle for Seniors, New York, Meals for Millions

Wallack, L. (1981) "Mass Media Campaigns: The Odds Against Finding Behavior Change," Health Education Quarterly, 8:209-260

Wartman, S., Morlock, L., Malitz, F., and Palm, E. (1981) "Do Prescriptions Adversely Affect Doctor-Patient Interactions," American Journal of Public Health, 71:1358-1361

Chapter 11

SELF-CARE AND SELF-HELP PROGRAMMES FOR ELDERS

Alfred H. Katz

TOWARD DEFINITIONS

Many discussions of self-help and self-care are confused by the lack of clear definitions. A precise definition of terms is essential to this increasingly popular field, which lacks standardised vocabulary and concepts.

I shall begin this discussion of some relevant issues by presenting and enlarging on self-help and self-care definitions that have seemed both useful and specific.

The term "self-help" is imprecise, but remains in use because it is popular and time-sanctioned. In common speech, the term is applied to diverse activities, from collective action by a social group to individual activity such as learning via a teaching machine. For scientific purposes, it seems better to limit the term to actions that occur in a group setting; in such usage, self-help is not or cannot be practised by the lone individual. "Mutual aid" is a preferable, substitute term since it implies ego's relationship with at least one alter. Some writers, e.g. Borkman and Silverman, use variant forms of the mutual aid idea to indicate this aspect in their references to "mutual self-help groups" (1) and "mutual help groups" (2). Although self-help activities can occur in ad hoc informal affinity settings, the organised self-help group is the most typical locus, since it is founded on mutual aid interactions. The most widely employed definition of such self-help groups was published in 1976 in my book, The Strength in Us:

Self-help groups are voluntary, small group structures for mutual aid and the accomplishment of a special purpose. They are usually formed by peers who have come together for mutual assistance in satisfying a common need, overcoming a common handicap or life-disrupting problem, and bringing about desired social and/or personal change. The initiators and members of such groups perceive that their needs are not, or cannot be, met by or through existing social institutions. Self-help groups emphasize face-to-face social interactions and the assumption of personal responsibility by members. They often provide material assistance, as well as emotional support; they are frequently "cause"-oriented, and promulgate an ideology or values through which members may attain an enhanced sense of personal identity. (3)

But self-care can be practised by the lone individual or with the aid of one or more others, including that of an organised self-help group. Self-care may be defined as "a process whereby a lay person functions on his/her own behalf in health promotion and prevention and in disease detection and treatment." (4) I will elaborate on this formulation later.

Some related distinctions and attributes that flow from these two definitions must be noted. Much difficulty regarding self-help and self-care arises from lack of clarity about the relationship of these activities to professionals and about professional instigation and direction of them. Thus, the well-known and generally useful survey of such programmes for the elderly, by Butler & al. (5) tends to lump the terms self-care and self-help together; they exemplify these terms by citing a wide range of programmes and activities -- some wholly initiated, conducted, and controlled by health professionals. An important example is peer counseling -- widely practised in self-help groups, where help and solutions are offered by persons who have experienced the problem themselves. We shall see later that peer counseling can also be set up under professional auspices.

As shown by the definition quoted above, such professional control does not fit the self-help group, an essential and distinguishing characteristic of which is that the group, whatever its origin, belongs to and is run by its members. Autonomy is, thus, a key defining characteristic of the self-help group -- that is, self-direction from within by members rather than direction by outsiders, i.e., professionals. This key defining criterion should be kept in mind whenever self-help phenomena are discussed.

An additional basic characteristic of both self-help and self-care is that they are chosen, voluntary behaviour. The individual practising self-care or participating in self-help groups is usually under no compulsion to do so from the State, professional authority, or any other source. A major reason in fact, for the growing popularity of self-help and self-care is that they enlarge the individual's ability to make choices about things important in life -- e.g., health status and the means chosen to maintain or improve it. Self-care programmes and self-help groups, thus, offer specific alternatives to the traditionally sanction-ed means of maintaining or improving health through the professional health care or other human service systems.

Arising from this enlargement of choices is the common theme and objective of empowerment, which is a major motivation, goal, and result of both self-care and self-help programmes. The individual -- often feeling powerless in relation to massive, impersonal social forces and bureaucratic service structures -- gains a greater sense of autonomy and control over his own life. Terms like "the activated patient" (Sehnert) and "the energized family" (Pratt) reflect this dynamic in self-care program-mes. Many personal testimonies of participants in self-help groups stress the positive feelings of personal confidence, identity, and strength gained from their participation. (6)

Conceiving the goals and results of self-care and self-help activity along these lines seems fundamentally at variance with the view of some writers such as the Kanes in this volume (Chapter 11), who state, "Self-help must be linked to the care giving system," and that self-care consists of "actions instituted by the individual in conjunction with health-care providers." In my view, this is a narrow and inaccurate conception that does not reflect the breadth and variety of current re-alities.

The definition of self-care formulated and employed in a current University of North Carolina School of Public Health study pulls together the various aspects we have discussed and, thus, usefully elaborates on the succinct definition of self-care presented earlier:

A self-care program is defined as a formal, structured set of activities whose primary purpose is to enable (medical) laypersons to effectively engage in self-care activities.

The focus of self-care enablement is generally (although not exclusively upon the individual. The locus of self-care activity is generally the enabled individual and his/her immediate family. However, the locus might range from the isolated individual ministering to another isolated individual (as in the application of first aid techniques to a stranger), to one's neighbors, fellow students or work associates.

The emphasis of this definition is upon consciously willed behavior change as well as the conscious learning of specific skills in voluntary joined programs rather than pre-scribed clinical programs. (7)

SELF-CARE AND SELF-HELP FOR THE ELDERLY

From these brief considerations of definitions and concepts let us now examine what can be said about the nature and extent of these two related phenomena in the elderly population. Our discussion will draw primarily on experiences in the U.S.

A discussion of this subject must avoid the common stereotypes of considering all persons over 65 (or 60) as a homogeneous population and seek to differentiate various groups among them for whom distinct problems and possibilities of self-care and self-help may exist and be appropriate. At least four groups should be distinguished: the well-aged, who are basically independent and as fully function-al as any segment of the population; the aged who have one or more chronic health problem, but are not significantly limited or disabled in their function-ing; the aged who have chronic, severely limiting conditions -- e.g., who are homebound; and the so-called "frail elderly," aged 75 or more, many of whom are in nursing homes or other institutions. The mix of problems encountered, of possible activities, of useful knowledge and skills, of involvement of relatives, is clearly different for each of the above groupings; therefore, the elderly population we are concerned with must be specified.

A quantification of the size, numbers, and growth trends in self-help group initiatives among the older population in the U.S. is difficult, since no firm data currently exist, only impressions or estimates. There are, of course, plenty of senior citizen organisations and educational service programmes on their behalf. Many States have Departments of Aging Services to encourage or organise the growth of such efforts. Likewise many local voluntary agency programmes -- Senior Centers, church and YM-YW sponsored groups etc. -- also have been set up. On a national scale, the American Association of Retired Persons (AARP) numbers more than a million members.

These membership organisations and social agencies and the programmes for seniors organised by them undoubtedly are useful and may stimulate or conduct some self-care activities, but do not meet the definitional criteria or operational principles of self-help groups. This is because they lack the crucial element of freedom from outside control basic to a self-help group. Furthermore, the membership organisations such as AARP do not emphasise personal participation and interaction, or personal responsibility by members. They may take some broad social and legislative actions, but these are conducted from above, don't arise from membership initiatives and usually do not involve individual members. As is the case with AARP, they may offer material benefits such as insurance policies or travel packages for members, but these are simple membership services, made possible by the large size of the organisation. Therefore, though significant socially, organisations of this type do not meet the criteria for self-help groups and should be distinguished from them.

SENIOR MEMBERS IN HEALTH SELF-HELP GROUPS

A recent research paper (8) by Borkman examined the question of what is known about the membership of older persons in existing health-related self-help groups. Are older persons found in these in numbers proportionate to the incidence and prevalence of the particular health problem? Borkman found the data exceedingly scattered and fragmentary; many self-help groups do not seem to have records regarding the ages of their member-participants. Borkman obtained access to eight national health self-help groups whose age data were "minimally sufficient to include in the analysis." These were: Alcoholics Anonymous (A.A.), Recovery Inc., International Association of Laryngectomees, United Ostomy Association, Mended Hearts, Make Today Count, Stroke Clubs, Women's Alternative Health Services, and Women's Consciousness Raising groups.

In all but the Women's Alternative Health Services and Consciousness-Raising groups, the data showed some representation of older persons. In only two organisations, however, A.A. and the Ostomy Association, did the representation seem proportionate to the estimated age distribution of potential members -- which in A.A. is thought to be about two percent. In Recovery, Inc., older persons were found, but were proportionately under-represented; in Mended Hearts and Make Today Count, the potential membership could not be estimated; therefore, whether or not the membership of older persons was proportionate could not be established.

Borkman summarises her findings as follows:

> Mutual self-help groups for heart surgery, stroke, life-threatening illness and dying, alcoholism, various cancers and mental troubles, were found to have older persons represented, on the basis of the often sparse empirical data available. The only exception was the lack of representation of older women in many self-help-health groups related to the women's movement. The reasons for this lack are unknown. Perhaps the young women in the movement perceive that the older generation's outlook is incompatible with theirs. Overall, these findings indicate that older persons join with others who have common afflictions irrespective of age. (9)

This limited but useful initial study of the problem -- admittedly tentative and subject to revision as more data become available -- would benefit from conceptual expansion.

Statements about the prevalence of and participation in self-help groups for health problems of the elderly ought to include the many self-help groups that have been formed by those, usually relatives, who are care-takers for elderly persons suffering from debilitating diseases. Thus, as more has become known about Alzheimer's as a clinical entity, self-help groups for Alzheimer's disease have recently sprung up in a number of localities. The disease clearly poses severe problems to family members. Huntington's Disease, for which several national organisations of relatives and sufferers exist in the U.S., organised on a self-help basis, is another example that should be included in order to give a more complete account of self-help organisations for health problems of the elderly. perhaps the most rapidly growing self-help group of the past decade is the National Alliance of the Mentally Ill, set up in 1979 as a federation of many local, State and regional associations of relatives and friends. The NAMI now numbers some 30,000 members in 90 groups in 48 states and maintains a legislative office in Washington, D.C. A major stimulus to its dynamic growth has been the de-institutionalisation of mental patients, which has obviously brought many "chronic" schizophrenics and other psychotic patients back to families and communities ill-equipped to take care of them. Here, too, age data are lacking, but evidently many of the returned "chronic" patients had spent years in mental hospitals and thus would be in older age groups. As a self-help consumer group, NAMI is concerned with strengthening the family as a support system, with "issues of stigma and misinformation," research, needed changes in treatment and service delivery, and the maintenance of adequate funding for federal and state programmes for the mentally ill (10).

Though not beamed especially to the elderly, a recent study by Giloth of the Patient American Hospital Association's Patient Education Division includes some suggestive findings (11). Her survey in 1981 showed that 48.3 percent of U.S. hospitals reported having one or more self-help groups in six specifically listed areas (stroke, post-heart-attack, ostomy, cancer, weight reduction).

Cancer support groups were the most numerous reported by 21 percent of the responding hospitals. Stroke groups ranked lowest, reported by only 9.9 percent of the hospitals. A follow-up questionnaire sent to a sample of initial respondents indicated that the survey had probably underestimated the actual extent of hospital relationships with self-help groups, both those formed within the institution and community groups.

This survey has some methodological problems and did not seek information pertinent to the elderly as such, but nevertheless provides useful evidence for the growth, usefulness and continuing stimulation and use of self-help groups by health professionals in hospitals. Elderly patients would clearly seem to be substantially represented among cancer, post-heart-attack, laryngectomy, ostomy and stroke patients in the reporting hospitals, but the extent of their actual participation in the self-help groups was not reported.

Both age-specific epidemiological data on the incidence and prevalence of health problems, especially chronic diseases, and reliable information on the extent of the elderly population's participation in formal self-care programmes and in self-help groups would be needed before any definitive, rather than impressionistic, general statements can be made.

Some organisations of a different type than those discussed earlier exist among the elderly population. Using the typology advanced in my self-help book (12), these are organisations whose predominant focus is on social action. The best-known of these is the Gray Panthers, an organisation of a true self-help character whose major goal is to combat "ageism" (social discrimination against the elderly) through public education, work for remedial legislation, and other social actions. The Gray Panthers are clearly interested in health issues, the reform of delivery systems, the defense and extension of public medical care programmes, health insurance, and the like. Their national office and Health Task Forces in local units are active on these issues. They have not yet exhibited comparable interest in promoting self-care educational programmes or participation in health-oriented self-help groups, but would seem to have the potential for doing so.

SOME PROGRAMME INNOVATIONS

Having briefly considered definitions, concepts, and the extent and nature of self-care/self-help activities for the elderly, let us turn to the discussion of some programme models for seniors that stand at the interface between self-care and self-help. I will present some information on the peer-counseling approach on the Sage project, and on a dramatically innovative self-care project at Yale.

Peer Counseling
An approach and method of counseling employed in a growing number of senior self-care programmes and senior self-help groups is peer counseling. Counseling by peers, of course, is not a novel idea; it forms part of our concept of self-help, being based on a relationship between persons of equal status

who face common problems. Peer counseling has been exemplified in recent years by many programmes for drug addicts, indigenous or "para-professionals" in community mental health, public health clinics for youth and so on. It is as clearly applicable to the elderly as to younger persons. Certainly, this has always been an important component of the informal support system of elderly persons experiencing distress or difficulties who find help by talking through their problems with a trusted peer.

Despite the denigrating attitudes held by some mental health and other professionals toward this kind of help, a noticeable establishment of peer-counseling activities has occurred by and in professionally-staffed agencies for the aged. The 1980 volume, Non-traditional Therapy and Counseling with the Aging describes several of these (13). ·

An outstanding programme of this type is that of the Santa Monica Senior Health Screening Center in California which was established in 1975 and set up formal peer counseling in 1978 (14). Peer counselors were selected from local volunteers, including regular clientele of the agency, and given two months training. The initial group of 25 trainees ranged in age from 50 to 82 years, with a mean age of 63; the group included 18 women and seven men from diverse educational, ethnic, and socio-economic backgrounds. Their two-month training course was in the psycho-social aspects of aging, counseling principles and methodology, and government and local community resources, and regular group meetings were held for supervision and "case" discussions. In addition to the formal 1-1 peer counseling provided in the agency, in other community settings, or in the homes of the approximately 50 percent of programme clients who were homebound, six community discussion groups were organised with the peer counselors taking a prominent role.

The success of the Santa Monica programme of professionally-organised peer counseling has exceeded all projections by its planners: in its first 16 months, 264 seniors were seen in individual counseling, and the rap groups had an attendance of more than 3,000 persons.

SAGE

Another prominent example in which professionals have organised or encouraged a self-help approach among the elderly is the SAGE (Senior Actualization and Growth Explorations) project in Berkeley, California (15). In the first phase of the project, professionals taught physical and mental self-care techniques to small groups of elders, who met weekly over a nine-month period. The techniques emphasised what people could do for themselves in diet, exercise, medication-taking, stress-reduction and so on. Participants were required to keep daily journals. Peer counseling was encouraged by the assignment of a partner for personal interaction, discussion, and support in between the regular group meetings. Intense personal involvement and a supportive network developed, and in subsequent phases of the programme, elderly participants or graduates began themselves to participate on the governing board of the project and to be group leaders, providing services that had previously been professionally offered. On the latter developments, Borkman comments "SAGE represents a case of deprofessionalisation, whereby the professionals are relinquishing some control by sharing it with the elderly participants." (16) Such a transfer does not occur in many professionally-organised programmes, but the potential for it is greater than usually believed.

Yale Self-Care Project
By far the most innovative recent programme is the Self-Care Education Project at the Yale School of Public Health, conceived and directed by Lowell Levin and supported by the Kellogg Foundation. As stressed earlier, many formal self-care education programmes for seniors and others have their content and formats devised exclusively by professionals; clients or recipients of the education have little or no input -- the professionals decide what the target populations need. This might account in part for the marked similarities found in many such programmes. Further, most self-care education programmes seem to be aimed at predominantly middle-class populations or at least at persons with a degree of education sufficient to master the technical written and oral materials that are usually presented.

In contrast, Levin and his co-workers proposed a project where the clients would decide the content, methods, and desired outcomes, on an heuristic basis.

Several applications of this philosophy in the

functioning of the programme are worth nothing. Firstly, it started with an emphasis on problem-posing rather than problem-solving techniques. With 75 percent of the study population at or below the poverty line, it was felt that participants themselves rather than professionals should define the chief problems affecting their lives. It was not assumed that these problems were necessarily the result of individual deficits or handicaps; environmental hazards or deficiencies in public programmes might be deemed the main culprits. This approach led to an implicit emphasis on collective action rather than on personal change in the participants.

Secondly, the project has shown awareness of great cultural differences in learning styles as well as in the techniques necessary for group change. Two of the four demonstration groups were based in neighbourhood health centers, with blue-collar and poverty-level people of Black, Italian and Puerto Rican origin. The third group was composed of an "ethnic" population of south-east Europeans, the fourth of a middle-to-high socio-economic population of Yale Health Plan members.

A third innovation is that the clients in the demonstration-study groups are very active in producing its evaluation data. Instead of a corps of professional researchers, there are "observation posts" in every setting, manned by clients who record quantitative and qualitative data for evaluation.

While the project has not been reported as yet in a formal publication, its originator, Professor Levin, summarised some findings in an informal presentation:

> What did we learn about the clients? We learned that the belief that self-care education belongs only to the middle class is an absolute myth. Interest varied but the level of interest was uniformly high. What we have to do is stop doing needs assessments and begin to do preference assessments. If we respond problematically to preference data, rather than needs data, we don't have to worry about motivation or the organization and the planning process being with people themselves. I would like to propose that we think about how one can organize program planning around preference rather than needs. Needs are the professional construction, preferences are the layman's construction ...

Lay people have already established an effective base of self-care skills ... they are a vast resource in health care. We learned that the process of identifying clients and getting their participation in the program means that you have to go with the flow of their preferences which are both individual and collective (17).

Although not specified in Levin's account, the Yale project includes many activities and groups for and of seniors. Their participation in determining the content, methods, and evaluation criteria has been just as active as that of the younger participants.

All the data on this project are not yet reported, but clearly it represents a fascinating, even revolutionary departure from other programmes, and constitutes what might be called an _in vivo_ experiment in self-care empowerment.

SOME RECOMMENDATIONS

Our brief excursion through a few aspects of self-care and self-help for the elderly was designed only to offer some supplementary suggestions and comments to the more extensive discussions in this volume. It makes no claim to being a thorough analysis of these contributions, or to advance systematic or completely thought-out alternative formulations. Nevertheless, a few recommendations, which have not been stressed in the other papers, would seem to be in order.

Most pressingly needed is education/discussion which can conduce to changing the attitudes of health professionals, including gerontologists, to self-care, self-help initiatives. At present, lay initiatives tend to evoke distrust among the helping professions. Whatever the reason -- whether economic self-interest, perceived threats to status, apprehension about the dangers of self-carers and self-helpers "going too far" -- such attitudes cannot hold back the dynamic growth of these approaches, since they arise as reflexive, popular responses to broader social developments, forces, and attitudes, not merely to the professional ones. But professional misconceptions, suspicion, and unwillingness to cede some elements of a monopolistic and privileged status by recognising the importance of the lay resources and transferring

295

some functions to it can inhibit the growth of a constructive, mutually-beneficial relationship with these important social resources. Not only can further programme initiatives be discouraged, but two other areas can be negatively affected: research and social policy, in both of which professionals are prominent and influential. There is no need here to expound on the importance of empirical studies regarding many aspects of how, why, and for whom self-care and self-help function or do not function and with what outcomes. These needs have been well set forth in other contributions to this volume. In a climate of stringency of support for behavioural research, research regarding the elderly is happily a partial exception. Clinical and field trials of procedures and methods, surveys of programmes and attitudes, cost-studies and many others are not only needed, but feasible in the present climate.

Data from an accumulation of such studies are required to influence social policy -- the other area where the views of the professionals' are important. Without conviction of the value or otherwise of these initiatives, professionals will not be in a position to make whole-hearted and responsible recommendations to policy-makers.

Self-care and self-help activities have grown apace and attract significant and growing professional interest, but are very little reflected in the curricula of professional schools in the human service fields -- in medicine, nursing, social work, clinical psychology, etc. Apart from courses in a few schools, there is little systematic presentation and analysis of the phenomena, in their many-sided clinical and organisational manifestations, their important embodiment of consumer interests and reactions, their significant implication for policy.

Thus the most timely, immediately pertinent and attainable recommendation that can be made here is that professionals who are convinced of the importance of understanding self-care and self-help apply pressure on the established training programmes in their professional fields so that current and new students will emerge from them with a broader knowledge and greater ability to relate constructively to this important part of social reality.

NOTES

(1)   T.   Borkman   (1982)   "Where   Are   Older Persons in Mutual Self-Help Groups." In A. Kolker and P. Ahmed (eds.), Aging, New York, Elsevier Biomedical, pp. 257-283.

(2)   P.   Silverman (1981) Mutual Help Groups, Beverly Hills, Sage Publications.

(3)   A.   Katz & E.   Bender (1976) The Strength in Us: Self-Help Groups in the Modern World, New York, Franklin-Watts, p. 9.

(4)   L.   Levin,   A.   Katz,   and E.   Holst (1979) Self-Care: Lay Initiatives in Health, New York, Prodist, 2nd ed., p. 11.

(5)   R.   Butler & al.   (1979-80) "Self-Care, Self-Help and the Elderly," Int'l. Jo Aging and Human Development, x.10, pp. 95-119.

(6)   A.   Katz   (1981)   "Self-Help   and   Mutual Aid," Annual Review Sociol. v. 7, pp. 129-155.

(7)   Self-Care study prospectus, mimeographed, pp. 2-3.

(8)   Borkman, op. cit.

(9)   ibid, p. 280

(10)   B.   Giloth   (1982)   Hospital   Involvement with Self-Help Groups, Chicago, Am. Hosp. Assn.

(11)   A.   Hatfield (1981) "Self-Help Groups for Families of the Mentally Ill," Soc. Wk. ≠26, pp. 408-413.

(12)   Katz & Bender, op. cit.

(13)   S.   Sargent   (ed.)   (1980)   Nontraditional Therapy and Counseling with the Aging, New York, Springer Publishing Co.

(14)   B.   Bratter & E.   Tuvuran,   "A Peer Coun- seling Program in Action." In S. Sargent (ed.), Nontraditional Therapy & Counseling with the Aging, pp. 131-145.

(15)   S.   Fields (1979) "The Greening of Old Age," Innovations, v. 4, pp. 2-21.

(16)   Borkman, op. cit., p. 263.

(17)   L.   Levin,   "Lay & Professional Involvement in Self-Care," presentation at Self-Care Symposium, Bauff, Health Promotion Directorate, Department of National Health and Welfare, Canada.

Chapter 12

SELF-CARE AND HEALTH POLICY: A CONFLICT OF INTERESTS

Ronald Liddiard and Roger A. Ritvo

INTRODUCTION

This chapter focuses on the potential conflicts
between the need for policies in health care and the
development of self-care programmes. Self-care
remains outside the domain of public policy in many
countries. As noted in previous publications (Ritvo
1982), policy development emerges from one of three
different perspectives. First, and most common, are
those policies and programmes developed in response
to commonly recognised problems. Community mental
health services and orphanages illustrate this
point. A second option for policy making lies in a
population focus. Here, the policy decision-makers
review the needs of a specific population and
develop services and programmes to fit these needs.
Mobile food programmes and disability payments
document this option. The third, and least clear
approach, is the geographic analyses. What are the
needs of a specific state, local authority, or
catchment ares? Land management and water conser-
vation efforts illustrate this approach. While we
would be remiss to leave the reader with the
impression that policy development is as rational as
these three categories imply, the model does have
validity.

- - - - - - - - - -

The views expressed in this chapter are entirely
those of the authors; they do not necessarily
represent those of either the City of Birmingham or
Cleveland State University.

Self-care does not fit into any of the three approaches. In many ways, self-care is outside the direct application of policy, since many policies emerge solely as a response to a known problem or political pressure. As we will demonstrate in this chapter, efforts to promote self-care may work. But, often they reach the same level of success as public health efforts to curb smoking: high visibility, massive expenditures, and modest results. This could lead to a conclusion that such efforts will never work. We hope not. An equally viable alternative is that the programmes thus far have only begun to work and long-term reinforcements are needed.

With this caution in mind, we will devote our attention to the challenges of the title. The answer to this question is found in the mosaic pattern formed by organisational interests, financial constraints, professional domains, client needs, governmental structures, and national ideologies. Each of these contributes on its own; each is affected by others. Our effort aspires to show the difficulty of developing clear policies in the field, but also to raise the hope that clear policies will be developed. They are needed.

Policy analysis can take many forms, depending on the perspectives of those conducting the analyses. At one pole lies the notion that policies develop out of a collective sense of the most efficient and effective paths to goal achievement. This model assumes that decision makers know the most relevant facts, understand and subscribe to social values and will, therefore, select the most appropriate policies to implement these aspirations. An alternative approach views policy as an outcome of an elite group's actions. Decisions reflect the interests of those who possess power. This form of social control is intended to keep the "haves" in control of the "have-nots." By extending this logic, a third model emerges: policy making by compromise. In this framework, policies represent a composite strategy to balance divergent points of view. Frequent changes, even if structured into a national system, encourage this process. Compromise differs from incrementalism, a form of decision making that allows policies to develop almost without attention to related events. This is seen where governments stress health promotion and disease-prevention efforts, while at the same time excluding payments for these services or providing cash benefits insufficient for good nutrition, adequate housing, and sufficient heating. Self-care falls into these last two categories. Self-care programmes rarely fit into policies; they remain outside the main interests of most of the populace. Providers using a medical model generally connect care with professional concepts; so do social workers. After all, self-care may challenge the competence or need for the professional.

Self-care refers to actions taken by an individual (or a family member on behalf of an individual with that person's knowledge and consent) in response to a known illness or presenting symptom. In the United States and many other western nations, "calling the doctor" seems most prevalent. This reflects a generation-long growth in the role, power, and control of the physician in the delivery of health care and, in some countries, the notion that the "Welfare State" will and should provide needed services. It also diminishes our own abilities to assist in or control the treatment process.

In this chapter, we will discuss health, social services, and related environmental factors that have an impact on self-care efforts. We argue for policies and programmes, for financial approaches and professional ideologies to recognise and support the development of self-care as a legitimate and integral part of the treatment options. We use a perspective that supports the philosophy of the World Health Assembly's 1983 recommendations. We believe "that health is not strictly a medical issue, but environmental, cultural, biological, social, and economic" factors must be considered. For self-care policies to have an impact, they must include these perspectives.

This disease-focused model of public health and human-service programmes and policy limits the effectiveness of self-care programmes generally and especially for the elderly. The situation becomes even more compounded when mean tests are applied. The United States uses means tests as a form of social exclusion: those with means, resources, and assets are not eligible for many public services. The British model has a greater attractiveness since eligibility is virtually assured. The means test is modified to assure that those who can afford services contribute some level of payment. This reversal effectively eliminates an important barrier to service delivery.

"The greatest potential for improving health lies in what we do and don't do for and to ourselves." (Fuchs 1974: 151) This expression of a neo-classical perspective gives (if not commands!) the individual to greater action, to increased self-reliance, and to reduced dependence on the health and medical establishments. This view is not inconsistent with the perspective that health care is a right (Ritvo & al. 1978) and that the public interest is served by policies and active programmes which set minimum standards of care and distribute resources to those who are "truly needy." This position does not deny the role of the individual; rather, it presents a framework for individual action within the context of strong policy initiatives to guarantee the health of a population. Strong national health care efforts are not necessarily antithetical to self-care efforts. The following sections explore how this can happen as well as the pitfalls and impediments to success. We illustrate mainly by reference to the USA and Great Britain, but the main themes are common in most advanced societies.

BACKGROUND

Great Britain has approximately 9.5 million people over retirement age (65 for men; 60 for women). But those over 75 represent the most significant demand for social and health services. The 75-84 year-old age group in general demands domiciliary and other support services. Those over 85 represent the most significant demand for residential accommodation in homes for the elderly, geriatric hospitals, or the so-called "very sheltered" housing. Of the 3.05 million people over 75 in Great Britain, 40 percent live alone. There are 552,000 people over 85.
    Since the beginning of this century, the number of people in Great Britain aged 60 and over has more than tripled, rising from 2.75 million in 1901 to over 10 million in 1981. By the 1990s the number in their 60s will have declined, while those aged 70 and over will have increased. In absolute numbers, the biggest expansion will be amongst those aged 75-84. These projections imply that in the 20-year period 1976-1996, the number of people 75 and over would increase from a quarter to a third of the total number of old people. This picture of the "graying of the nation" holds true in general for all developed societies, and the phenomenon will be even more marked in the less developed nations, as medicated survival at all ages becomes the norm. The frail and dependent, including the mentally infirm,

comprise a disproportionate percentage of those over 75. Against this demographic background, the social work and other social services for the elderly must be viewed.

Social mobility has become more central to the life-style of many modern families as a result of which families tend to be geographically scattered, making it more difficult to extend help to old people in the family and increasing the potential call upon statutory services.

The shift from independence to increasing dependence typically occurs between the ages of 75 and 84 with the decline in social contacts, health, mobility, and the ability to perform personal and domestic tasks. After 85, this decline generally accelerates. Failing health is a particularly common cause for elderly people to move into the household of a married son or daughter. Only a small minority of the elderly fail to get any help from at least one of their children. It is much more common to find children striving to help their ailing parents until they die, sometimes at considerable physical and/or financial cost to themselves. A small number of elderly people exhaust even the most loving and generous care of their relatives. Usually this would be a female suffering from incontinence and brain failure. Loss of sleep, long-term care needs, and incomprehension of the old person's extraordinary behaviour leads typically to a rejection of the elderly relative and referral to the statutory health or welfare services, often the local authority.

A BRIEF GLANCE AT THE HISTORY OF THE "WELFARE STATE"

The rapid post-war development of the health and welfare services in Great Britain is popularly believed to have resulted from the Beveridge Report of 1942. But Lord Beveridge himself said "The scheme proposed ... is in some ways a revolution, but in more important ways it is a natural development from the past -- it is a British revolution." Over the pre-war years, a slow but significant education of opinions took place which, under the combined shock of total war, mass evacuation of children, and the suffering of bombardment altered public opinion. The revelation of proudly concealed poverty among old people provoked The Times in 1940 to comment on "The remarkable discovery of secret need." (1) When the Beveridge Report appeared, a change of opinion so radical had taken place as almost to promote a new approach. It was Lloyd George's notion of "social pity" carried forward.

The actual term "Welfare State" was probably coined by the Oxford scholar, Alfred Zimmern, but was objected to by Beveridge, who preferred the idea of a "Social Services State." In 1944, a Government White Paper entitled "A National Health Service" recognised the anomalies and inequalities of the existing services and proposed a comprehensive cover for health provided for all people alike. The Beveridge Report showed that on the basis of pre-war conditions, it would have been possible to re-distribute income so as to put most urgent needs first. As Beveridge himself expressed it succinctly on the eve of his lecture tour to America, "Bread for everyone before cake for anybody."

The plan, therefore, substituted existing arrangements with an insurance-based scheme aimed at removing all taint of the poor law or means test, while ensuring adequate support in times of need without making extravagant demands on the State. Following the White Paper of 1944, a series of proposals emerged from the Government in what Beveridge himself called the "White paper Chase." Beveridge's interests were wider than health. They concerned social insurance and full employment in a concerted attack on inequality of opportunity in the nation. The Labour Government of 1946 made a cautious modification introducing a broad subsist-ence basis which has subsequently been abandoned except for certain minimum rates in relation to social security which are widely held to be inadequate.

This illustration documents one of the central differences between policy making in the U.S. and in the U.K. The U.S. tends to focus on problem-solving policy making, while the UK's history lies more in a population-based approach. Means tests are but one of many eligibility requirements used to exclude, to stigmatise, and to control potential recipients of service. The British have moved toward undoing these barriers by using a population-focus on human needs rather than a problem-focused policy process. Recent announcements, however, may have revealed a policy shift towards the American model, with emphasis on the virtues of privately purchased care, family support, and community self help. The U.S. model understates the potential value of self-care. Since self-care is not a solution to any commonly recognised problem, it tends to receive lip-service.

And, it is not rooted in the "high-tech" aspects of medical care!

In the period since the remarkable series of British social legislation of 1944-1948, increasingly stronger professions have been emerging. In the health field, the para-medical professions have been developing rapidly. The advent of the Seebohm Committee in England gave a political and financial power base to social work, something which it had hitherto lacked. From a professional and organisational point of view the major differences were, first, that social workers in the health setting were no longer responsible to doctors for their work and, second, that a bureaucratisation of the profession was bound to take place.

THE SOCIAL SERVICES IN LOCAL GOVERNMENT

Local authorities in England have a degree of independence which is quite different from what is found in many other nations. Therefore, the place of personal social services within this context gives rise to a wide variety of responses.

Central government attempts to control variations by a combination of advice, exhortation, and fiscal requirements. Overall, it claims to be reluctant to interfere with the priorities of local government. Thus, monies voted at the national level may be diverted to other purposes locally; for example, the percentage of the "rate support grant" earmarked for social services in any particular local authority may be altered, even though objective measurement of the criteria relating to that population's needs may indicate the contrary.

Quantifying needs and earmarking funds to meet them is a task which perplexed many nations. The size of the problems, the methods of setting priorities and the difficulty of defining measurable outcomes are much greater in the human services than in some other fields. There is public concern about perceived inefficiencies in the public social services. Nevertheless, whatever measures are available merely demonstrate that they are underfunded, but not to what degree. The British government has now abandoned its own social services guidelines to local authorities -- principally because they were so much higher than average in achievement throughout the nation. The general financial climate indicates a virtual standstill in local government expenditures over the next few years, although published data indicates a rising demand for services.

No examination of the performance of Social Services can be divorced from the economic and political context in which it operates. With customary British ingenuity, a number of different systems have been established for various aspects of social services. Unlike many countries, Britain specifically decided to separate the provision of cash assistance from social work and personal services. This happened in 1948. The Poor Law -- for 350 years the only defense people had against destitution -- was abolished. The Children's Act of 1948 required local authorities to provide for children in need of care and the National Assistance Act gave them the duty to provide residential and other services for elderly, handicapped and homeless people. This ended the era of the workhouse and the public assistance institution as they had developed.

The objective was to provide services available to rich and poor alike by removing the shadow of the Poor Law and making it unnecessary to prove or imply poverty in order to receive personal services. Stigma would be removed. Many would argue today, however, that this has never been successful; the stigma still remains, although less so than in some countries.

In practice, personal social services are still mainly directed at the relatively poor. As in education or health, the more affluent can purchase services and so rely less on the public services. Where they require services, this more articulate and powerful section of society obtains a disproportionately large share. If recent trends are continued, this dichotomy will become more pronounced. This example shows how policy often reflects the needs and aspirations of the rich and more powerful sectors of society.

ORGANISATION OF SERVICES

Arising from a typical British compromise, three different service delivery systems have been established; one for Northern Ireland; one for Scotland; and one for England and Wales. In each case health, income maintenance, and personal social services are accountable separately. Accountability systems are radically different for the three arms of public help.

What is popularly called the National Health

Service is delivered through a network of Regional Health Authorities, of which fourteen are found in England and Wales. In 1982, these regional health authorities became directly responsible for the delivery of health services throughout a network of 192 district health authorities. The previous 90 health authorities in England, whose areas were in most cases identical with those of the local authority, were abolished. In some cases the District Health Authority's boundaries fit those of the local authority; in others, the two did not match at all. Within the boundaries of some large local authorities are found several general hospitals and several health authorities. Sometimes boundaries overlap, and to add to this confusion, catchment areas for hospital medical specialities do not necessarily match either! District Health Authorities are funded through the Regions by central government.

Membership of each District Health Authority includes four representatives nominated by the local authority in whose area it operates.

Primary Care (non-hospital) services are organised differently. Family practitioner services are organised on approximately the same basis, but they have their own structure. Family physicians are not employed by the National Health Service; they are independent contractors paid either on a capitation fee, on a fee-for-service basis, or a combination of the two. In theory, the capitation payment system is analogous to the health maintenance organisations (HMO) in the United States. These systems place a higher priority on self-care and prevention than do the fee-for-service providers. By using resources in a wellness model, the hope is to reduce the costs of care. Very many of the U.S. health care traditions are rooted in receiving payments for treatment of the ill. This needs to be changed if self-care is to expand.

At best, in England the two systems -- local government and the health service -- connect together only loosely. The degree of cooperation often rests on the motivation and personalities of those involved at service delivery level. Perhaps the variety and initiative shown in many sections of the country owe their origin in part to the fact that very few people understand the entire kaleidoscope!

The third Arm is the personal social services. These are delivered by local authorities, metropolitan districts, non-metropolitan counties, and

London boroughs. Social services departments were created in 1971, under the Local Authority Social Services Act 1970, by an amalgamation of the previous welfare and children's departments together with certain aspects of the work of health departments. This reorganisation followed the lines of the major recommendations by the Seebohm Committee (1968), set up to recommend to the government whatever changes were necessary to achieve "an effective family service."

The Committee, chaired by the banker Frederic Seebohm, concluded that three main faults troubled the then-fragmented system of social care. They were: 1. lack of information and research; 2. lack of coordination, leading to gaps and overlaps in services; and 3. lack of political power in social services.

Therefore, they recommended a new, powerful committee of the local authority (counties, metropolitan districts and London boroughs) with statutory protection for its activities. A combined social care department, headed by the Director of Social Services, would be a mandatory requirement. There would be "one door upon which to knock" for service. Thus, the faults would be overcome.

Theoretically, local authorities are independent of central government, although in practice they are severely constrained by legislation, by government financial policy and by the fact that they receive about half their income from that source.

The personal social services continue within local control, a method which produces variety and local ingenuity, but also wide variations in types, standards, and quality of service.

So there are three completely different systems, all reporting to the Secretary of State for Social Services. One is directly funded and directly managed by Central Government. (Social Security). One is indirectly funded and indirectly managed (Social Services). One is directly funded and indirectly managed (Health). All three have separate systems, hierarchies, recruitment, training, and traditions. It would have been difficult to devise a system which had more possible problems inherent in it. However, it is remarkable how closely the systems can, in fact, work together when the local personnel set out to achieve that goal.

Of the three systems, local government is the most independent. Its politics, financing, and planning grow from the assumption that it is separate from central government, although subject to audit, advice and, in extreme circumstances, direction by central government. This tradition is normally upheld by central government, which encourages and cajoles local authorities while retaining its inspectorial powers. But recently, new legislation has enabled central government to control the overall expenditure of local authorities and to constrain their property tax ("rates") income. However, central government has still not attempted to define exact amounts of expenditure on individual services, though it publishes a calculation of the theoretical total amount each local authority should need to spend, based on a combination of measurements of need and the historical spending patterns.

Much of the legislation governing the operation of Social Services Departments is discretionary. Certain services must be provided for those in need. The local authority is responsible for determining whether the need exists. There are minimum statutory requirements laid down by law which are more codified in the case of legislation concerning children and young persons.

One unfortunate effect of the dramatic curtailment of local government expenditure in the last few years has been the degree to which innovative projects have been restricted. New initiatives are now severely restrained unless existing services are curtailed or more cost-effective methods devised. In such a climate, public rhetoric about self-care is heard, but without appropriate provider or policy efforts to make it a reality. This reinforces one common theme regarding self-care: it is often a luxury of public sector finances. In difficult economic times, the "harder," more traditional services receive top priority.

Much of social services departments' money and energy for elderly clients goes into providing relatively straight-forward services -- meals-on-wheels, home visits, homes for the elderly. But those who seek personal counselling or casework are likely to be seen by an unqualified assistant unless their case is an emergency. For those reasons, additional personal social services were provided from health service funds. These monies, called "joint financing," were to be spent by the local Joint Consultative Committee, a body set up to ensure cooperation between local authorities and the health services. Initially, the money was intended for social services projects which had a beneficial effect on health services. The rules have gradually been widened and the method of funding changed to meet the demands of a slack economic climate.

The relative responsibilities of British health and social services for the elderly rest on the assumption of a division of duties between the family, the social services, and the health services. The relative responsibility of the departments were defined by law. Broadly speaking, local authorities are expected to provide services, including residential care, for those persons who would otherwise be capable to being cared for by their family with appropriate support from the domiciliary support services, including visiting general practitioners (family physicians). This has eroded over time due to a number of factors, the principal one being the development of specialised geriatric services which are geared to rehabilitation and away from long-term care (except in certain highly constricted categories).

Thus the burden of residential care for the highly-dependent elderly has shifted to local government. This has major implications for the design of residential accommodation, its equipment and staffing, and for the training of practitioners and care-givers in the field. However, a greater burden has also been thus placed on those families which are prepared to look after their elderly relative. Unequivocally, the entrant to an old persons home in England and Wales today is the kind of person who would probably have been regarded as a hospital case 20 or even 10 years ago. The kind of disabilities that are coped with by local authority housing departments throughout the country represents the typical entrant to an old persons home of the same era. The social services provide the appropriate resources to maintain such dependent old persons in their own accommodation. Because of the restricted resources available, the implication is that other care-givers will assist on a voluntary basis.

Typically, the entrant to local authority residential accomodation may be very frail, confused, enuretic, wheelchair bound. Increasingly, hospitals will only care on a long-term basis for the bed-bound, extreme behaviour disturbance, intractable double incontinence, and the totally confused, with their major emphasis increasingly on rehabilitation and treatable illness.

INTERDEPENDENCE OF SERVICES

That these separate systems of service do not have clear and defined boundaries must be recognised. Neither is the knowledge base of each profession totally exclusive. Furthermore, the traditional health and welfare approaches to care of the elderly can only succeed in a social and economic context which allows the full contribution of professionals involved.

It is interesting to compare the British approach with the results of the 1981 White House Conference on Aging which ranked issues of housing, social security and inflation as having dramatic impact on care of the elderly. The top recommendation was for the preservation of the financial integrity of the social security system through emphasis of the "earned right principle." This holds true for the United Kingdom, but is being eroded by inflation.

The second priority was to develop a U.S. national health policy which would guarantee full and comprehensive health services involving all levels of government and the private sector. The current difficulty of the U.K. health service in meeting the demands upon it would be very relevant in this context. This has particular poignancy when one considers the length of waiting lists in many parts of the country for such relatively simple, but important services to the elderly as chiropody, occupational therapy, physiotherapy, and other medical services.

One of the major philosophical and pragmatic concerns for the elderly in the United States lies in the Medicare programme. Since the U.S. is on record as providing a minimal level of financial security for its elderly, the approach reinforces a sickness-disease-dependency model. In other words, payments for allowable costs have generally excluded until very recently many activities that focus on self-care, non-institutionally based programmes, health promotion, and consumer education efforts. Such a model of action ultimately disappoints the proponents of self-care activities.

Self-care in U.S. policy is rooted in an illness/disease model. Often connected with long-term care, rehabilitation programmes, chronic or terminal illness, self-care becomes a mechanism to decrease dependence on the provider or the institution.

Under the new U.S. government prospective

payment system, diagnosis-related groupings, there are institutional incentives to adopt programmes, services, and attitudes which may reduce in-patient lengths of stay. An ironic outcome could be an increased interest in self-care. Ample evidence already exists that home care and nursing home placements are options for hospitals to control in-patient days. This form of payment gives hospitals incentives to experiment with cost reduction programmes. If self-care can be documented to improve quality of care, assist in discharge planning, or reduce expenditures or costs, it may find a strong advocate among a group which has been somewhat reticent: the hospital's administrative staff.

The next choice was to endorse the social security system as the foundation of economic security for all Americans, with cost of living increases. A very substantial number of elderly, through pride or ignorance of the benefits involved, do not in fact apply for their financial rights. There are some issues of stigma, accessibility, ease of understanding and, information which are relevant here.

Another recommendation concerned elimination of mandatory retirement and the spreading of work for older people on part-time temporary or shared basis. Such flexibility of employment and of retirement age is in our view a major factor. In particular, so many men die within the first year or two of retirement that there is a major health and self-care issue connected with the psychological and self-perceived status of elderly people which is or should be of major concern to public policy makers.

Among the top-ten recommendations was a call for adequate assistance for low-to-moderate-income renters. Provision of appropriate housing, modified as necessary to facilitate continued living in their own environment by persons who might become heavily handicapped is an issue which is exercising many minds in Great Britain at the moment. It has particular relevance now that social services departments are finding it difficult to meet the on-going revenue costs of their capital schemes -- quite apart from the human factors involved in deinstitutionalisation of the services and the desire of many elderly people to remain "behind their own front door." There is a distinct advantage in public policy terms in putting together a package of services to support individuals in their own home. A principal component in this package is the assurance of continued occupancy through health and social crises as well as the financial assistance necessary to guarantee permanent residence.

The ninth ranked recommendation called for expanded home help and in-home services based upon individual needs with more flexible eligibility requirements and simpler administration. We would all say amen to that: However, in both the U.S. and the U.K. -- and indeed in many other countries -- a jungle of administrative complexities remain. Some authorities have attempted to remedy this by the appointment of specialist welfare rights advisers to guide people to their entitlements and, where necessary, to act as advocates on their behalf.

We can see that the twin evils of poverty and bad housing still rank high in the consciousness of many nations. Self-care is vastly facilitated when a good warm home and a satisfactory income are assured. Without these necessities health and welfare services fight an uphill battle; apathy and resignation can result, self-care diminish, and neglect predominate.

THE CARE GIVERS

The tendency of large agencies -- whether private voluntary or statutory -- to make largely undifferentiated provision for a wide-ranging client group militates against self-care. Local flexibility and variety of provision is essential if there is to be a realistic attack upon what has recently been called the "Rising Tide," a title applied by the British Health Advisory Service to the increasing incidence of mental illness in old age. Their report recommends a local framework of cooperation of concerned professionals. In our view, it is typical in that it still restricts its vision to health and welfare services. Professions and governmental organisations must create an environment to value and integrate the elderly with society, not to separate and categorise them.

As the balance of the population changes, and more people move into advanced old age, it is essential that they should retain their health and mobility as far as possible. Physical and social as well as psychological separation is to be overcome.

About 95 percent of old people in Britain are estimated still to live outside institutions. Thank heavens that is so! Otherwise the health and welfare sectors would be completely overwhelmed. A good number of these elderly people either look after themselves or may rely upon a middle-aged or elderly care-giver. It follows, therefore, that services should be organised in order to facilitate this process. Services should also be most appropriate.

Liddiard & al. (1982) stressed that many workers in health and social services see their task as the provision of practical direct services. When the old person moves into full-time care, the task approximates to guardianship. In residential care and geriatric hospitals, there are many dedicated, hard-working individuals, but many basic human values are overwhelmed by the primacy of the institution. As yet, relatively little has been achieved in terms of rights of the individual in such settings. For example, in Social Services Departments, many units have hardly begun to use skills of group processes or residential care such as individual assessments involving the residents, agreed setting of goals, the maximum degree of choice, involvement in decision making, the chance to achieve, the maintenance of family relationships, the understanding of loss and bereavement and the dangers of labelling. Many would argue that we create dependency confusion and incontinence in institutional care regimes.

Some experiments show that those suffering a substantial degree of senile dementia can still retain values which are meaningful to them. Essential are the breakdown of total care patterns of living, the creation of small groups, rehabilitation of those thought to be totally institutionalised, the taking of risks in pursuance of better social functioning and the creation of communities of old people who are much more self-determining. Continuing education of health and social staff has made it possible with varying degrees of success to influence changes in residential and departmental routines -- in particular, the promotion of support and interest groups, the setting up of small group living situations for the elderly, occupational therapy and home-finding schemes in the community. Of equal importance are the formalised interprofessional review groups which can exert pressure, having identified inadequacies and short-comings in style, equipment, organisation and location of both hospitals and local authority provision for the elderly.

However, it is difficult to overcome the attitudes inculcated in professional training. Some examples are: the notion that the doctor is the unquestioned leader of the team whose word must be followed without question; the old fashioned "ward round," where teams of people stand at the foot of the bed and discuss the patient's condition; the hierarchical structure of the nursing profession which may emphasise the virtues of cleanliness and order rather than some of the more humane aspects of care; and the adherence to techniques which sometimes result in the discharge of elderly people into the community before adequate arrangements have been made for their care and welfare at home.

Professionals trained in this way and acculturated to these norms tend to take their values outside the institution when they are transferred to community care settings. We must beware of inadvertently reducing self-care capabilities of the elderly by these attitudes.

The development in some fields of specialisation in care of the elderly might be noteworthy here. In medicine, the emergence of the geriatrician over the past few years has been a major step forward.

The physician can assume a more central role in self-care activities of a patient. With a conscious plan to share information, the medical practitioner can direct and support such activities. But as Schulte (1984) points out, this group "... needs insight and understanding of the political and economic context of patient initiatives and self-care practices, as well as sensitivity toward those aspects of health care ..." (p. 33). We believe this commentary holds true for most nations and practitioners, not just for the author's native homeland, the Netherlands. This assertion supports the finding in a study (1977) conducted by Anderson & al. Self-care practices were not significantly different in outcome than physician-initiated treatments in a selected sample of British subjects. A series of other research results support this conclusion. (See Dean 1981 for a thorough analysis).

Potentially important for enhancing self-care has been the widespread development in Britain of the health visitor -- originally a local-authority employed visiting health monitor and counselor with a nursing qualification and advanced training. Such persons have often specialised in geriatric health visiting, a sub-specialty which still exists. However, they are regrettably few. In health visiting and nursing -- as in social work and other professions -- the boundary lines and methods of cooperation between the specialist and generalist workers have yet to be worked out fully. This is remarkable when one considers that 60 percent of all hospital beds in England and Wales (no matter what the specialty) are occupied by persons in the retirement age group. Such interprofessional rivalry is likely to lead to competition for "custom" and away from the encouragement of self-care behaviour.

We believe that much greater emphasis on the problems and, more important, the solutions to the care of the elderly is needed in the training of all professionals, but perhaps this is most noticeable in the fields of general medicine, nursing, and social work. In particular, more curriculum time should be given to methods of enhancing self-care behaviour. Perhaps financial incentives might help in attracting high quality entrants to gerontological careers in all the professions.

DEMOGRAPHIC CHANGE AND THE FAMILY

The growth of the multi-generation family has altered the view of what might realistically be expected from other family members. Liddiard has already noted that social mobility has not yet resulted in the volume of increased demand for services which might realistically have been expected, though it is increasing. It is interesting to conjecture what the next generation of senior adults will demand. Persons who have been accustomed to receiving a certain degree of public service throughout their lives will not easily acquiesce to shortage.

Social mobility will increase in the future. The medicated survival of large numbers of very old people will have an important impact on the ability of care-givers to go on coping. Many care-givers will themselves be in the retirement age group and looking after an extremely elderly old person (or more than one!) In developed societies the proportion of persons in the retirement age group is already above 16 percent -- in the less developed countries it is 5-6 percent. The problems experienced over the last half century in relation to the growth of the numbers of old people in developed societies, and their relative demands, will be mirrored in the less developed societies within 20 years. Thus, this is a world-wide problem on the scale of a pandemic. At the same time the willingness and ability of neighbours, friends, and families to provide the significant degree of care needed will decrease. Maximisation of self-care strategies and mutual aid groups are essential.

ATTITUDES TO CARE

As already noted, the attitudes of the very old to state provision are at best equivocal. We are dealing with a generation brought up to regard charity as an anathema. Welfare and many public health and human service programmes retain the long shadow of dependence and stigma. The elderly value personal pride, dependence, and self-sufficiency. Sometimes the headlines proclaim the isolated old lady who has been found dead in her own home after a few days, having rejected all offers of help in spite of manifest need. Such attitudes will change with time: The aged of tomorrow will <u>demand</u> help. They will not be grateful for small mercies -- they will seek a range of caring services. They will expect to remain in their own homes. They will seek to ensure their own comfort and independence and security. They will demand a choice between family and state provision which is now not available. They will be right.

CONTINUITY OF CARE - THE BASIS FOR POLICY

There is widespread agreement in the international community of scholars, gerontologists, and researchers that continuity of care remains an abstraction that has not yet been implemented. Fragmented services are not only costly and often inefficient, but also represent a potential source of harm. Care of the elderly requires links between the three major locations of service: the home, the community, and the agency/institution.

The home is the ideal location for care. Independent living arrangements maintain family, peer, and social stability. Whether outreach counseling, meals-on-wheels, or books-on-wheels, these programmes maintain stability and decrease dependence. Community-based programmes range from outpatient medical services to day-care programmes to recreational services. While still allowing maximum freedom of choice, such programmes begin a process of dependence. Institutional arrangements, whether congregate living, nursing homes, or mental health care facilities represent a dependent, controlled environment.

Policy development fails to incorporate this movement from one level and locus of care to another. The major reason for this failure lies in the programme and institutional focus of policy makers. It is both politically strategic and fiscally sound to fund the myriad programmes and organisations. The assumption is that the client-in-need has the information, ability, courage, transportation, and supports needed to negotiate "the system."

Both policies and programmes can be enhanced if a more generic approach were used to the provision of health and social services for the elderly. A clear point of entry facilitates this process. For example, the Danish use of the family practitioner illustrates one way to connect a person-in-need with services. The experimental use of social workers in the non-hospital health system augments continuity. Similar experiments will aid in the development of this process.

Control is a central theme of institutional care for the elderly. Organisations grow, both in size and services. They develop systems to retain control over their clients. James D. Thompson has written extensively on this theme. One of his most cogent propositions stresses that control in a changing or turbulent environment is to bring more "inputs" into the system. The demographics in most "western" industrialised countries point to a sharp rise in the number of people over the age of 65. This trend line further documents that this group will also become an increasingly large segment of the population in the next quarter century. And there can be little doubt that new organisations will emerge offering new services, often paid for by governmental funds. Even in the U.K., this trend is already evident.

Many experimental demonstration efforts il- lustrate this concept. EDCON is an acronym for Elder Day Care Organisationed in Neighbourhoods, an unusual approach for adult day services. While a most successful programme in its infancy, its purposes became subverted when nursing homes saw its participants as a new market to fill their empty beds. As these institutions expanded their domain to encompass the elderly not-yet-in residence, the programme lost its vitality and support. Instead of a day service, it became an extension of the nursing homes marketing efforts for new clients. For the chief executive officers, it became a new source of referrals; for the new residents who lost a vital programme, EDCON became a welcome mat to a new address.

This poignant vignette illustrates the growing complexity of coping with the needs of the elderly. Few would argue that independent living arrangements are preferable to institutional care. Institutions can not provide the same love, respect, and warmth that a family or friendship network does. Institutional living must, by definition, exert some control over the lives, the routines and indeed, the needs of their residents. Without rules, anarchy exists in any society even if that society is a home for the disabled elderly veteran. And the most subtle but dangerous form of control is the unwritten rule!

Yet, as we become a more mobile society, fewer nuclear families will be able to provide for their parents. As more social programmes pay for some of the health, welfare, and retirement costs, reduced incentives will lead to a greater demand for some form of institutional care unless programmes are carefully constructed and specifically targeted to avoid it.

This argument, that social institutions exist to meet human needs, receives additional reinforcement from the fact that all developed countries have social programmes to care for the aged. Some of these efforts are less for care than for the payment of care. Since government cannot fully mandate and nationalise an elderly care system (and we believe it should not), then its role is to provide funds for such care. And as the provider of revenue, government tends to enact programmes and procedures to assure the quality, quantity, and appropriateness of this care. But it does not always provide adequate staffing or funding to assure it.

Suddenly, in this labyrinth of programmes, services, funding patterns, and organisations, the incentives for self-help, independent living are almost lost. It is easier to "give-in," to retire from a life of contribution, of family, civic, and corporate responsibilty to an institution. This serves neither the needs of the individual nor the goals of society.

A coordinated philosophy of care is essential. Without it, a jungle of unrelated programmes will jostle for popularity, superiority, and available resources of manpower and money. Such a philosophy should reinforce the attitude and behaviour that aid self-care; it should resound through the training and practice of all professionals. But most important, it should enlighten the attitudes and actions of all governments, local and national.

NOTES

(1) Quoted in Coming of the Welfare State, Bruce, 1968.

REFERENCES

Anderson, J., Buck, C., Danaher, K., and Fry, J. (1977) "Users and Non-Users of Doctors," Journal of the Royal College of General Practitioners, Vol. 27
Beveridge, William (later Lord) (1942), "Social Insurance and Allied Services," HMSO
Dean, Kathryn (1981) "Self-Care Responses to Illness: A Selected Review," Social Science and Medicine, Vol. 15A
Fuchs, Victor (1974) Who Shall Live? New York: Basic Books
George, Lloyd (1911) Quoted in "The Coming of the Welfare State," Bruce 1968
Liddiard, & al. (1982) Evidence to the Barclay Committee (Appendix), "Social Work for the Elderly Association of Directors of Social Services"
Ritvo, Roger A. (1982) "Strengthening Health and Social Service Links: International Themes," In Hokenstad, M. and Ritvo, R., Linking Health Care and Social Services, Beverly Hills: SAGE
Ritvo, Roger A, Edward McKinney, and Pranab Chatterjee, "Health Care As a Human Right," Journal of International Law, Spring 1978, Vol. 10
Schulte, M.A. Brenner (1984) "Medical Education in Relation to Self-Activity of Patients," Education for Health, Vol. 1, No. 1
The Times (1940) Quoted in "The Coming of the Welfare State," Bruce 1968
Thompson, James D. (1967) Organisations in Action, New York: McGraw-Hill

Chapter 13

THE BEHAVIOURAL COMPONENT OF HEALTH PROMOTION:
KEY PROBLEMS AND RECOMMENDATIONS

Kathryn Dean, Tom Hickey, and Bjørn E. Holstein

The focus and conceptualisation of self-care vary
from chapter to chapter in this book, but the
unifying theme is the central and crucial role of
self-care behaviour in the continuum of care. The
differences in focus arise principally from the
varying disciplines and work responsibilities of the
contributors. This variety is both natural and
important. It provides a breadth of focus which
underscores the importance of self-care in health
promotion, education, and planning and in the
delivery of health and social services.

Dean (Chapter 4) focuses on the individual
behavioural components of self-care, with emphasis
on understanding the range and determinants of self
health care as a necessary knowledge base for
effective policy and programme development. Kane and
Kane (Chapter 10) reserve their concept of defensive
health behaviour to those strategies that maximise
the benefits and decrease the costs that older
people incur in interactions with the health care
system. Katz (Chapter 11) sees self-care as a social
movement which enlarges the individual's ability to
make choices, leading to an empowerment which he
considers the goal of self help programmes. Liddiard
and Ritvo (Chapter 12) focus on health and social
services as a means of supporting effective self-
care.

Differences in definition relate essentially to
the scope of behaviour ascribed to the concept of
self-care. For example, in one of her studies, Haug
(Chapter 9) defined self-care as intentional behaviour in response to health problems or symptoms and
excluding professional contacts, whereas Hickey
(Chapter 1) and Dean (Chapter 4) include preventive
actions as well as responses to illness in the
concept. Most authors include the intention to

promote health and function in the concept, although
sometimes this is not made clear. Dean considers it
important to include decisions regarding professional care seeking in the concept of self-care
not only in order to understand the determinants of
behaviour and the interface of components of care,
but also because aspects of self care are involved
at all levels of the continuum of care.

Care provided by others in the social network
is sometimes included in discussions of self-care
behaviour. A conceptual issue then would be whether
self-care is behaviour which individuals undertake
for themselves or whether the concept includes what
one does for family and friends. Katz (Chapter 11)
maintains, "Self-care can be practised by the lone
individual, or with the aid of one or more others,
including that of an organised self help group."
This interactive component would seem to be appropriately included in the concept of self-care, while
to avoid conceptual confusion and fuzziness, care
provided by others might more appropriately be
defined as lay care or network care.

Conceptual differences have implications for
understanding health-related behaviour and its role
in shaping health status. However, differences are
to be expected in the process of conceptualisation
of a long neglected subject. A consensus will evolve
from the exchange of ideas and accumulation of
knowledge. In the meantime, while we know little
about the range and determinants of self-care,
sufficient information is available to identify
important issues related to the subject of self-
care.

In this final chapter, we will attempt to draw
together major problems and issues concerning
self-care and aging. Thereafter, recommendations
will be formulated which on the basis of existing
knowledge are relevant for health policy, professional and public education, health care services
and research.

A growing body of epidemiological evidence
points to the importance of individual behaviour in
the preservation and promotion of health. The
effects of health-damaging life-style behaviour
begin to accumulate early in life. At the same time,
it is now well documented that individual decisions
regarding care and self-treatment account for the
bulk of all care during illness. Therefore, self
health care behaviour over the life course is an
important determinant of health and functional
capacity in old age. As Holstein illustrates

(Chapter 3), physiological changes which reduce resistance to disease and may retard the body's restorative processes increase the importance of promoting health and functional capacity with advancing age.

The subjects of health promotion and self-care have received considerable attention over the past few years. Unfortunately, however, as Liddiard and Ritvo point out (Chapter 12), public rhetoric about self-care has not been followed with the policy and funding support necessary to develop effective self-care programmes. Indeed, the past few years have witnessed a restriction of innovative programmes rather than the development of initiatives designed to improve and facilitate the health care capacities of individuals and communities.

There have been a few spectacular programmes where massive expenditures are directed at changing particular habits - e.g., dietary practices and/or smoking behaviour. There is also a growing market of self-care materials and appliances. These initiatives are generally narrow or fragmented approaches arising from a disease model of health. The social and psychological determinants of behaviour are ignored as well as the limitations of programmes directed at individual behavioural change. With regard to the elderly, as documented repeatedly throughout this monograph, the pathological model of aging described by Johnson (Chapter 2) is a major constraint to effective self-care both in the preservation of health and in its restoration during episodes of illness.

Motivation for health-enhancing self-care is influenced by expectations and perceptions of the possible. These, in turn, are shaped by cultural concepts and stereotypes and by the social situation in which the individual must function. Health enhancing life-styles and responses to illness focused on the cause of symptoms rather than their simple alleviation are unlikely unless one believes in the possibility of maintaining fitness and expects to have a meaningful future. It is important, especially -- but not only -- for old people, that these perceptions are possible in the face of chronic illness and functional impairment. As Rakowski points out (Chapter 5), it is important that old people can distinguish between health protective and "compliance" or "illness" behaviour. Passive attitudes toward health, excessive faith in and dependence on professional treatment, and belief that loss of function is inevitable inhibits or precludes such distinctions.

Eve (Chapter 8) cites evidence that old people do not want prescriptions for medications as often as doctors think they do. Anderson and Cartwright (Chapter 7) document that while medication prescribing has dropped for young people, prescribing for old people continues to increase. Old people are less likely to be aware of the side effects of drugs and more often get repeat prescriptions without face-to-face contact, despite that they are more vulnerable to drug-caused iatrogenesis. At the same time that the elderly are in greatest danger from the polypharmacy they experience, they are least prepared to challenge it. The evidence presented in several chapters of this monograph suggests that at least for cohorts of people already old, there are serious contraints to the type of doctor-patient relationships proposed by Kane and Kane (Chapter 10). Haug's work (Chapter 9) provides evidence that older people more often feel that physicians should determine care decisions and that older, less knowledgeable people are less skeptical of the efficiency of medicine. Similar findings regarding age differences in faith in the role of medical treatment in protecting health have been found in Danish investigations of self-care behaviour.

Since, as pointed out by several of the contributors, professional care systems deal with health selected segments of elderly populations, the risk is that the already existing tendency of professional caregivers to underestimate the self-care potential of older people is constantly reinforced. The elderly apparently are given less time in consultations, examined less carefully, receive less health information and fewer explanations regarding treatment options. Technologically oriented health care systems give time and resource priorities to acute conditions or to those conditions for which sophisticated diagnostic and curative interventions have been developed. As suggested by Haug (Chapter 9), these priorities may preclude or diminish the type of services and the type of integrated service systems which support effective self-care and the preservation of functional capacity of people coping with chronic conditions.

The structure and functioning of professional care services undoubtedly influence self-care behaviour. Yet, with the exception of findings from a few investigations of the effects of doctor-patient communication on "compliance," we know very little

323

about the effects of services on health-related behaviour. In fact, we know very little about the factors and processes that shape any of the components of self-care behaviour. Even consultation behaviour, the subject which has been studied most extensively, is poorly understood. As Ford points out (Chapter 6), most multivariate analyses have succeeded in explaining only about 20 percent of the variance. He posits a social model of health-related behaviour which focuses attention on the preconsultation stage, the context in which illness occurs rather than the illness itself. Dean's model of self-care behaviour based on her findings from studies of self-care behaviour in Denmark are consistent with this prospective of analysing the social situation of context of illness and illness behaviour.

The overriding issue concerning self-care and aging relates to the effects of self-care on the incidence and progression of chronic disease and functional capacity. In order to understand the role of self-care behaviour in shaping health, research investigators must move from simple studies of individual risk factors to face issues of multiple causation, chains of causation, and clarification of the influence of mediating variables which may exert health protective effects.

SUMMARY AND RECOMMENDATIONS

In summary, we may conclude that the health status of most older people in industrialised nations is better than ever. Nonetheless, the risk of chronic impairment is age-related: The probability that older persons will experience chronic illnesses and related problems increases with age. How much chronic impairment is due to preventable loss of fitness is unclear. The limitations of a disease model of health and of technologically oriented curative treatment services, however, are quite apparent. Moreover health systems which reinforce negative stereotypes based on a pathological model of aging contribute to an undesirable disengagement of society from the individual. It is not surprising that health care professionals and policy experts have begun to question the relevance and capability of traditional medical care delivery systems to provide leadership for the care and support of growing elderly populations. The types of care needed by these populations are much broader than medical treatment. The care and support provided by family members, friends, and neighbours as well as the care which older people can provide for themselves are critical factors in the effectiveness of health care services and delivery systems for the elderly.

Three premises guide our choice of recommendations: 1. health behaviour and positive self-care of older persons should be mobilised in interaction with formal care-giving systems; 2. self-care efforts should be in harmony with the cultural values land-rooted in the perceived needs of the local community; and 3. resources should be targeted to areas of the greatest need and potential for promoting health and effective self-care.

HEALTH POLICY RECOMMENDATIONS

1. New Health Care Initiatives for the Elderly Should Emphasise Preserving and Expanding Functional Capacity through Programmes and Incentives which Support and Enhance Effective Self-Care

It is important that definitions of health promotion and prevention go beyond the present emphasis on disease-screening. Life-style variables, environmental determinants of health and self-care behaviour, and supportive networks need to be incorporated into the development of health promotion policies.

2. A Comprehensive Health Care Policy for the Elderly Should Recognise Levels of Need, thereby Encompassing:

1. A broad range of health care services in the social context in which people live, and

2. Special efforts to cope with the complexity of chronic illness and its interaction with personal aging.

This policy recommendation implies a range of health and social services including services which provide support in the community, enhance health preservation, and provide an appropriate continuum of professional care. Present policy, which in many nations allocates the majority of health care resources for medical services, must be shifted to more balanced fiscal appropriations that.assure the needed range of professional care support services.

Research investigations have repeatedly documented discrepancies between physical condition and level of functioning. Some individuals become seriously impaired and limited in their daily functioning in the presence of less than serious physical problems, while others with major chronic disorders can function at exceptionally high levels. The traditional focus on medical screening and physical assessment must be broadened considerably to encompass functional health status, health perceptions and behaviours, and the social situation of the individual.

3. Service Entitlement and Care Expectations Should Be Based on Changing Need and Functional Capacity rather than Determined by Chronological Age

Aging has become a convenient label to denote socially constructed attitudes in a given context of time and culture. Many dangers are inherent in such a labelling process including the possibility of disenfranchising an entire population group from the power structure. Another danger entails erroneous classification of a wide range of conditions and experiences. What is known of the heterogeneity of older people clearly argues against such a labelling process. Older persons' capacities for self-care, their expectations of informal care and support from others, and their entitlement to services can only be determined by their functional status and care needs.

The absence of disease or clinical symptoms forms the basis for a medical model of "good health." However, such an approach does not explain behavioural capability or overall health status. On the other hand, a functional approach accounts for the personal and social meanings of symptoms in defining health status as a relative and dynamic phenomenon. This functional-adequacy approach is essential to understanding the health status of older people as individuals and as a group.

4. The Responsibility for Health Care and for Promoting Effective Self-Care Behaviour Needs to Be Shared by Lay People and Professional Caregivers. This Means that Older Persons Should Be Full Participants in Decisions about Their Health Care and about the Options and Choices Available to Them. It also Means that Providers Should Accept Promotion of Effective Self-Care as a Part of their Responsi-

bility

Major aspects of medical care decision-making are controlled by physicians. When applied to the elderly, there are serious problems with this traditional health care decision-making process. The nature and complexity of chronic illness and the influence exerted by and on the social environment requires a broader range of participation and expertise in decision-making regarding care regimes. The significance, and often permanent effects, of treatment decisions require the full participation of those individuals, who must live with the outcomes.

No individual or organisation is presently charged with the task of assisting older people to develop and use health information and skills on their own behalf. Clear lines of responsibility for promoting positive health behaviour need to be identified and programmatic endeavours supported sufficiently for effective implementation.

5. The Design and Implementation of Self-Care Programmes and Policies Should Be Based on Valid, Empirically-Tested Criteria which Achieve the Desired Outcomes

Self-care and self-help initiatives, to be effective, must build on the existing knowledge, values, and priorities of the people for whom they are developed. They should recognise lay concepts of health and disease, the importance of behavioural options, and opportunities for coping.

6. The Promotion of Self-Care Behaviour among the Elderly Should Be Recognised Internationally as a Health Care Issue which Transcends National Policy or System Differences

As noted in the introduction to this book, recent international discussions of health care for the elderly have been notable for their emphasis on the social and personal context of care. Various efforts of the World Health Organization as well as the 1982 World Assembly on Aging have stressed the importance of programmes of informal support and care, including self-care, peer support and mutual aid, health education, and other means of promoting effective health behaviour. It is also notable that these distinguished international forums have emphasised the necessity of avoiding the technological and institutional medical models of the past.

As discussed by Hickey (Chapter 1), the demographic case for recognising the international character of this subject has been well documented. The problems associated with the growth in numbers of very old people at greatest health risk are shared worldwide.

Many countries have shown interest in learning from the efforts and programmes of other lands. Of course there are crucial differences in the problems faced by developed and developing countries. For the former, major problems exist regarding the reorientation of health systems to effectively enhance and utilise lay care resources; for the developing countries, the very availability of formal health care services may be the overriding concern.

RECOMMENDATIONS FOR PROFESSIONAL EDUCATION AND SERVICES

1. In Order to Enhance Self-Care Capacities of Lay Elderly the Training of Professionals working in Health and Social Care Systems Should Include Courses Dealing with:

1. Lay decision-making in health related matters;
2. Communication with older persons;
3. Communication among professionals;
4. Skills for integrating self-care meaningfully into an integrated continuum of care.

The rationale for this recommendation is based on numerous reports and studies of the relatively poor communication between professional providers of care and old people. A prerequisite for effective communication is openness to patients' perceptions and future perspectives, as this can provide a basis to enhance motivation for active health promotion and illness responses which protect function.

Liddiard and Ritvo (Chapter 12) point to the generally recognised fact that continuity of care remains an abstraction, and that fragmental services are not harm. Health and social services can effectively meet their goals of improving health and well being only if they supplement and complement each other in supporting the care needs of the population.

2. Medication Prescribing for Old People Should

Receive Special Attention in Medical School Curricula. Topics to be Considered Should Include:

1. Regular assessment of all drugs being taken by old people, so as to discontinue any that are not absolutely necessary;
2. The special dangers for old people of side-effects and drug interactions;
3. The range of treatment options which might be preferable to the use of medications for illness.

Medicine use by the elderly involves not only greater frequency, but also greater danger than is the case for young people. Therefore, prescriptions should be time-limited to assure frequent reassessment of necessity as well as identification of other drugs being used simultaneously. Options which would be preferable to the use of psychotropic drugs include self-help support groups such as the Alzheimer's support groups and groups of persons coping with some other particular illness or problems such as the loss of a spouse.

3. Health Promoting Professional Services Should Focus on Older People's Functional Capacities and Well-Being Rather than Only on Disease

The potential of professional services for supporting and enhancing effective self-care is best realised by focusing on the maintenance and expansion of:

1. Intellectual functions including memory;
2. Social interaction;
3. Feelings of belonging, usefulness, and security;
4. Autonomy and independence;
5. Sensory stimulation;
6. Safe locomotion;
7. Control over bodily functions.

4. Practitioners Working to Enhance Self-Care Should Base their Efforts on the Wide Range and Changing Needs of Elderly Populations

Actual needs and capacities should be identified through a continuous dialogue with the elderly. A range of self-care programmes are needed to support effective health related behaviour, including self-help groups dealing with health-related issues.

329

Needs change over the life course, sometimes unpredictably. Periods of increasing and decreasing needs due to acute disease, social events, and other changes in life situations characterise late life. Assessment of old people's needs for services, however, tends to be rigid and not responsive to changes in old people's life situations.

Care for the elderly sometimes is based on the philosophy that functions should be maintained, but the capacity for improving functions is rarely considered.

5. Professional Services Should Provide an Opportunity for Chronically Ill Elderly Persons, their Relatives, and Professionals to Participate Jointly in Designing Care Plans

The chronically ill are often in a disadvantaged social and psychological situation, without the same "rights" as the acutely ill, e.g. to complain about their situation, expect interest and care from their friends and relatives, or receive opportunities to use their capacity for intellectual growth. When old people lack a future time perspective and are unaware of these problems, self-care behaviour is probably negatively affected.

Thus, self-care strategies need to be carefully designed to recognise the living situation and include full participation of people in decisions regarding their care, treatment, and daily living.

6. W.H.O. and Other Interested Groups Should Facilitate Communication and Dissemination of Information about Education and practice of Self-Care and Preventive Health Behaviour. Programmes, Materials, and Services Should Be Designed to Enhance the Opportunities for Elderly Persons, Family Members, and Professionals to Participate in Designing Care Plans

RECOMMENDATION FOR EDUCATION FOR HEALTH

1. Health Education Programmes for Older Persons Should:

1. Be rooted in the local culture, priorities, and values so that they build on the competence of the people and on their concepts of health, disease, and effective care;
2. Utilise carefully planned mass media programmes to present images of healthy and active aging, increase awareness of self-care, and reinforce health enhancing self-care practices in populations;
3. Concentrate on subjects especially important for old people such as protecting functional capacity; maintaining social contact and the availability of mutual aid groups; effective interaction with health care systems; and safe use of drugs.

Such a strategy of enlightening the public, includes education about the health system, about how to avoid learned helplessness, how to avoid inappropriate use of services, and improve communication with their physicians.

Decisions about living arrangements in cases of sudden breakdown are often made when the situation is most chaotic. Important benefits can be expected from awareness of alternative options and their unanticipated consequences prior to crisis situations. Vehicles for this type of education and support include advocacy programmes, voluntary organisations, or self-help groups for dealing with these issues.

2. Health Education for Caregivers (Family Members, Friends, and Neighbours) Should:

1. Be based on the assumption that functionally dependent elderly persons are full participants in the process of care;

- - - - - - - - - -

The recommendations in this section draw heavily from those developed in a WHO scientific consultation on Health Education in Self-Care, Possibilities and Limitations (WHO, 1984)

2. Teach caregivers how to support the dependent elderly to maintain and expand functions;
3. Teach care techniques, preventive health care, and the importance of intellectual stimulation and social control.

The social support network - by which we mean the family, relatives, neighbours and friends that old persons perceive as an important part of their social life - can either effectively stimulate or negatively affect the old person's health behaviour by: 1. the amount of social interaction with the old person which influences happiness as well as intellectual and mental functioning; 2. helping the old person too much or too little, which affects capacity; 3. influence on the old person's contracts with providers of health care and social service; 4. attitudes and behaviour in relation to chronic disease or impairment which can influence the feelings of self-worth of the old person and the capacity to cope with functional decline; and 5. influencing major decisions regarding the future (housing, living arrangements, medical treatment, etc.).

3. Health Education Endeavours Should Include a Life-Course Perspective in Programme Development By:

1. Teacher training programmes which include education for the teaching of self-reliance and self-care skills at all levels of formal education systems;
2. Education programmes which offer opportunities to learn and practice self-care skills and decision-making;
3. Using work sites, medical facilities, religious centres and other community settings for education in health promotion and illness related components of self-care.

Self-care capacity and skills can be improved at any age, but the greatest potential for enhancing health and functional capacity in old age is to be gained from effective health promotion over the life course.

RECOMMENDATIONS FOR RESEARCH

Our basic knowledge about self-care and aging is so limited and the research issues arising from the discussions included in this book so numerous that a detailed and exhaustive list of recommendations is beyond the scope of this chapter. However, basic social science studies, health services research, and research for policy development are all needed to establish a knowledge base in self-care.

1. Basic Social Science Studies Are Needed in Three Distinct Areas: Healthy Aging, Patterns of Chronic Disease, and the Influence of Self-Care Behaviour on the Incidence and Progression of Chronic Conditions
Effective gerontological policy and programme development is limited by large gaps in our knowledge regarding health behaviour and functioning of old people. A great deal of faulty information and misconceptions exist regarding aging. Carefully collected and analysed information in the areas mentioned are prerequisites to the development of effective approaches to enhance the self-care behaviour of old people. Studies concerned with normal adaptive aging are essential in order to identify factors associated with maintaining functional capacity in old age. Research in aging must shift from problem-centered approaches and pathology models of old age to approaches which identify the factors and processes shaping health and health-related behaviour.
     Research investigations need to concentrate on problems of causal interaction. Recent work in social epidemiology has begun to address the complexity of multiple causation and this type of research should, therefore, be expanded. Moreover, a broader range of variables should be included in the search for causal interaction. Studies of the impact of situational stress and the role of social support are important advances in this regard and should be expanded. Also, the role and importance of health and social services, both the mix and the content of services, need investigation.
     Research investigations charting the content and scope of health-related behaviours and the factors which shape these behaviours must also be given priority e.g.

     1. Studies which identify the factors associated with alternative patterns of self-care

in elderly populations;
2. Identify the factors promoting and the
   barriers prohibiting effective self-care
   practices and health maintenance in elderly
   populations;
3. Examine the impact of structural changes in
   society, especially the content and amount
   of time spent engaged in work on the
   content of self-care behaviour; and
4. Examine the influence of health services on
   self-care decisions in illness.

2. Health Services Research Is Needed to Study the Influence of Services on Self-Care Behaviour and the Most Effective Content and Mix of Services, in Support of Health Promotion and Effective Health Related Behaviour

A critical examination is needed of the assumptions,
values, and perspectives underlying professional
concepts and constructs and how they affect health
care as it functions in contemporary settings.

Studies of the content of health care (self-
care, lay care, and professional care) should be
conducted to determine the aspects of caring most
beneficial for different health problems and conditions.

We also need to achieve greater knowledge and
understanding regarding the content and range of
self-care and which practices and life-style patterns produce better health and more optimal
functional capacity in old age. The results of
studies of incentives and methods which produce
behavioural change and enhance learning will be
necessary for the development of effective teaching
materials and programmes.

Research investigations should identify service
gaps and the appropriate mix of health and social
services which most effectively support people with
varying levels of functional capacity and social
support. An extensive amount of medical consultation
is taking place for non-medical reasons. Unmet need
for social support appears to be an important
factor. The elderly are especially vulnerable to
these weaknesses in our care systems. The data
presented by Anderson and Cartwright indicate that
the administration of psychotropic drugs is a
frequent response to the psychological and support
needs of old people.

Experimental studies and demonstration projects
should, therefore, identify appropriate mixes of

services and resources which best support people with varying levels of functional capacity and informed social support.

3. Studies which Develop Operational Criteria to Achieve Self-Care Goals Need to Be Conducted

Persons responsible for political and administrative decisions need clearly defined objectives to reach social goals and testable indicators to measure the progress made toward the achievement of social goals. High quality and effectiveness of service are goals which everyone can agree upon, but limited resources always entail cost constraints and the need to reach a balance in the allocation of resources which can achieve the best possible outcome.

Therefore, it is important to develop methods of weighting goals and developing indicators of success in achieving the goals in order to test decision-making models and the amount of resource inputs which will achieve desired outcomes. Policies for this purpose need to be intersectoral in character, recognising that the prerequisites to health and optimum functional capacity lie outside the medical sector.

Finally, we would like to add a few words on research methodology. Johnson (Chapter 2) has discussed the importance of establishing better criteria for defining cohorts. The biographical method, for instance, is effective for identifying variables, generating hypotheses, and improving understanding of behavioural processes. Similarly, other process-oriented methodologies such as the methods of social anthropology are important tools for the evaluation of health services and programmes.

However, carefully designed quantitative survey investigations of populations are crucial to achieve the research goals outlined in this chapter. Recently developed statistical techniques provide more effective tools than those used in many past investigations. Research problems of multiple causation and causative interactions can be addressed with these newer analytic models.

As discussed by Ford, the more complex models needed in the study of illness and illness behaviour might be more effectively developed and tested in cross-national research investigations. It must be emphasised that more effective and consistent testing of research models and theories is essen-

335

tial. Just as the development of testable theories and models is important to advance knowledge, so is the discarding of incorrect or inappropriate theories and models essential to avoid non-productive and costly research that does not advance knowledge and understanding.

The contributors to this book have discussed the process of aging in two ways: 1. as a highly individual process with immense variability - often with considerable potential for improvement of health and function, and 2. as a social construct where the dangers of discrimination and ageism have often replaced knowledge as the basis for public attitudes and social policies.

Similarly, self-care has been characterised as a multi-faceted phenomenon. It includes the individual's health-related motivation and actions. It also can function as a defense against ageist views and behaviour. Likewise, it includes the autonomous individual's cooperation and interactions with others to enhance health. The importance of self-care for the process of aging has been stressed.

The focus of the recommendations, then, has been on the responsibility of policy-makers and professional caregivers to enhance the capacity for self-care in elderly populations and to improve the cooperation between the complementary levels of health-care, both lay and professional.

LIST OF CONTRIBUTORS

Robert Anderson
Institute for Social Studies in Medical Care
London

Ann Cartwright
Institute for Social Studies in Medical Care
London

Kathryn Dean
Institute of Social Medicine
University of Copenhagen

Susan Brown Eve
Department of Sociology and Anthropology
North Texas State University, Denton

Graeme G. Ford
Medical Sociology Research Unit
Medical Research Council, Glasgow

Marie R. Haug
Center on Aging and Health
Case Western Reserve University, Cleveland

Tom Hickey
Institute of Gerontology and School of Public Health
University of Michigan, Ann Arbor

Bjørn E. Holstein
Institute of Social Medicine
University of Copenhagen

Raymond Illsley
Center for Social Policy Analysis
University of Bath

337

Contributors

Malcolm L. Johnson
Health and Social Welfare
The Open University, England

Robert L. Kane
School of Medicine and School of Public Health
University of California, Los Angeles

Rosalie A. Kane
The Rand Corporation
Santa Monica

Alfred H. Katz
School of Public Health
University of California, Los Angeles

Ronald Liddiard
"White Friars"
Birmingham

William Rakowski
School of Public Health
University of Michigan, Ann Arbor

Roger A. Ritvo
Graduate Program in Health Administration
Cleveland State University